A Colour Atlas of
Dental Analgesia & Sedation

Graham J. Roberts
BDS (Lond), Phd (Lond), FDSRCS (Eng), MDS (Lond), Reader in Paediatric Dentistry, United Medical and Dental Schools of Guy's and St. Thomas's Hospitals, London

Norman L. Rosenbaum
BDS (Lond), General Dental Practitioner and Senior Clinical Lecturer in Department of Oral and Maxillofacial Surgery, United Medical and Dental Schools of Guy's and St. Thomas's Hospitals, London

Wolfe Publishing Ltd

Published by Wolfe Publishing Ltd, 1991
Printed by Hazell Books, Aylesbury, England
ISBN 0 7234 0920 X

A CIP catalogue record for this book is available from the British Library.

This book is one of the titles in the series of Wolfe Atlases, a series that brings together the world's largest systematic published collection of diagnostic colour photographs.

For a full list of Atlases in the series, plus forthcoming titles and details of our surgical, dental and veterinary Atlases, please write to Wolfe Publishing Ltd, 2–16 Torrington Place, London WC1E 7LT, England.

CONTENTS

Part 2 INTRAVENOUS SEDATION

By Norman L. Rosenbaum

FOREWORD

In all fields of scientific endeavour progress and change go hand in hand and time brings many changes. The provision of dental treatment without pain or the awareness of unpleasant procedures has been the goal of dental surgeons for more than one hundred years — since Wells, in the United States of America, first demonstrated the use of nitrous oxide for the extraction of a tooth. Analgesia, in those early days, was imperfect but it soon became considered, by anxious patients, as a gift from heaven, gratefully received.

Recent advances in technology and pharmacology have provided dental surgeons with a facility to eliminate pain and an awareness of dental treatment with an unparalleled degree of safety and effectiveness.

The authors of this excellent atlas have combined to present, with great professional competence, the knowledge and technical training which should be acquired by all dentists who wish to use the techniques of relative analgesia and intravenous sedation in all aspects of dental practice. The essentials of effective application of local analgesic techniques, used in association with the techniques of allaying apprehension and memory of the procedures, are reviewed with admirable clarity.

Such is the safety of the techniques described that collapse in the dental surgery, using these methods, should be a most unlikely event. Nevertheless, the authors, quite properly, have addressed the fundamental skill of resuscitation with brevity and accuracy. Practitioners who follow the concepts described in this volume should be most unlikely to find themselves burdened by the problem of litigation; to avoid the unexpected occurrence of medico-legal complications all who administer these techniques should be familiar with the preventive procedures advocated in the conclusion to this practical and most professional volume.

Complete freedom from discomfort for the patient and perfect operating conditions for the dental surgeon, with complete safety, have, in the past, been considered unobtainable ideals; the authors of this volume have presented procedures which, if practised to the letter, should make these ideals achievable! The book should be essential reading for both undergraduate and postgraduate students who wish to achieve competence in the demanding, but satisfying, field of pain and anxiety control in dental practice.

David Poswillo CBE, DDS, DSc, MDhc, FDS, FRACDS, FRCPath, FIBiol, Hon FFDRCSI

PREFACE

This important new book looks at the whole spectrum of pain control in dentistry – including local analgesia, inhalation sedation and intravenous sedation – the aim being to provide the aspiring practitioner with sufficient knowledge of the basic procedures to carry them out him- or herself. (On the question of the sex of the practitioner, etc.: to avoid never ending 'she or he', 'he or she' repetition, dental surgeons are referred to as 'he', dental surgery assistants as 'she', and patients as 'he' throughout the book – unless accompanying illustrations make this plainly ridiculous. No sexual stereotyping is intended.) Each vital technique is considered in turn, the simple step-by-step instructions being accompanied by over 300 full-colour photographs and artworks, and many illuminating diagrams, tables and graphs. Helpful hints and technique variations are also included, to enable the practitioner to choose the sedation technique to suit the needs of the individual patient.

Considerable emphasis has been placed, throughout the book, on the safety of the patient. Possible complications are carefully described, as are preventive measures, and – where these prove unsuccessful – remedial action. The monitoring of the patient and the duties of the Second Appropriate Person receive particular attention.

The section on cardiopulmonary resuscitation should be essential reading for any dental surgeon or doctor, dental surgery assistant or nurse, contemplating the use of inhalation and/or intravenous sedation techniques in general or hospital practice.

The knowledge contained within the pages of this book, correctly applied, and combined with the benefits of a recognized training course and with the experience to be gained working under the supervision of an experienced colleague, must make for the safer practice of inhalation and/or intravenous sedation – which has got to be in the interests of not only the patient, but also the whole dental team.

ACKNOWLEDGMENTS

We are indebted to many people for assistance in the preparation of this book. Worthy of mention are Pentax (UK) Ltd. for the provision of photographic equipment, and Agfa-Gevaert for the film used for many of the illustrations appearing in Part 1.

I wish to record my special thanks to my dental surgery assistant, Beverley Hart, for much forbearance and help during work on the clinical aspects of this atlas. Of all the others who offered help, I would like to mention Ian Nelson, Meg Skelly and Peter Longhurst, who gave me much useful advice.

During the preparation of such a text one inevitably draws upon sources too numerous to mention. However, I would like to thank Miss Usher Desai, the Dental Photographer at the United Medical and Dental Schools of Guy's and St. Thomas's Hospitals, London, for much of the photography appearing in Part 1, and Victoria Roberts for her line drawings. Also, Professor Andrew Lumsden for figures 2 and 3 in Chapter 1. We are particularly indebted to Norma Whyte, who typed and retyped the numerous redrafts.

I must thank Nesor Dental Equipment and Matrx Medical for their financial support.

Finally, thanks must go to my patients, whose generous cooperation enabled me to carry out the clinical photography.

Graham J. Roberts

I would first like to acknowledge the support of Professor D.E. Poswillo and all of my colleagues at the United Medical and Dental Schools of Guy's and St. Thomas's Hospitals, London, including Mrs H. Jenrick, Mr. R. Raj, Miss M. Skelly, Mr. I. Nelson and Mrs C. Osborne-Smith; also Professor M. Brookes and Mr. G. Bridgeman of the Department of Anatomy at Guy's Medical School; also Mr. R. Ellis, Director of Dental Photography at Guy's Dental Hospital, and his staff, Mr. N.R.P. Taylor, Miss U. Desai, Miss J. Hodgkin and Miss A. Talbot, for their high-quality photography.

I would like to acknowledge the supplementary photography carried out by Mr. R. Hutchings; and the contribution of Miss D. Savva, Medical Artist of Guy's Medical School. In addition, I would like to thank my colleague, Mr. R.I. Hintzen, and dental surgery assistants, Miss G. Irwin and Miss R. Nagi, and all the other members of staff at my dental practice.

I would also like to mention Dr. R. Shah, Consultant Anaesthetist, North Middlesex Hospital, for his helpful suggestions and Mr. J. Perez, Director of Holly House Hospital, and his hospital staff for the facilities made available to me.

I would like to thank KabiVitrum Ltd. and Roche Products Ltd. for their financial support; also Dr. M. Wagner, Dr. P. Hooper and Miss K. Watson for permission to use some of their pharmacology material. And St. Mary's Hospital Medical School in London for permission to use figure 322 in Chapter 16. Also the World Life Saving Association for the use of some diagrams.

Finally, I would like to thank my wife, Eve Rosenbaum, for all her support and help in producing the manuscript for this book.

Norman L. Rosenbaum

PART 1
LOCAL ANALGESIA AND INHALATION SEDATION

1 GENERAL CONCEPTS

The spectrum of patient management

In general terms, the less traumatic or minor procedures – such as the scaling and polishing of the teeth – can be carried out without any special strategy, apart from behaviour management, being adopted by the dental surgeon. Other procedures, the conservative treatment of teeth or simple extractions, for example, require that local analgesic methods are used. When more serious measures prove necessary – the removal of impacted third permanent molars, say – it is common practice for the patient to be given a general anaesthetic to overcome the discomfort and fear of being subjected to such procedures whilst fully conscious.

Concern at the cost of full hospital general anaesthesia – which, with its associated risks, is considered unacceptable anyway by many dentists – has led to the development of alternative methods of sedation which enable patients to submit themselves to traumatic procedures with equanimity.

In **1**, the vertical axis indicates the frequency with which a given management strategy is used, and the horizontal axis the relative degree of trauma occasioned by a particular procedure. The problem of dental anxiety introduces a paradox into this logical scheme. Many patients who are quite fit and well, and of normal intelligence and behaviour, will nevertheless refuse even the simplest dental treatment because they are frightened of needles and/or the drill. These patients can usually be treated successfully using either inhalation or intravenous sedation supplemented by local analgesia.

1

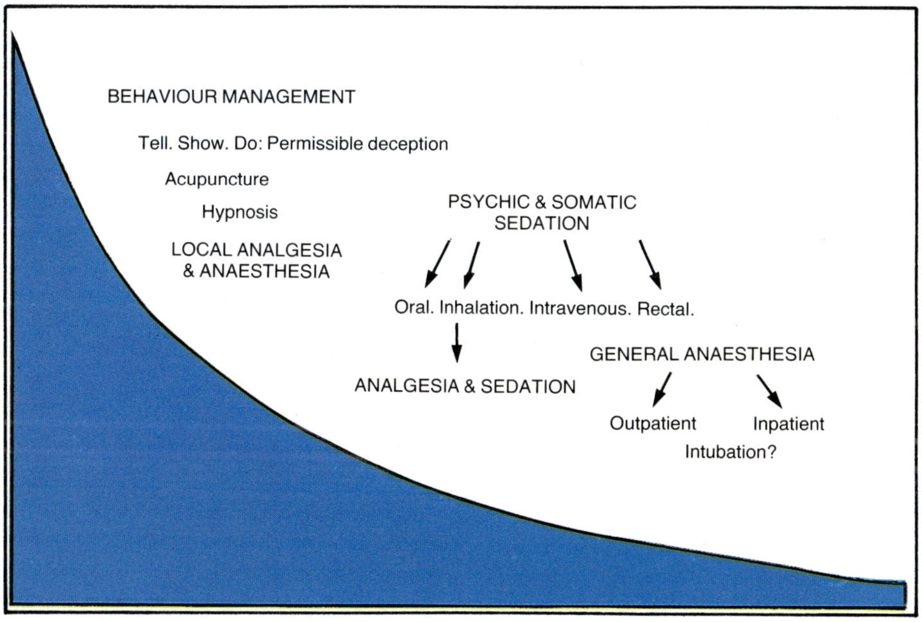

1 The spectrum of patient management

The nature of pain

When a patient is suffering from pain he is experiencing an emotional disorder caused by the stimulation of a specific receptor system. Thus pain as it presents is essentially an abnormal affective state that is caused by the activity of a specific sensory system. Many things can affect a patient's perception of pain, among them psychological factors, the sex of the patient, personality traits, previous experience, ethnic differences, and current state of health.

Assessment of patients

Dental surgeons generally assess patients according to a number of criteria:

Age. This important factor clearly influences the choice of pain-control technique. For example, small children and adolescents will be unsuitable for intravenous sedation using benzodiazepines, while young, middle-aged, and elderly patients can all be treated using oxygen: nitrous oxide sedation.

Sex. In general terms this has little effect on the choice of sedative technique, both sexes responding equally well to inhalation sedation or intravenous sedation.

Medical status. This can significantly affect the pain control and sedative technique chosen. Each patient's medical history must be carefully considered before it is possible to plan the treatment and management strategy.

Degree of anxiety. The level of anxiety felt and/or displayed by the patient will obviously influence the choice of technique. Patients with a phobia of needles may need to be sedated with oxygen and nitrous oxide before they can be given a local analgesic. Some patients have a fear of masks and may be more suitable for treatment using intravenous benzodiazepines.

Dental experience. When considering a patient's history, the dental surgeon should make a note of anything which might adversely affect the patient's future response to treatment. For example, a child who has suffered an unhappy 'dental gas' experience might well fear the prospect of an inhalation mask. Similarly, an elderly patient who has had an unpleasant intravenous experience in the past may be reluctant to submit to a further intravenous sedative.

Patient's choice. Whilst the final decision about which form of pain control to use is made by the dental surgeon, it is not unusual to go along with a patient's own preference.

General considerations. Although it is common for patients to demand a particular method of pain control and sedation, it is the dental surgeon's duty to ensure that that chosen will prove effective, consistent with minimum risk or hazard to the patient.

Handicapped patients. This group requires special care. There is a tendency to resort to a general anaesthetic for any treatment, irrespective of the individual circumstances. However, many such patients can be successfully treated using sedative techniques.

Psychological aspects of pain control

Most dental surgeons would agree that a patient's perception of pain is considerably influenced by his state of mind. Adequate psychological preparation of patients about to undergo dental treatment can therefore be of significant benefit.

Put simply, this means that patients should be provided with sufficient explanation during assessment visits to enable them to cope more effectively with the subsequent treatment. During treatment, simple psychological techniques such as distraction, suggestion and diverted attention can be employed to great effect in the case of individual patients – for example, when a local analgesic is being administered. In more general terms, hypnotic suggestion can play an important role. Approximately 15 per cent of the population are highly susceptible to hypnosis. Whether hypnosis leads to the achievement of a special, unique state of consciousness or simply to a heightened susceptibility to suggestion is a matter of considerable controversy. Without doubt, however, it can be an invaluable aid in the practice of effective pain control.

It is known that many drugs, too, including nitrous oxide and the benzodiazepines, can markedly influence the suggestibility of patients. This is especially true of nitrous oxide, used in relative analgesia for its pharmacologic effect.

Although no single therapy alone is regarded as being 100 per cent effective, combinations of them do have a cumulative effect: hypnotic suggestion, distraction, pharmacotherapeutic sedation and local analgesia constitutes a good example of 'multiple convergent therapy' to control pain. It is these strategies, often utilized together, that can be used so effectively in general dental practice.

2 ORO-DENTAL PAIN

The anatomical basis of pain

Impulses originating in the nerve endings of the teeth come from the **dentinal tubules** and **subodontoblastic plexus.** Other nerve endings are derived from the **periodontal ligament,** the **alveolar bone,** and **soft-tissue plexus** of nerves, which merge into the maxillary and mandibular divisions of the fifth cranial or trigeminal nerve. Thus whether the pain comes from the teeth, supporting bone, oral mucosa, or muscles, all nerve impulses, painful or otherwise, end by passing through the **trigeminal ganglion.**

Innervation of the teeth and periodontium and soft tissues

A **terminal branch** of either the maxillary or the mandibular division enters the tooth through the **apical foramen.** About half of the nerve fibres are myelinated fibres (A) and half are terminal nerves (C). These form a **subodontoblastic plexus** of nerves which gives off nerve endings entering the **dentinal tubules** (2 and 3). The terminal branch gives off a branch to the **periodontal ligament.** In addition, other branches enter the periodontal ligament from the alveolar bone to form a plexus of nerve endings in the periodontium.

The soft tissues surrounding the dento-alveolar structures are innervated by a **soft-tissue plexus** derived from branches of the maxillary and mandibular divisions.

2

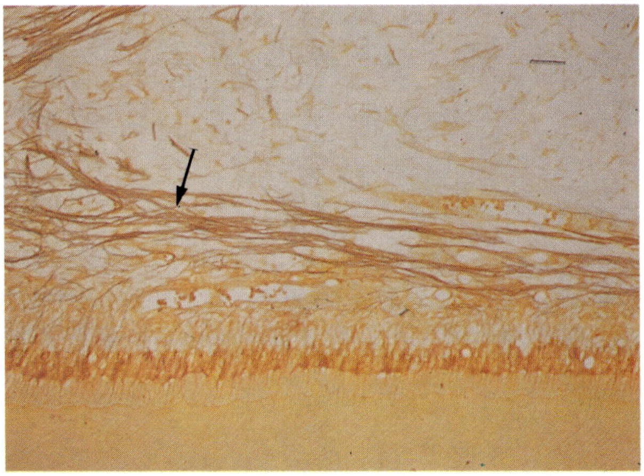

2 The plexus of nerves visualized histologically using a silver stain (arrow indicates nerve fibre)

3

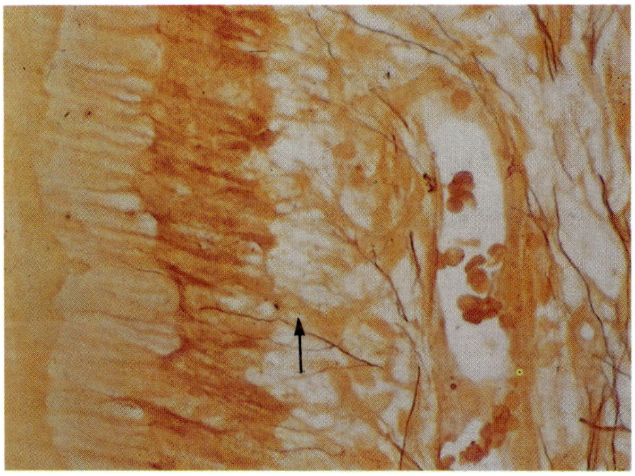

3 Nerve fibres from the plexus enter the predentine, whence they continue into the dentine to provide dentinal pain perception (arrow indicates nerve fibre)

Propagation of the nerve impulse

The sensory supply to the hard and soft tissues consists of both **unmyelinated** (C—fibres 0.25–25μm in diameter) and **myelinated** nerve fibres (A—fibres 2–5μm in diameter). The pulp of an upper incisor tooth, for example, contains approximately 500 myelinated fibres and 40–150 unmyelinated fibres. The nerve membrane is a multi-layered structure with a control band sandwiched between two layers of protein. It maintains an electrical potential of approximately 70mv by keeping sodium ions extracellularly and potassium ions intracellularly. When a nerve impulse passes along the nerve it becomes depolarized by causing sodium to flow into the nerve fibre and potassium to flow out. Once this occurs there is a flow of current in a **local circuit** ahead of the active region. This depolarizes the resting membrane and becomes a self-propagating impulse, thus passing along the nerve branch to the trigeminal ganglion.

In unmyelinated nerve fibres the impulse moves from the area of initial depolarization to the contiguous segment of nerve. Myelinated nerve fibres have prominent **nodes of Ranvier** at which sodium flows from the outside to the inside of the nerve. Consequently, the nerve impulse appears to jump from one node of Ranvier to the next.

The administration of a local analgesic solution which permeates the tissue around the nerve fibre inhibits the passage of potassium and sodium ions through the nerve membrane, thus preventing depolarization and propagation of the nerve impulse.

4

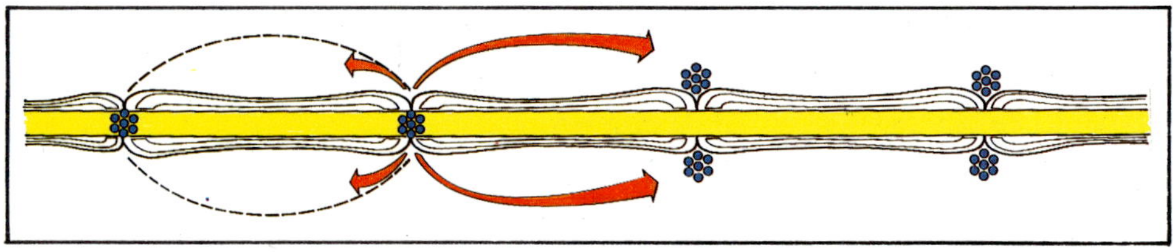

4 Propagation of the nerve impulse

Distribution of maxillary and mandibular branches of the trigeminal nerve

The branches serving the maxilla and mandible originate from the **trigeminal ganglion** in the middle cranial fossa.

Mandibular division

The sensory and motor roots of the **mandibular nerve** leave the cranial cavity through the foramen ovale and unite to form a single trunk. Four large branches are given off from the trunk. The first of these is the **long buccal nerve**, which passes between the two heads of the lateral pterygoid muscle, then forward deep to the coronoid process, to appear on the face on the surface of the buccinator muscle. It supplies the skin and mucous membrane of the cheek as far forward as the angle of the mouth.

The second major branch is the **inferior alveolar nerve**, which is at first deep to the lateral pterygoid muscle, appearing at its lower border in front of the inferior dental artery and on the lateral surface of the medial pterygoid. It enters the mandible on the medial surface via the **inferior alveolar foramen**. Within the mandible it travels via the inferior alveolar canal, giving off branches to all teeth posterior to the canine. At the level of the **mental foramen** it divides into the **incisive nerve** and the **mental**

nerve. The former travels forward to supply the lower canine and incisor teeth. In the midline there is some overlap of innervation with the contra-lateral incisive nerve. The mental nerve passes through the mental foramen and divides into several filaments which supply the skin and mucous membranes of the lower lip.

The **lingual nerve** lies in front of the inferior dental nerve on the surface of the medial pterygoid muscle deep to the mandibular ramus. It enters the floor of the mouth between the styloglossus medially and the body of the mandible laterally. It innervates the anterior two-thirds of the tongue, the floor of the mouth and gingivae on the lingual side of the lower teeth.

5

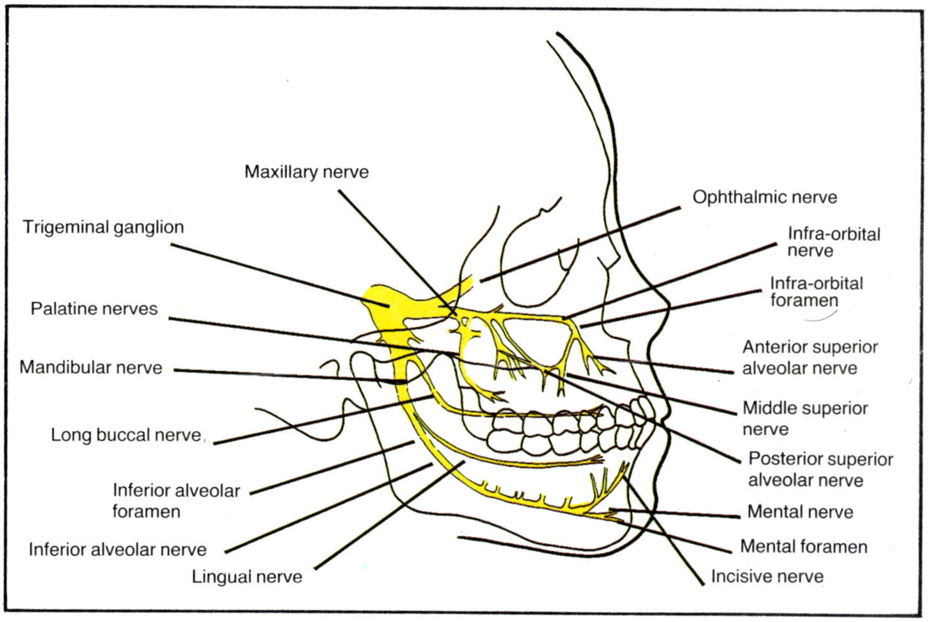

5 Distribution of maxillary and mandibular branches of the trigeminal nerve

Maxillary division

The **maxillary nerve** leaves the cranial cavity through the foramen rotundum to enter the upper part of the pterygo-palatine fossa. It crosses the fossa to leave it anteriorly as the **infra-orbital nerve,** which runs on the floor of the orbital cavity in the infra-orbital groove and canal. It leaves the maxilla by way of the **infra-orbital foramen.**

Within the infra-orbital canal the **anterior superior alveolar nerve** is given off the infra-orbital nerve to run in a canal which passes close beneath the infra-orbital foramen. Near the nasal aperture the nerve descends towards the apices of the incisor teeth. Posterior branches communicate with the **posterior superior alveolar nerve.**

Central connections of the trigeminal nerve

The nerves from the maxillary and mandibular branches of the trigeminal nerve have their cell bodies in the **trigeminal ganglion.** The central processes of these connections enter the brain stem through the root of the trigeminal ganglion, whence they turn caudally to be gathered together in the superficially placed **spinal nucleus of the trigeminal nerve.**

From here connections lead to the **bulbo-thalamic tract,** which ascends anteriorly to the **ventrolateral nucleus** of the **thalamus,** whence impulses are dispersed simultaneously to four regions:

- The **inferior paracentral region of the cerebral cortex.** Activation of this somatotopically organized projection system leads to the patient's recognition of the anatomical site of the pain and of its physical nature.
- The **orbital surfaces of the frontal lobe.** Activation of this projection system gives rise to the specifically unpleasant emotional disturbance associated with the pain and which causes the patient the most distress.
- The **temporal lobe cortex.** It is here that the major memory storage system is located; activation of this system builds up the memory store of past painful experiences.
- The subjacent and adjacent **hypothalamic and reticular nuclei** in the brain stem – this group includes projections from the bulbo-thalamic region, too. Through these projections visceral nervous reflexes, endocrine responses, and reflex changes in respiration accompany a painful stimulus.

6

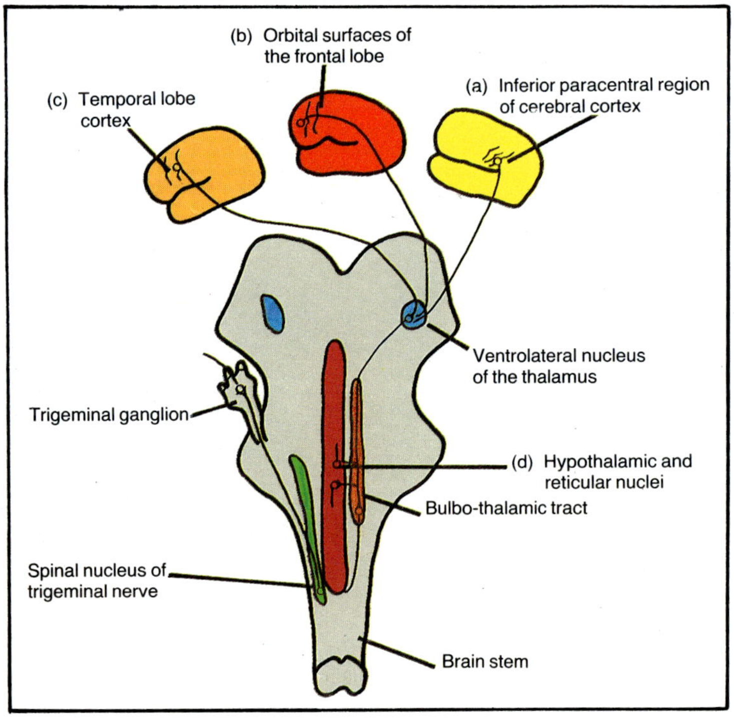

6 Central connections of the trigeminal nerve

Reticular projections of the trigeminal nerve

The **reticular system** extends the whole length of the brain stem. Cells in the upper reticular system receive collaterals from all the afferent fibres of the **bulbo-thalamic tract** as they traverse the brain stem on the way to the **thalamus.** Thus painful stimuli are projected, in part, via the reticular system upwards to nearly all areas of the cerebral cortex by the **ascending reticulocortical projections.** These ascending systems are continuously active and function as an alerting or activating mechanism for the cerebral cortex. The prevailing degree of awareness will influence the intensity of any sensory experience, including pain.

From the caudal part of the reticular system **descending reticulo-inhibitory projections** to the **spinal nucleus of the trigeminal nerve** control the flow of sensory impulses from the periphery to the brain by inhibiting – and, therefore, reducing – the number of nerve impulses eventually reaching the four-fold projection system leading to the experience of pain.

Projections are active throughout life and, on

a moment to moment basis, influence the amount of pain experienced. Almost anything can affect reticular system activity, e.g. emotional relaxation or drugs, and in so doing can increase or decrease the awareness and perception of pain.

A simple example in the dental field is the counter stimulation caused by the finger and thumb retracting the cheek prior to the insertion of a needle for a buccal infiltration. By distraction, influencing cognitive control, and activation of the inhibitory effect of the large fibres which are stimulated by the finger pressure, a simple local analgesic can be given painlessly. In a patient who is extremely anxious there is likely to be a total failure of cognitive control and, therefore, a lack of inhibitions – leaving the 'gate' wide open (see 'The gate theory of pain perception', below). The minor stimulus of a needle being inserted is perceived and experienced by the patient as being very painful.

7

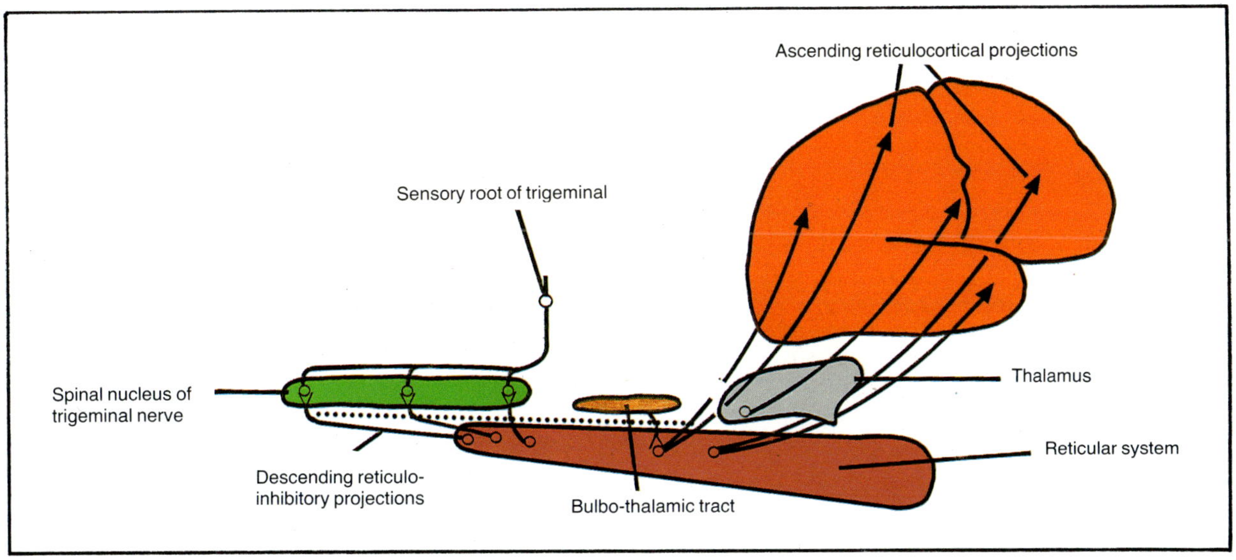

7 Reticular projections

The gate theory of pain perception

In general, the gate theory of perception states that, in its passage from the periphery to the central nervous system, a nerve stimulus associated with a 'painful' event is modified by a special gating mechanism situated in the region of the dorsal horns of the spinal cord. If the gate is open, painful stimuli are transmitted to the brain. If the gate is partially open or closed, the pain is felt less or is even not experienced.

The gating mechanism is in the substantia gelatinosa (SG), which extends the length of the spinal cord. Injury produces signals which are transmitted by **small-diameter fibres**. These enter the dorsal horns of the spinal cord and activate transmission (T) cells, which project the nerve signals to the brain. The latter is the **action system** which initiates the complex sequential patterns of experience and behaviour characteristic of pain. The small-diameter fibres also link up with the substantia gelatinosa, and successive bursts of activity in these fibres can cause increasingly larger bursts of nerve impulses from the transmission cells.

Impulses from the transmission cells are inhibited by large-diameter fibres either directly or via connections to the inhibitory cells of the substantia gelatinosa. In addition to the simple loop of inhibition versus stimulation existing between the large and small fibres, there is the

8

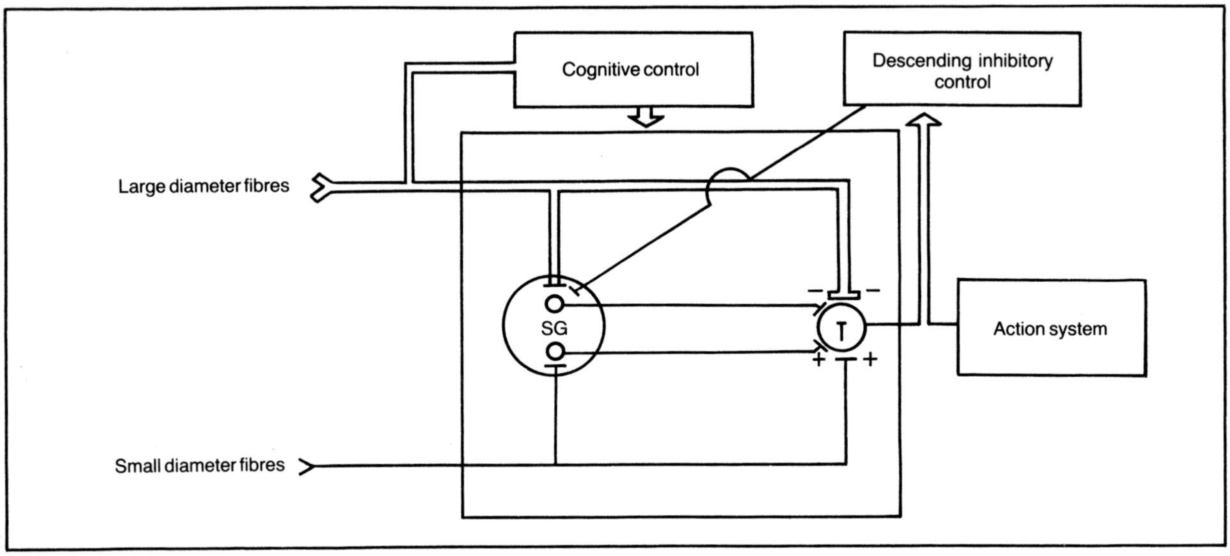

8 Gate control system

effect of descending influences. Cells in the brain stem exert a powerful influence on afferent fibres to the transmission cells via the substantia gelatinosa, a process known as 'descending inhibitory control'. Cognitive or 'higher central nervous system' processes – such as attention, anxiety, past experience and anticipation – also exert profound inhibitory effects on the transmission cells through the substantia gelatinosa.

3 LOCAL ANALGESIA

Introduction

Local analgesia has undoubtedly been a great boon to dentists and dental patients alike. Millions of operations are carried out each year with a remarkably low number of complications. So infrequent are these complications that when they do occur there is an element of surprise.

When considering pain control there are:

1. Local considerations – the distribution of sensory nerves in the tissues to be traumatized during operative dental surgery.
2. General considerations – the central connections and inter-relationships of the peripheral nerve supply as it connects up with the central nervous system.

Types of local analgesia

It is convenient, from a practical point of view, to consider local analgesia as a spectrum of closely related techniques. The common factor is that local analgesia solution is deposited on or in tissues to bring about the analgesic state.

Topical analgesia (surface analgesia)

If a certain local analgesic (e.g. lignocaine) is applied in a gel to the intact mucous membrane, it passes through the epidermis and makes the nerve endings analgesic. This is used clinically to make mucous membranes analgesic, prior to the administration of a deeper or infiltration analgesic. The surface analgesia prevents the pain of the needle penetrating the mucous membrane.

Submucosal infiltration

This is used on particularly nervous adults or children where the dental surgeon believes that the pressure caused by injecting subperiosteally is too uncomfortable for the patient to tolerate. The analgesic solution is deposited around nerve filaments in the submucosa, thus causing the submucosa and the periosteum to become analgesic. Because of the relatively dense nature of the periosteum the local analgesic solution does not penetrate or diffuse through the bone, so this type of local analgesia is inadequate for simple conservation or extractions. It should be regarded simply as a preliminary local analgesic, enabling the dental surgeon to administer a subperiosteal local analgesic.

Subperiosteal infiltration

Subperiosteal infiltration is necessary to ensure adequate analgesia for conservation or extractions. The technique requires that the tip of the hypodermic needle is inserted under the periosteum. Quite a lot of pressure must be applied to the plunger to deposit solution in this way, which can be very uncomfortable for the patient unless the periosteum is first made analgesic by means of a submucosal infiltration.

9

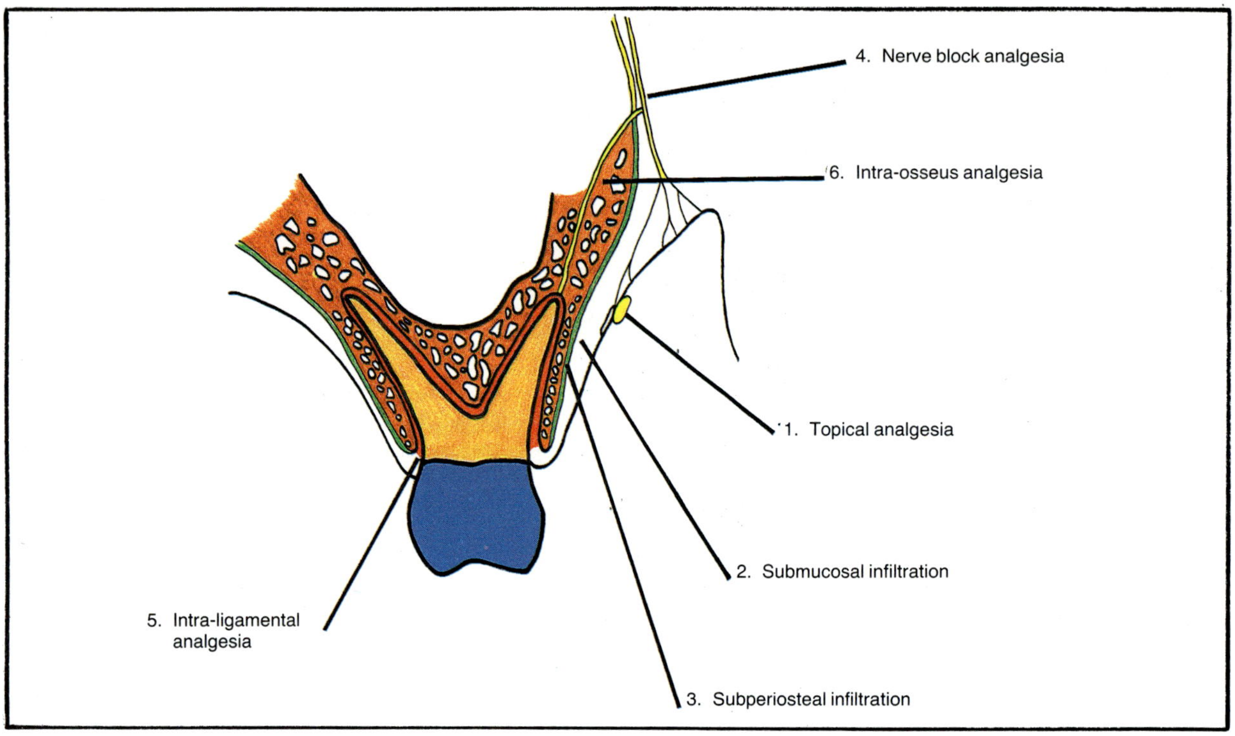

9 Types of local analgesia

Nerve block analgesia

The tip of the hypodermic syringe is inserted near an anatomically discrete nerve bundle and local analgesic solution is deposited around the nerve bundle. Provided this is done accurately the analgesia is profound and extends over the area served by the nerve bundle, e.g. the inferior dental block or superior posterior dental block.

Intra-ligamental analgesia

Of comparatively recent origin, this method provides analgesia localized to a single tooth. The tip of a 30-gauge (extremely fine) needle is inserted into the coronal part of the periodontal ligament and local analgesic solution is injected under very high pressure.

Intra-osseous analgesia

This is used only when other methods of local analgesia have failed. The mucosa and periosteum have already been made analgesic but there is insufficient analgesia to allow conservation, extraction of a tooth, or perhaps extirpation of an inflamed pulp. A small hole is drilled through the mucosa and the bony cortex to allow the insertion of a needle directly into the bony medulla, enabling the dental surgeon to produce profound deep analgesia around a group of teeth.

Because of the risk of high blood levels of local analgesic solution being taken up from the intra-osseous site of local analgesia into the blood stream, this method is indicated only when all other forms of local analgesia have failed.

Equipment for local analgesia

The equipment available for the preparation and administration of local analgesia has been developed to ensure 100 per cent sterility and ease of use in everyday practice. All procedures should be carried out with both the dental surgeon and the dental surgery assistant wearing sterile rubber gloves.

Topical analgesia

This requires merely a tube of topical analgesic paste or ointment and a sterile cotton roll. A small amount of the analgesic paste – a blob about the size of a large pea – is squeezed onto the cotton roll. The ointment contains five per cent lignocaine, and also hyaluronidase – the latter to aid penetration of the mucosa.

An alternative presentation is liquid topical analgesic: this is sprayed onto the sterile cotton roll before being placed on the mucosa.

Other forms of local analgesia

These all have the same essential requirements: a sterile needle, a sterile cartridge of local analgesic solution, and a suitable sterile syringe. The individual demands of the clinical techniques of infiltration analgesia, nerve block analgesia and intra-ligamental analgesia have resulted in appropriate variations in design, but the basic concept remains the same: a local analgesic solution is deposited by means of a hypodermic needle which has the solution forced through it by a manually operated plunger on the syringe.

Sterilization

Although pre-sterilized disposable equipment – i.e. needles, local analgesic cartridges and plastic syringes – can be purchased, for economic reasons it is usually necessary to have a reusable metal syringe which can be sterilized after each use. Pre-sterilized equipment such as needles is prepared using gamma radiation.

'In surgery' sterilization. In a general dental practice this usually consists of steam

10

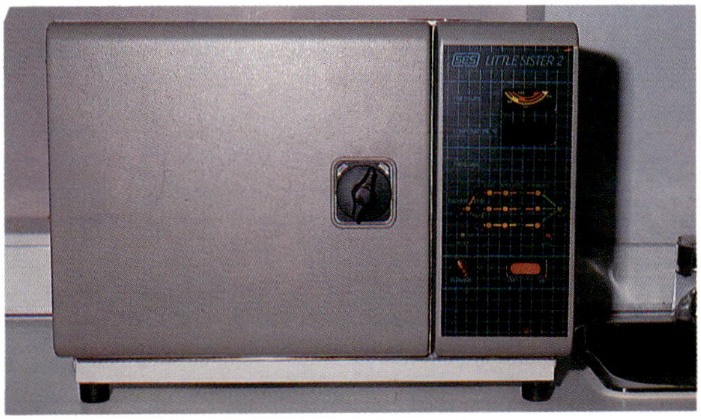

10 A steam autoclave, for 'in surgery' sterilization

11

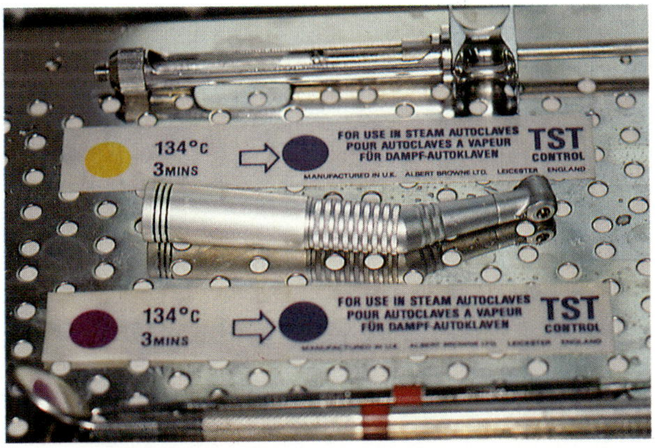

11 An **unused** TST strip (yellow and purple discs) above a **successful** TST strip (purple and purple discs) illustrates the change that occurs with sterilization

sterilization in a suitable autoclave. The latter is a high-pressure boiler which can give a cycle of 120 seconds' high-pressure steam for 210 seconds (a Time Steam Temperature – or TST – Cycle). Modern autoclaves have several cycles, e.g. 115°C for 30 minutes, 121°C for 15 minutes, and 134°C for three minutes; the most efficient of these is the last.

The instruments are placed unwrapped on a stainless steel tray and subjected to the 134°C cycle for three minutes. It is important that the dental surgeon should be able to verify that the autoclave is sterilized effectively, so TST indicator strips are used for the first sterilization cycle of each morning.

Some institutions require reliable documentation of the efficiency of the TST cycle, in which case an electronic pen recorder is linked to the autoclave to provide a written record of the cycle (**12**).

If instruments are wrapped in paper bags (autoclave paper), it is necessary to evacuate the chamber to ensure that the steam penetrates to the surfaces of the instruments.

For occasional use – for example, if there is a machine or power failure – it is necessary to have available a two per cent solution of glutaraldehyde for the purpose of emergency sterilization. Several instruments can additionally be stored in this fluid until they are needed (**14**); they must be rinsed thoroughly in sterile water before use, however, as glutaraldehyde is an extreme irritant of the skin. Alternatively, if the instruments are paper-wrapped they can be stored thus until use.

12

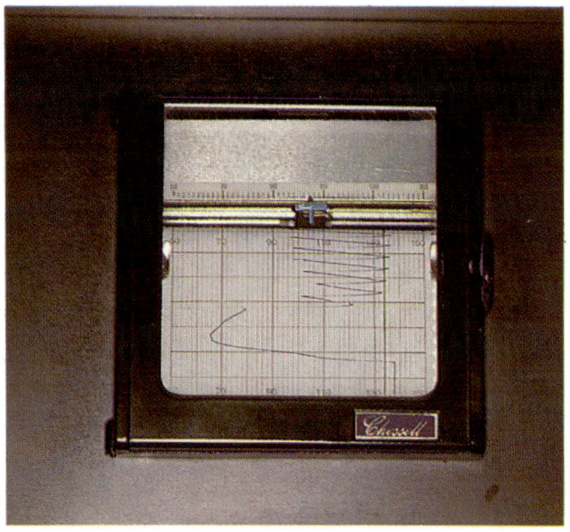

12 Electronic pen recorder – the first recording shows a cycle for unwrapped instruments of three to five minutes at 134°C

13

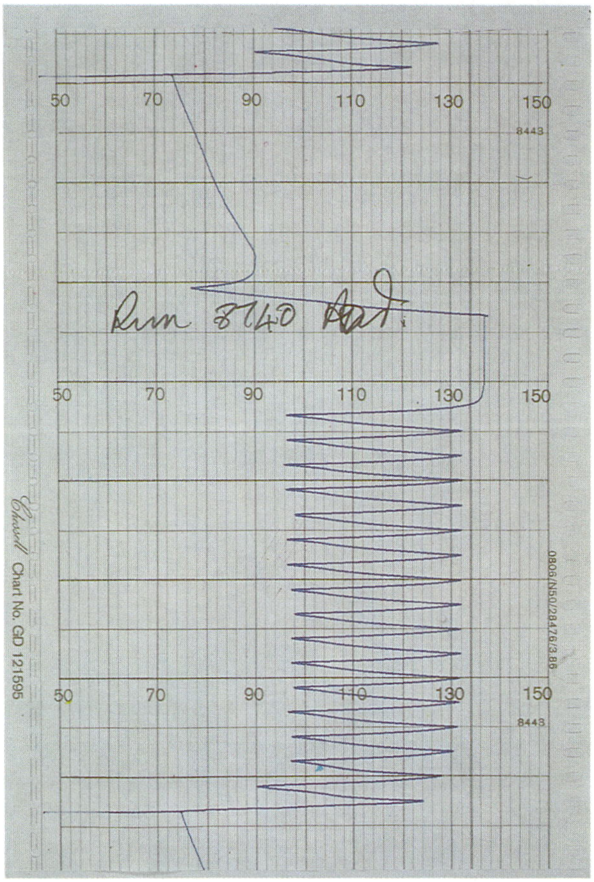

13 The second recording shows the TST cycle followed by over ten evacuations of the autoclave chamber

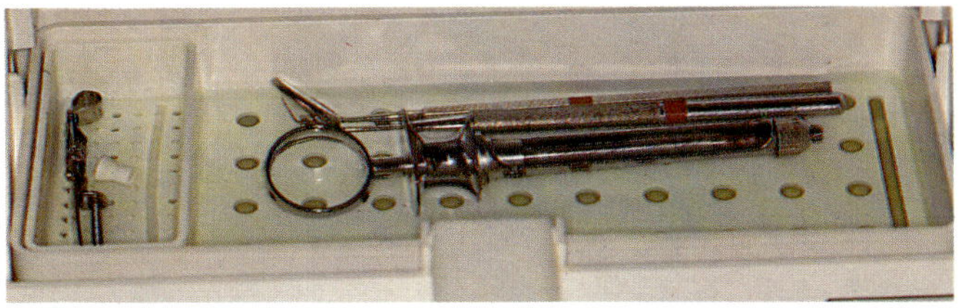

14

14 Instruments can be stored in a two per cent solution of glutaraldehyde prior to use

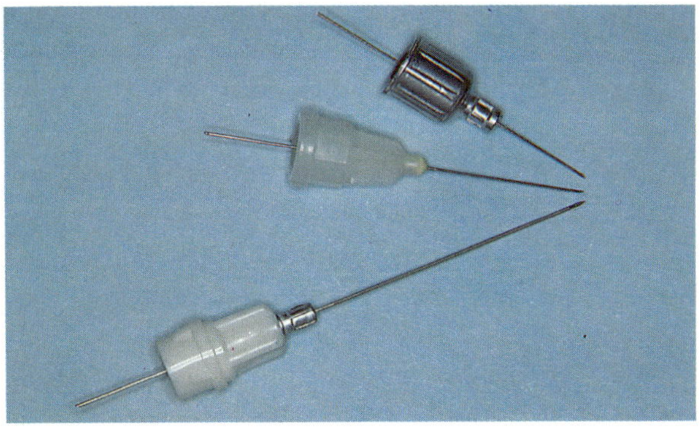

15

15 A 32mm 28-gauge or 'long' needle, used for nerve block analgesia; a 20mm 28-gauge or 'short' needle, used for infiltration analgesia; and a 15mm 30-gauge or 'extra fine' needle, used for intra-ligamental analgesia. Intraosseous analgesia is achieved with either the long or the short needles

Needles

These come in several sizes, are double-ended, and have a plastic or metal screw hub which attaches to the end of the syringe. The shorter end of the needle penetrates the rubber diaphragm of the local analgesic cartridge, and the longer end penetrates the tissue for delivery of the local analgesic solution.

The needles illustrated are for single use only and come fully sterilized in plastic containers. These are made in two parts: a coloured body which covers the longer part of the needle, and a cap which covers the shorter part. Before breaking the cap it is essential to see that the 'heat seal' is intact; if it is not – if the seal is broken – the needle must be discarded.

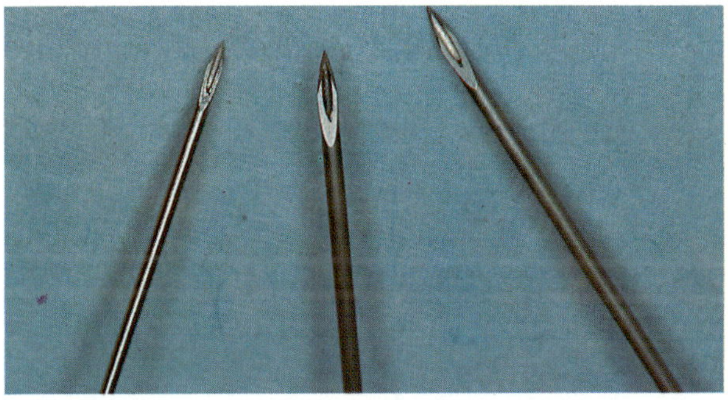

16

16 Examination of the tips of the two 28-gauge needles and the extra fine 30-gauge needle reveals a long bevel with an additional bevel near the tip, which provides for easier penetration of tissues. These needles are for single use and come ready sterilized in plastic containers (**17**)

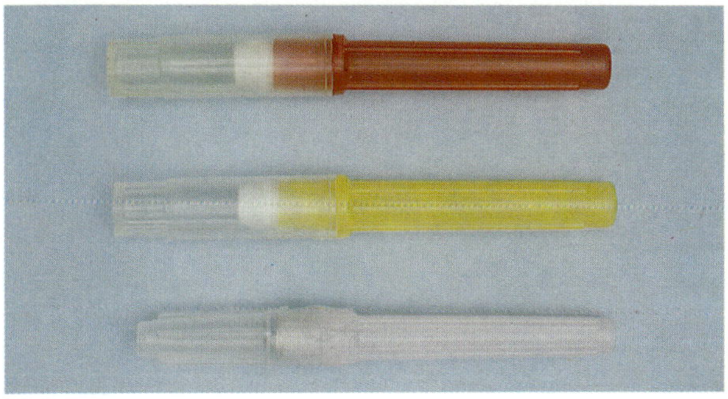

17

17 The yellow container holds a long needle, the red one a short needle, and the purple one an extra fine needle. (*Note*: Colour coding by manufacturers is *not* standardized.)

18 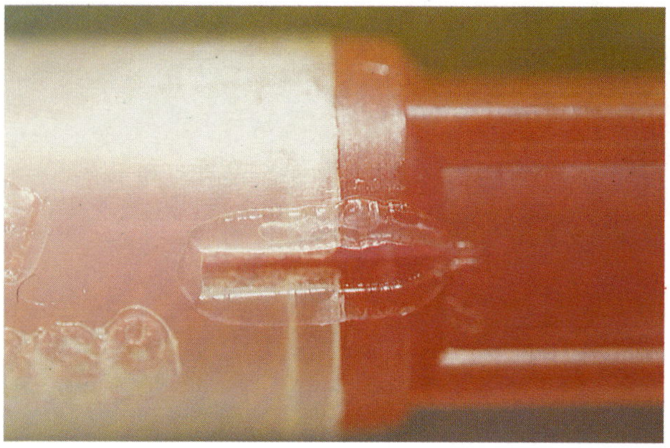 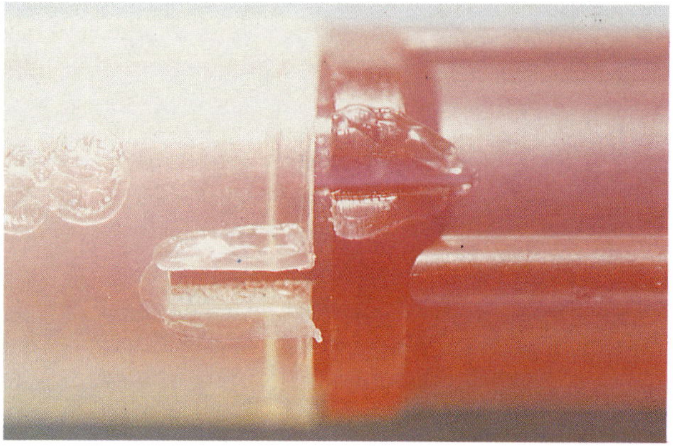 19

18 and 19 The 'heat seal' on the cap joining the coloured body of the needle container must be intact prior to use (**18**); if it is broken (**19**), the needle must be considered to be contaminated and discarded

Syringes

Figure **20** illustrates the most widely used local analgesic syringe currently available. It is sterilized using a suitable TST cycle in an autoclave after every usage. It consists of a chromium-plated or stainless steel metal barrel with a large window at the side to enable the dental surgeon to see the contents of the local analgesic cartridge. On the bottom is the thread onto which the hub of the needle is screwed. At the top is a hinge which allows the cartridge retainer to swing back so that the cartridge can be placed in the barrel. The flat-ended plunger is encased in a cylinder which guides it during movement. The handle is gently shaped to enable it to fit comfortably into the palm of either a left- or right-handed dental surgeon.

Another very common design of syringe is illustrated in **21**. Again, it has a stainless steel or chromium-plated barrel which must be sterilized after each use. The major difference from the syringe in **20** is the design of the plunger: this consists of a double barb which engages the rubber bung after slight pressure, enabling aspiration to be carried out. The other end of the plunger has a large ring attached, to allow the plunger to be pulled out and aspiration to be achieved. The advantage of this aspirating syringe is that it can be used with conventional local analgesic cartridges.

The first design of an intra-ligamental analgesic syringe incorporated a pistol grip similar to that illustrated in **22**. The purpose of this grip is to enable the dental surgeon to generate the high pressure necessary for the technique of intra-ligamental analgesic. At the tip of the syringe is a conventional steel barrel with a screw thread for the extra fine needle. At the other end is a screw thread to attach it to an assembly with a spring-loaded ratchet which prevents the high back pressure from reversing the movement of the rubber bung. The pistol grip underneath is to the right and the spring-loaded trigger attached to the ratchet is to the left. A plastic sleeve which fits closely around the glass local analgesic cartridge can be seen through the window in the barrel. This syringe is also TST cycle sterilized.

A more recent – and elegant – design of an intra-ligamental syringe is the Cito Ject (**23**). On the left is a steel barrel. The screw thread at the end is angled to enable angulation of the needle into the periodontal ligament when injecting. A plastic sleeve marked in 0.18ml gradations can be seen through a window in the barrel. The plunger and ratchet are in a separate part of the syringe on the right: after sliding the cartridge into the barrel, they are joined together by approximating two lugs to an L-shaped cut-out and twisting together. The whole assembly is held in a pen grip. Sterilization is achieved by disassembling, careful washing and an appropriate TST cycle.

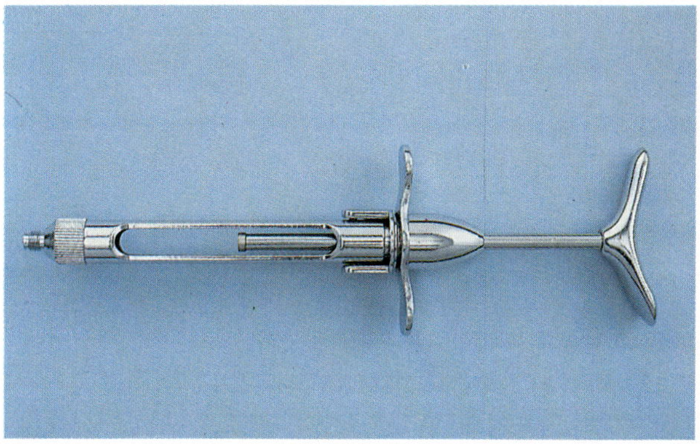

20

20 The most widely used local analgesia syringe

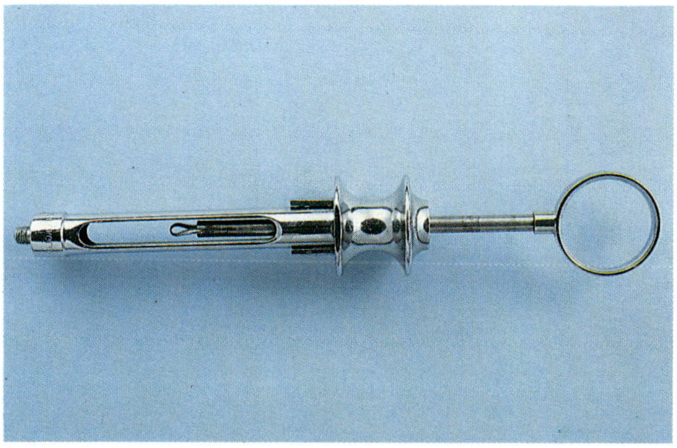

21

21 Another very common design of syringe

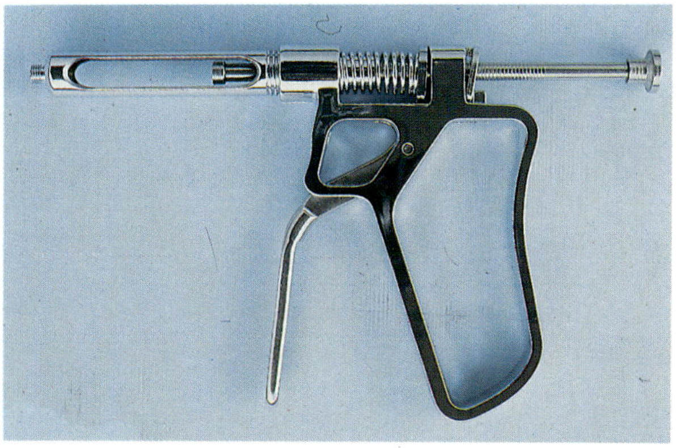

22

22 Intra-ligamental analgesia syringe complete with pistol grip

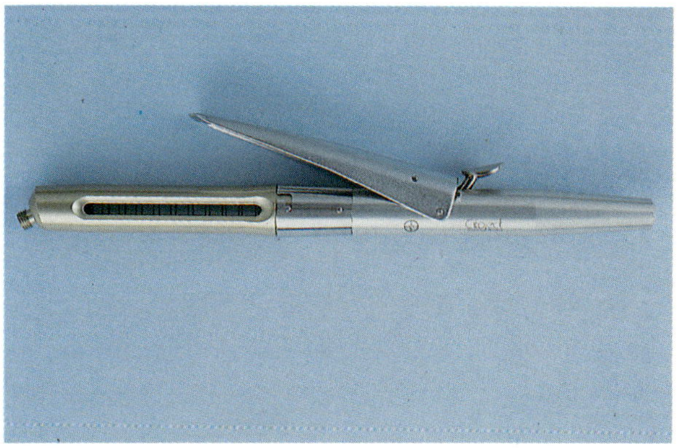

23

23 The Cito Ject – a more recent intra-ligamental syringe

Drugs for local analgesia

The plant alkaloid, cocaine, was isolated in 1860, but has since fallen into relative disuse in medical and dental practice because of its addictive properties.

Procaine, a synthetic aminoester, was discovered in 1905 and was used extensively in the early part of the 20th century. However, a major rival which proved to be stable in solution was synthesized in 1943. This was lignocaine (or lidocaine), an amino-amide. It has been used successfully in clinical practice for over 40 years now.

Further development of amino-amide molecules led to the development of prilocaine, which has a lower level of systemic toxicity.

The chemical structure of the last three drugs is shown in **24**. The latter two local analgesic drugs are now widely used, and appear in a range of strengths of solution with various concentrations of vasoconstrictor agents, e.g.:

- two per cent lignocaine and 1:80,000 adrenaline
- two per cent lignocaine
- three per cent prilocaine and 1:300,000 felypressin
- four per cent prilocaine

The site of action of these local analgesic agents is generally believed to be a specific receptor, near the sodium channels on both the external and internal surfaces of the nerve cell membrane.

Vasoconstrictor agents such as adrenaline (1:80,000) and felypressin (1:300,000) enhance

24

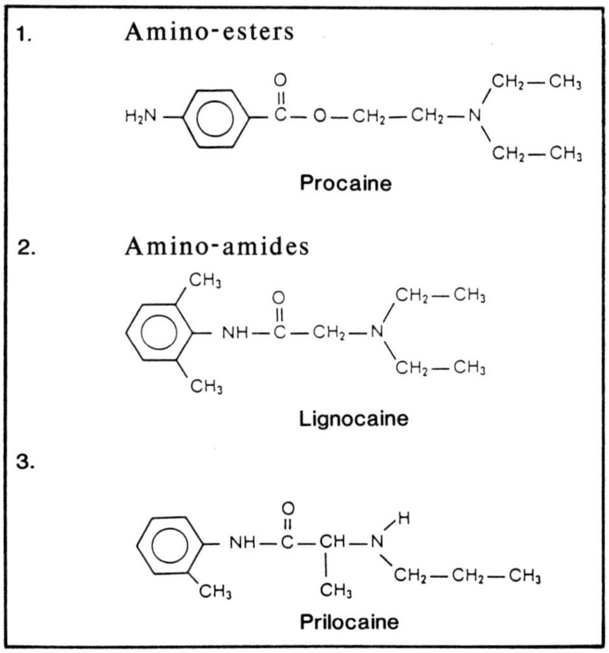

24 Local analgesic drugs

the effect of the drug by constricting local blood vessels and so reducing the rate at which the drug is removed from the injection site.

Elimination of local analgesic is by biotransformation followed by excretion of both active and inactive metabolites. Approximately 20 per cent of lignocaine is excreted unchanged, the remaining 80 per cent being broken down into its metabolites. Prilocaine is excreted in its metabolite form, which constitutes about 75 per cent of the original dose, while around 25 per cent is excreted unchanged.

Local analgesic cartridges

For all practical purposes, local analgesic solution is supplied in alkali- and pyrogen-free glass. It is pre-sterilized and comes 'loose' in boxes of one hundred. However, most local analgesic solution is available in cartridges containing 2.2ml each. The cartridges are usually sold in sealed packs of ten – which means the whole cartridge remains sterile until immediately before use.

The sealing cap of the cartridge comes in a variety of designs, the most common comprising a metal cap with a thin rubber diaphragm (**26**). When loading the syringe care must be taken to ensure that the needle penetrates the centre of this rubber diaphragm. The rubber plunger at the other end of the cartridge is in the form of a solid bung, or else it has a tapered socket to allow the plunger to be inserted and enable aspiration to take place (**27**).

Local analgesic cartridges have the name of the particular drug, its concentration, and also the name of the vasoconstrictor, printed in coloured paint on the outside. An important piece of information which must be checked before each cartridge is inserted in the syringe is the expiry date (also printed on the outside – usually in the style of the 'EXP OCT 89' etc. seen in **28**).

25

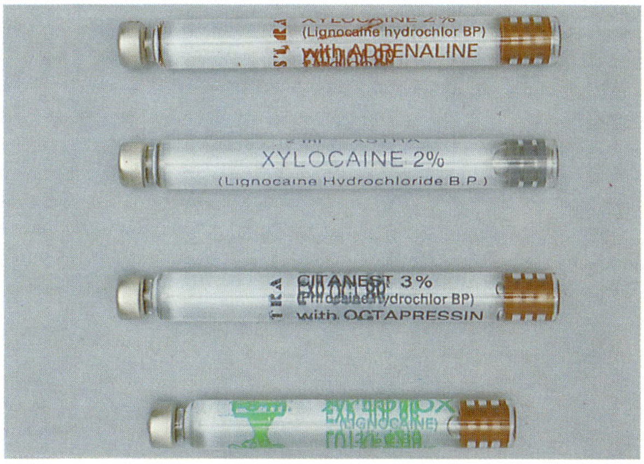

25 Four popular formulations of local analgesic solutions: from the top, two per cent lignocaine with 1:80,000 adrenaline (red ink and red bung); two per cent lignocaine plain (blue ink and blue bung); and three per cent prilocaine with 0.03 international units of felypressin (blue ink and red bung). At the bottom is a smaller 1.8ml cartridge (green ink and red bung) containing two per cent lignocaine with 1:80,000 adrenaline

26

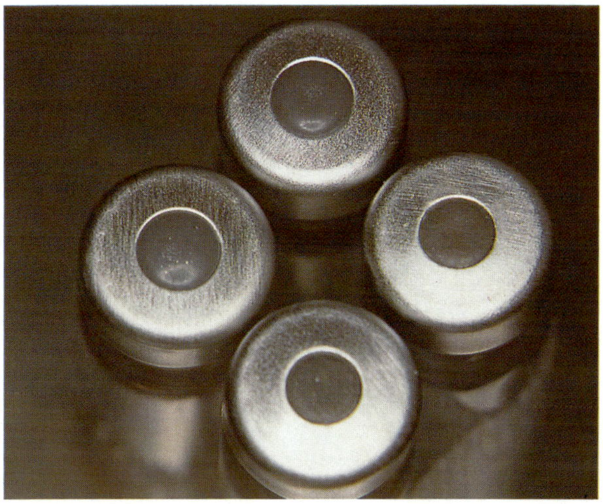

26 Metal sealing caps, with thin rubber diaphragms, atop local analgesic cartridges

27

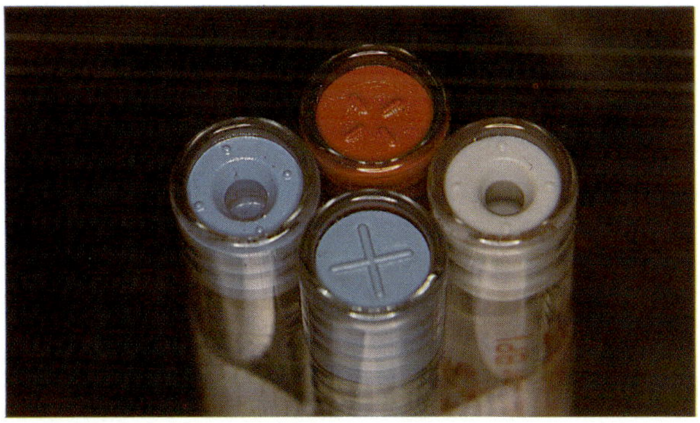

27 Rubber plungers at the other end of the local analgesic cartridges

28

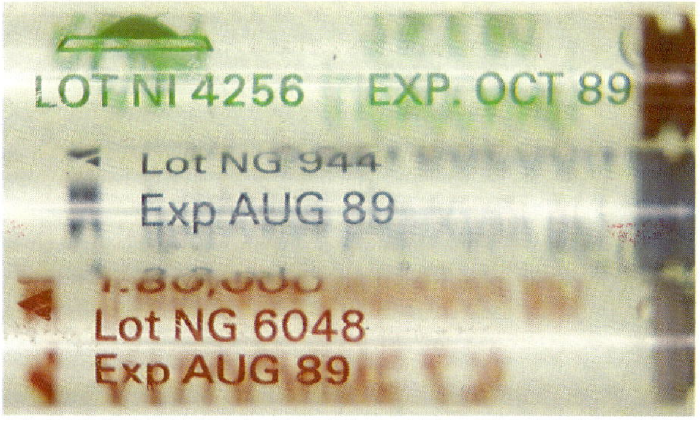

28 Expiry dates are clearly indicated on the sides of the local analgesic cartridges

Résumé of local analgesic syringe assemblies

Non-aspirating

When the component parts illustrated in **29** are assembled, the cap of the needle is kept for recapping the needle when removed. The syringe is placed on the work top, or bracket table, when ready for use, with the yellow sheath to prevent 'needle stick' injuries (see below, under 'Replacing the plastic sheath . . .').

Aspirating

When assembled, the double barb on the plunger is twisted into the rubber bung to engage it. The protective sheath is also left on the hypodermic until immediately before use. This assembly is particularly suited for nerve block analgesia when aspiration is carried out.

Pen-grip intra-ligamental

The same components are assembled as in the case of the pistol-grip syringe, but the ratchet mechanism is oriented so that the dental surgeon can grip the assembly as he would a fountain pen (**31**).

Pistol-grip intra-ligamental

When assembled, the gradations on the plastic sleeve can be seen through the window in the screw-in steel barrel (**32**).

29

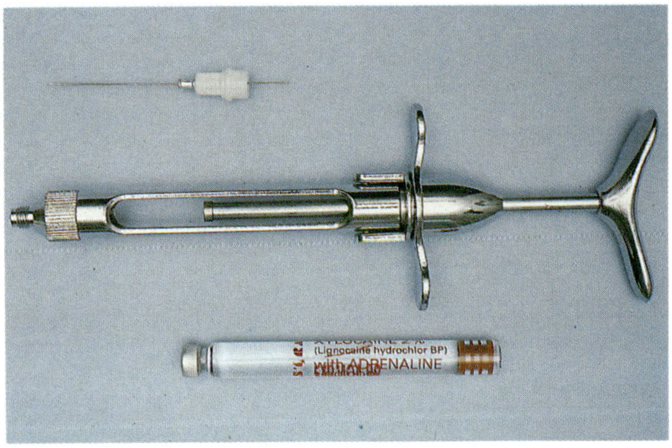

29 Component parts of the non-aspirating syringe: needle, local analgesic cartridge, and syringe

30

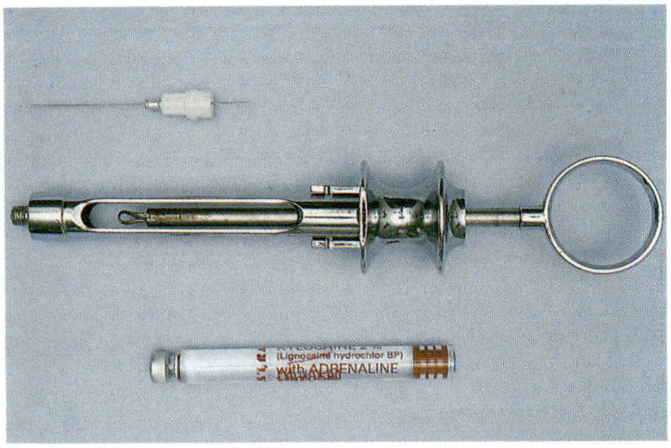

30 Aspirating syringe: needle, local analgesic cartridge, and syringe

31

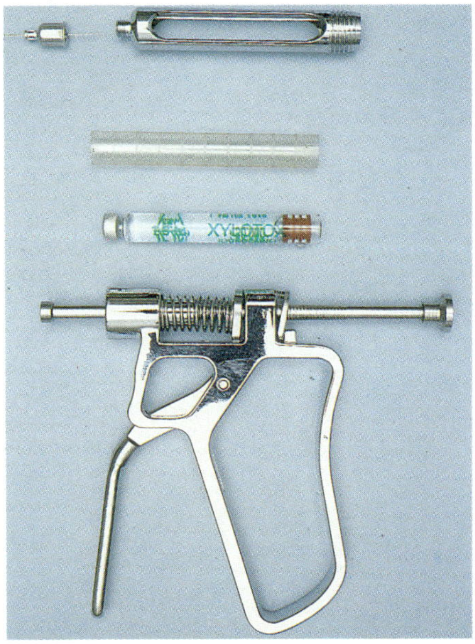

31 Pistol-grip intra-ligamental syringe: needle, screw-in steel barrel, plastic sleeve, local analgesic cartridge, and pistol-grip ratchet mechanism

32

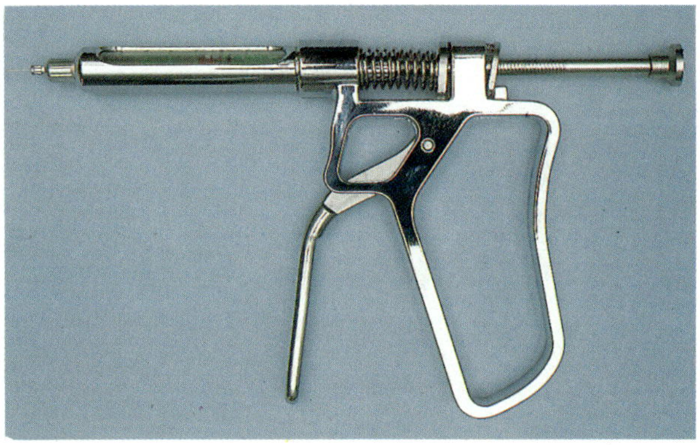

32 Pistol-grip intra-ligamental syringe, assembled. The gradations on the plastic sleeve are visible through the window in the screw-in steel barrel

33

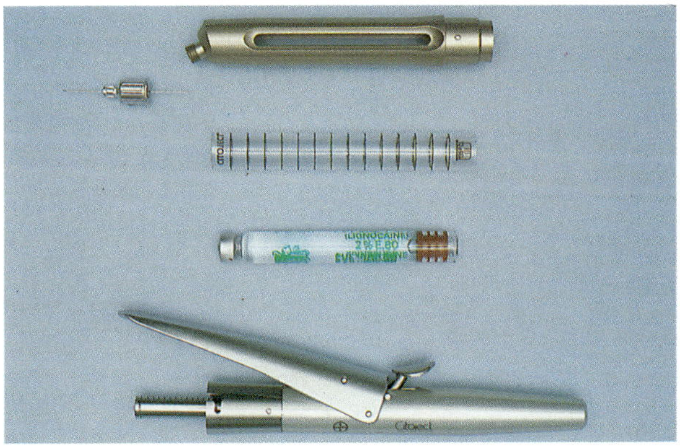

33 Pen-grip intra-ligamental syringe: screw-in steel barrel and needle at top, plastic sleeve, local analgesic cartridge and fountain pen-like ratchet mechanism below

34

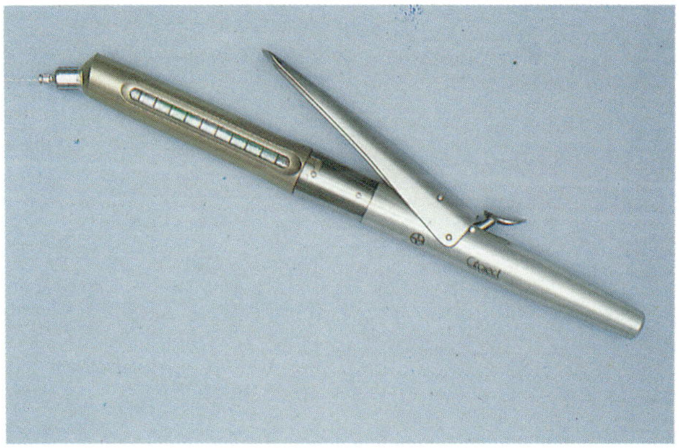

34 Pen-grip intra-ligamental syringe, assembled. The gradations on the plastic sleeve are clearly visible

Replacing the plastic sheath using a 'Sharpsafe' technique

The potential dangers from a needle stick injury are well documented: it takes only a tiny amount of blood from a patient with hepatitis B to transmit the infection. Therefore, when replacing the plastic sheath on the local analgesic assembly, special care must be taken by both the dental surgeon and the dental surgery assistant, each of whom should concentrate on the immediate task at each stage of the procedure:

1. The local analgesic assembly should be placed on the flat work top surface and held still with the fingers extended.
2. The plastic sheath should be moved slowly and carefully over the needle tip until it is held by the friction grip of the sheath on the plastic or metal hub.
3. The plastic sheath should be pushed firmly onto the hub of the hypodermic.

Local analgesia techniques

Topical analgesia

A small quantity of topical analgesic paste or ointment is placed on a sterile cotton roll by the dental surgery assistant. Meanwhile, the mucosa is dried by the dental surgeon using another sterile roll, discarded after use.

The topical analgesic is then placed on the mucosa at the proposed puncture site and left for two minutes to take effect (35). Care must be taken to prevent it spreading elsewhere in the mouth as this would be unpleasant for the patient. Excess 'topical' is wiped away immediately before administration of the local analgesic.

35

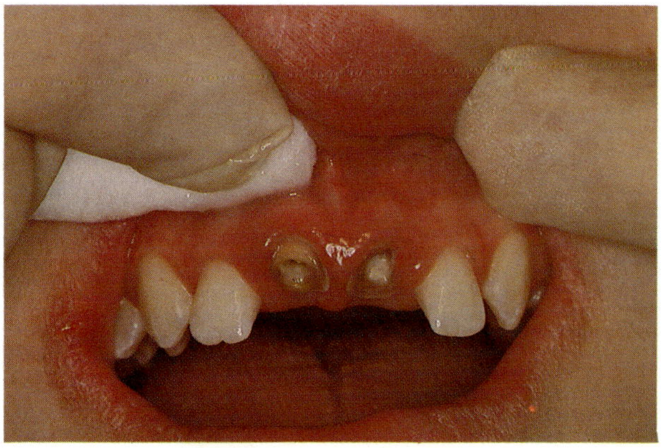

35 Topical analgesic paste is placed on the mucosa at the proposed puncture site

Infiltration analgesia: supraperiosteal and subperiosteal

The supraperiosteal and subperiosteal variations of this technique differ only in the fact that, in supraperiosteal infiltration, the tip of the needle is placed beneath the submucosa in elastic tissue. This allows the dental surgeon to administer a local analgesic to a very apprehensive patient, as the submucosal infiltration can be achieved with the minimum of discomfort. The disadvantage of submucosal infiltration is that the analgesic solution takes a long time to penetrate the periosteum and make the nerve bundles entering the apical foramina of the teeth to be conserved analgesic.

To ensure adequate analgesia by the infiltration technique it is necessary to insert the needle beneath the periosteum. This is likely to be perceived as extremely painful by an anxious patient, in which case it can be preceded by the less discomforting submucosal infiltration, which will make the periosteum analgesic. In the case of non-anxious patients, the dental surgeon can proceed directly to a subperiosteal infiltration if he thinks this is appropriate.

THE MAXILLA: CENTRAL INCISORS, LATERAL INCISORS, AND CANINES

Infiltration analgesia on the upper central incisor. The upper central incisor can be made analgesic using the technique of infiltration analgesia. The mucosa is pulled taut and the needle – which should preferably be a short one, in a non-aspirating syringe – is inserted about 8mm apical to the gingival margin. It is then pushed gently upwards, passing beneath the periosteum (unless it is decided to carry out a submucosal injection first), until the tip of the needle – with the bevel towards the bone – is over the apex of the tooth. A useful guide to positioning is to place the tip of the needle approximately 21mm from the incisal edge: thus, the hub of a short needle should be just apical to the incisal edge. The correct alignment and positioning of the needle can be seen in relation to the skull illustrated in **36**. The mucosa is pulled taut and the needle is passed through it with a deliberate forward motion. Approximately 1ml of local analgesic solution is deposited.

When inserting the needle for lateral incisors, account must be taken of the shorter root (**37**). In addition, because of the relative palatal position of the apex of the lateral incisor root, it is often necessary to administer a naso-palatine block to ensure adequate analgesia of the tooth. Do not forget that, where canines are concerned, the root is usually some 25mm long. A useful guide to placement of the needle tip is the canine eminence.

36

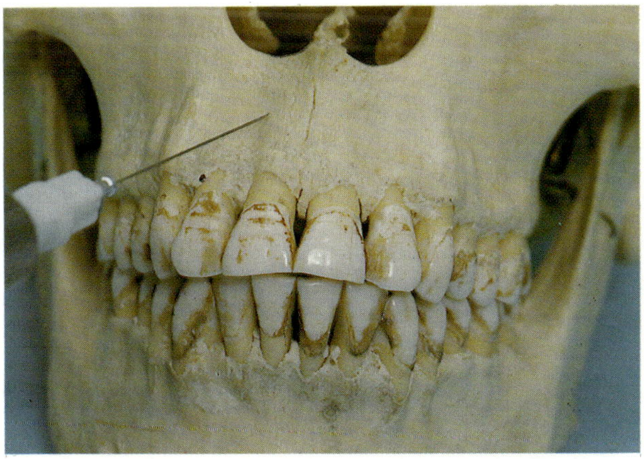

36 Infiltration analgesia on the upper central incisor. Note the position of the needle

37

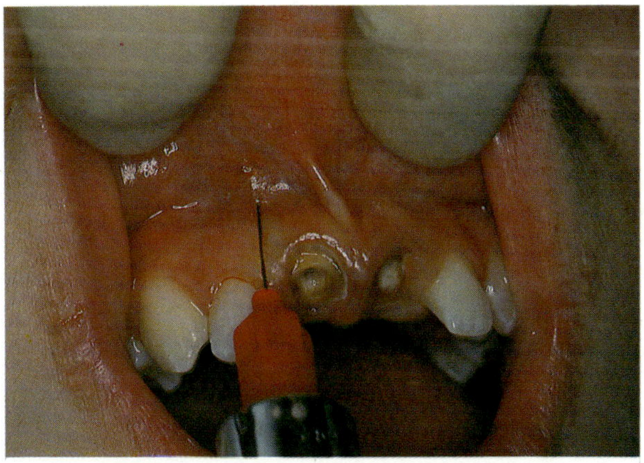

37 Infiltration analgesia on the lateral incisor. The shorter root must be considered when inserting the needle

Infiltration analgesia on the upper second premolar. The same basic technique as for incisors and canines is used (**38**). The mucosa is pulled taut and the needle – again, preferably a short one – is gently inserted, bevel towards the bone until the tip is over the apex of the tooth to be made analgesic (**39**). The canine eminence and the base of the zygomatic process of the maxilla are useful guides to positioning the needle. For the first premolar the needle should be placed distal to the canine eminence and approximately 22mm from the tip of the buccal cusp, while for the second it is placed mesial to the base of the zygomatic process and about 21mm from the tip of the buccal cusp.

A palatal infiltration is administered to the first, and occasionally the second, premolar (**40**), to ensure that analgesia (especially of the soft tissues) is sufficiently profound for operative procedures.

38

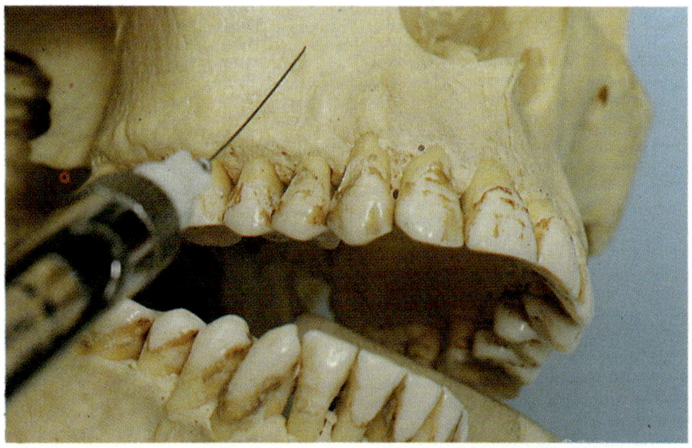

39

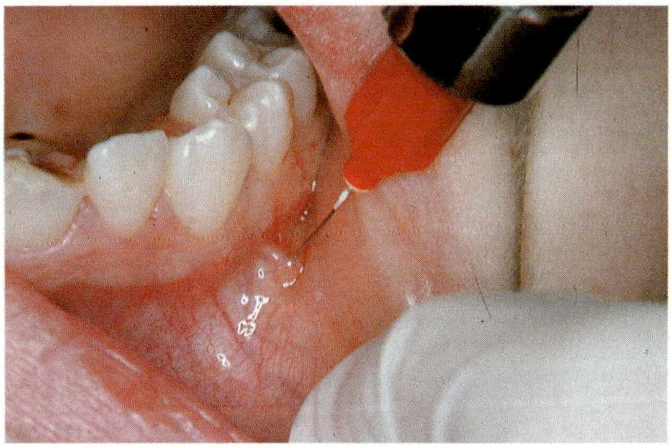

38 and 39 Infiltration analgesia on the upper second premolar

40

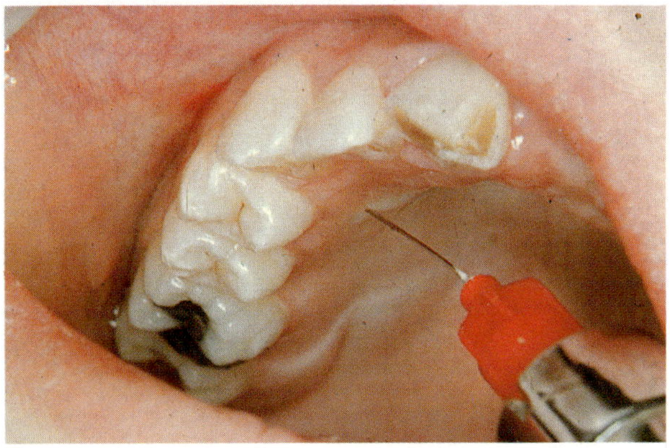

40 Infiltration analgesia: palatal infiltration is administered to the first, and occasionally the second, premolar

Infiltration analgesia on the upper first permanent molar. The upper first permanent molar can be made analgesic by means of a buccal infiltration (**41** and **42**). A short needle in a conventional assembly is preferred. The presence of the zygomatic process of the maxillary bone means that it may be necessary to administer two infiltrations, one mesial to the zygomatic process for the mesio-buccal root and one just distal for the disto-buccal root. For the mesio-buccal root the needle tip should be about 23mm from the mesio-buccal cusp, while for the disto-buccal root it should be slightly distal and approximately 21mm from the disto-buccal cusp (**43** and **44**).

The palatal root is so far away from the buccal cortex of the maxilla that a separate palatal infiltration is needed. To achieve this a short needle is used, approximately 3–4mm being inserted into the palatal mucosa, roughly 8mm apical to the gingival margin (**45** and **46**). Because the palatal mucosa is very firmly bound to the bony palate the dental surgeon must take care to inject gently to minimize the discomfort to the patient. On pressing the plunger, the increased pressure within the tissues will result in saliva being expressed from the minor salivary glands in the palate. In addition, the tissue will blanch – indicating the area of infiltration of the tissue.

41

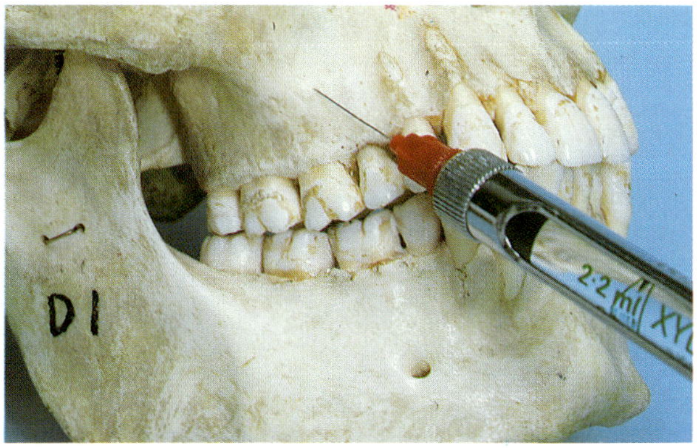

42

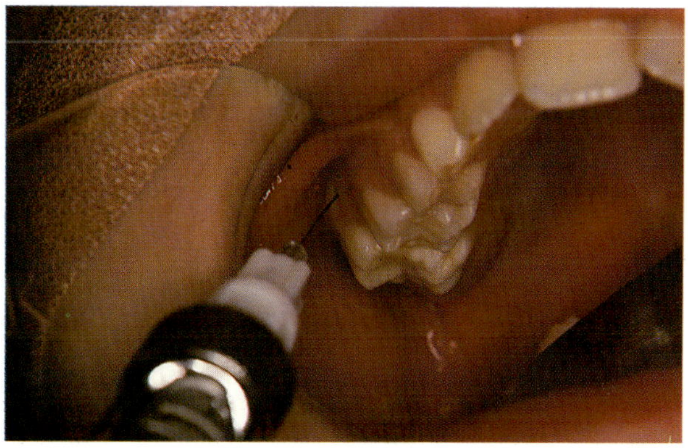

41 and **42** The tip of the needle is placed deep in the buccal sulcus to lie over the apices of the upper front and/or the second molar(s)

43

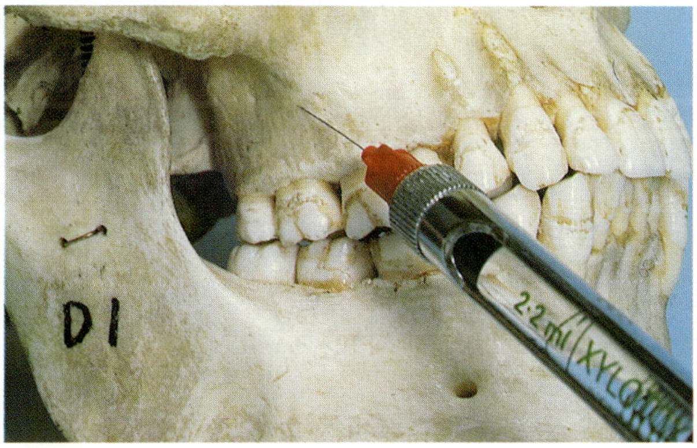

44

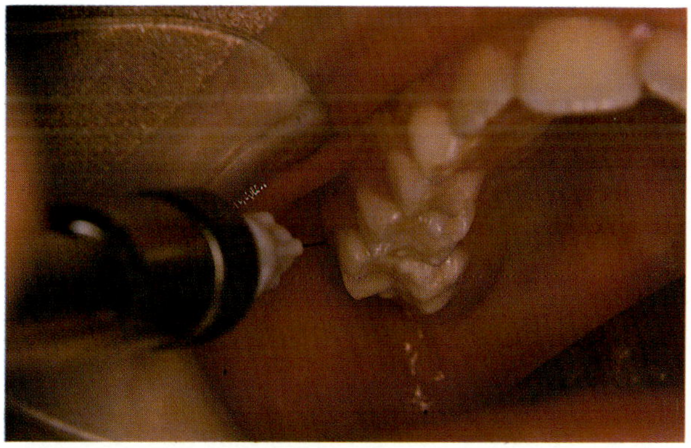

43 and **44** The tip of the needle is placed distal to the zygomatic eminence onto the tuberosity

45 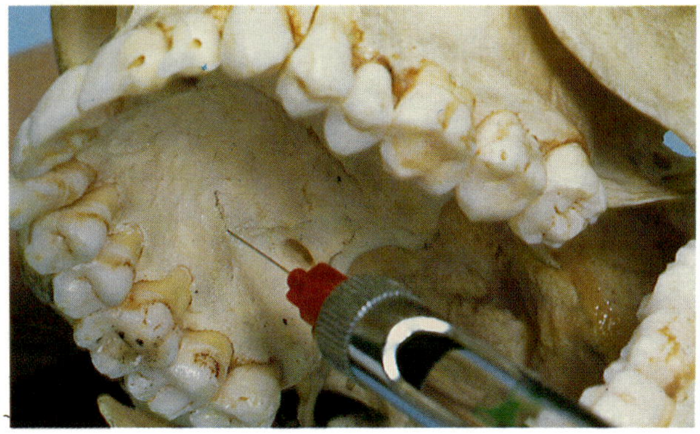 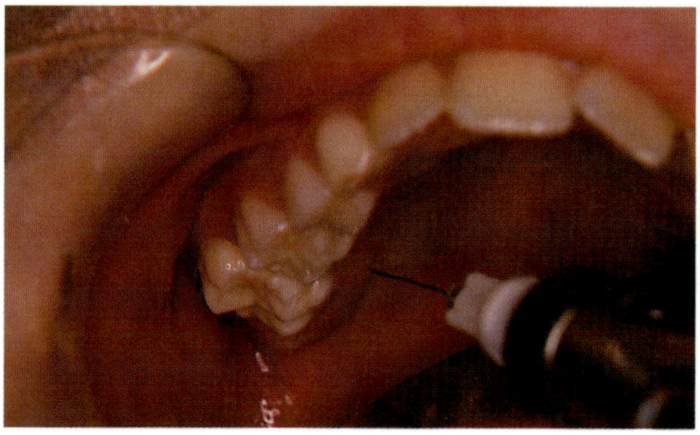 46

45 and **46** Injection into the palatal area causes blanching of the mucosa

THE MANDIBLE: CENTRAL INCISORS, LATERAL INCISORS, AND CANINES

47 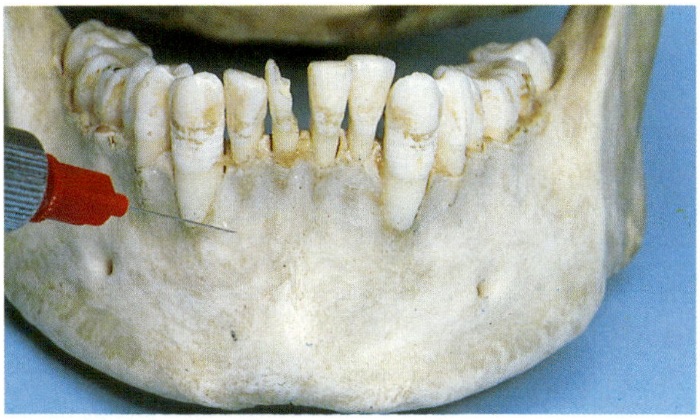

47 The needle is placed so that the tip is approximately 18mm from the incisal edge

48 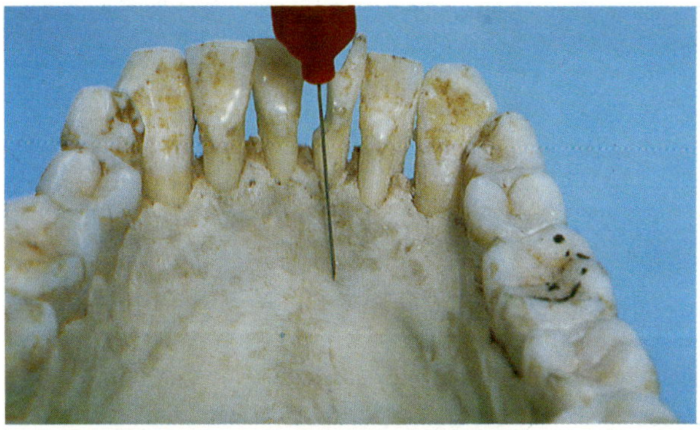

48 Clinically, the needle is placed deep in the labial sulcus, and the tip inserted beneath the periosteum. Approximately 0.75–1ml is injected

49 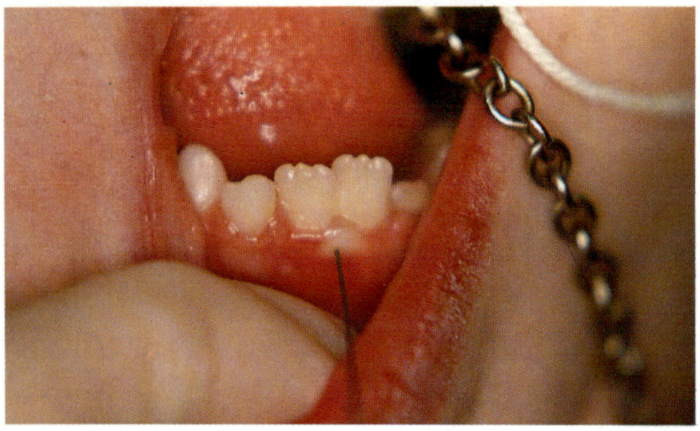

49 A variation on the infiltration technique is to give a simple infiltration into the interdental papilla

50

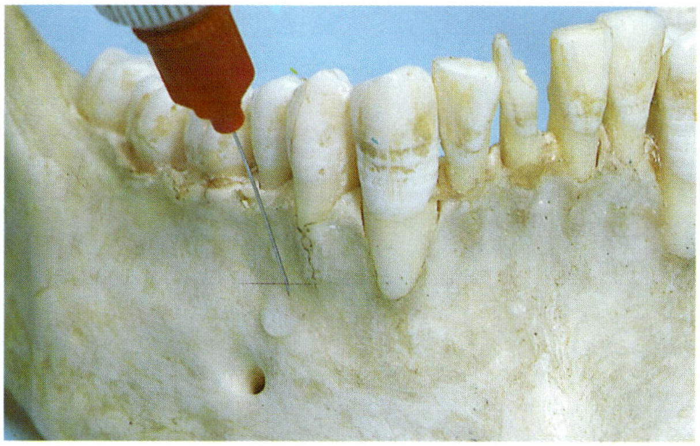

50 and 51 The tip of the needle is placed in the buccal sulcus, close to the apex of the teeth concerned

51

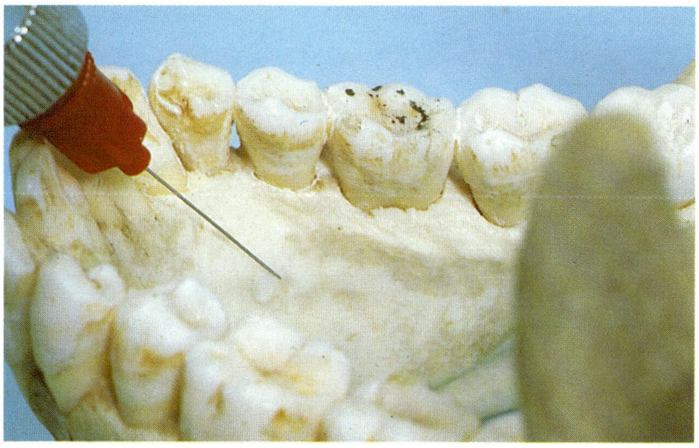

52

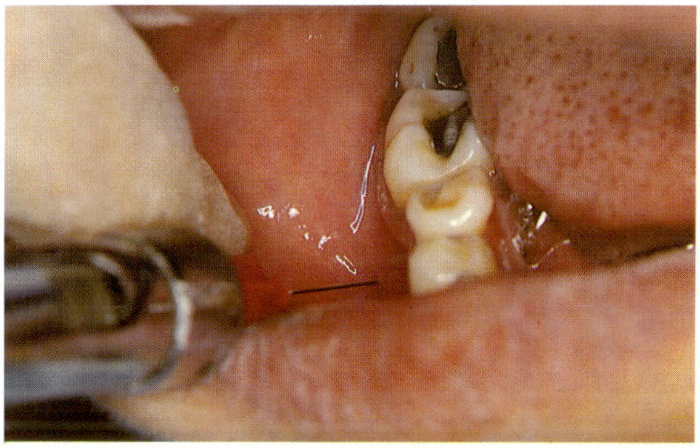

52 and 53 The mucosa is pulled taut and the tip of the needle placed subperiosteally with the bevel towards the bone. Between 1 and 0.50ml of solution is deposited on both the labial and the lingual aspects

53

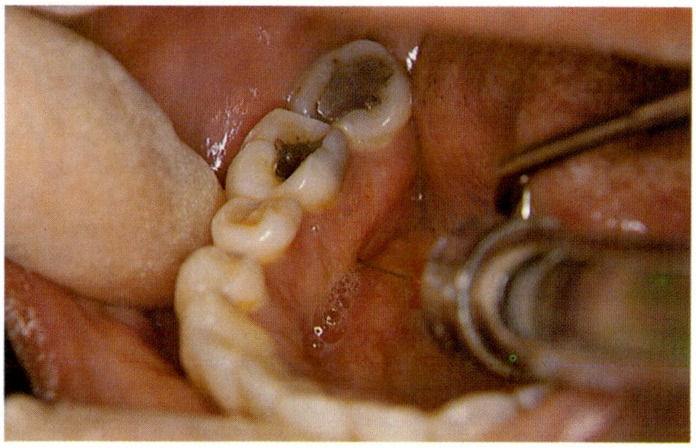

THE MANDIBLE: FIRST, SECOND AND THIRD PERMANENT MOLARS

The basic technique here is the same as for premolars, apart from the obvious position of the needle in relation to the teeth involved.

54 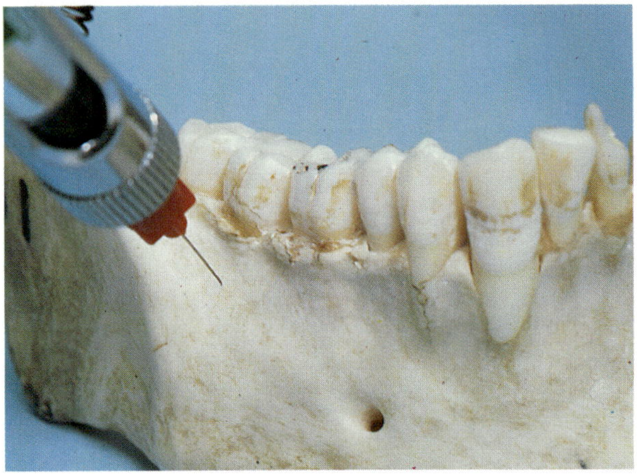 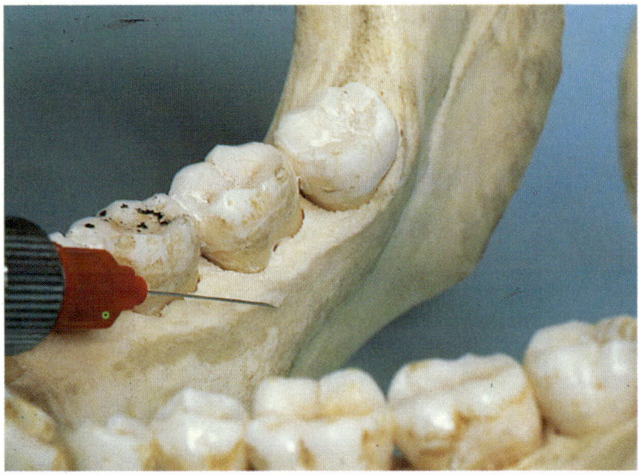 55

54 and 55 The tip of the needle is placed in the sulcus adjacent to the apices of the tooth. The broad shelf of bone buccally means that penetration of the solution takes a relatively long time

INFILTRATION ANALGESIA: MODIFICATIONS FOR YOUNG PATIENTS

The smaller size of young patients' jaws in comparison to older patients' means that, when administering infiltration analgesia, the dental surgeon should not insert the needle as far. The amount of solution injected should likewise be correspondingly reduced. Because of the greater tendency of child patients to react adversely to painful stimuli, more use should be made of submucosal infiltrations prior to the administration of a subperiosteal infiltration analgesia.

INFILTRATION ANALGESIA: MODIFICATIONS FOR OLDER PATIENTS

The techniques for older patients are virtually identical to those employed for young adults. However, since many such patients have chronic periodontal disease, the depth of the sulcus is often reduced. The risk of potentially serious medical complications is also greater in older patients, either because of the medical problem itself or as a result of the drugs being used. Furthermore, such patients are often emotionally frail: behaviour management may require special consideration and more care may be necessary in the presentation of post-operative instructions.

Nerve block analgesia

The basic principle of local analgesia applies as much to nerve block analgesia as to any other technique: a local analgesic solution is deposited close or adjacent to a bundle of nerve fibres to achieve analgesia of the tissues served by that neurovascular bundle. The major difference in the case of nerve block analgesia is that considerably larger quantities of the local analgesic solution are required to ensure that local analgesia is adequate. Furthermore, the anatomical size of the neural bundle means that the solution will usually take longer to penetrate to its centre; thus, more time must be allowed to elapse before operative procedures can be started.

THE MAXILLA: POSTERIOR SUPERIOR ALVEOLAR NERVE BLOCK

The upper third molar, second molar, and the disto-buccal and palatal roots of the upper first molar are supplied by branches of the maxillary division of the trigeminal which form the posterior superior dental nerve.

The posterior superior alveolar block is achieved by inserting the needle distal to the last molar, upwards and medial at about 45°, to enable the deposition of approximately 1.5ml of solution on the disto-buccal aspect of the maxilla (**56** and **57**). A common complication of this technique is when some of the vessels of the pterygoid venous plexus are ruptured, resulting in a haematoma. Since modern local analgesic drugs have become widely used, infiltration techniques – involving the deposition of only 1ml of solution – have been employed instead.

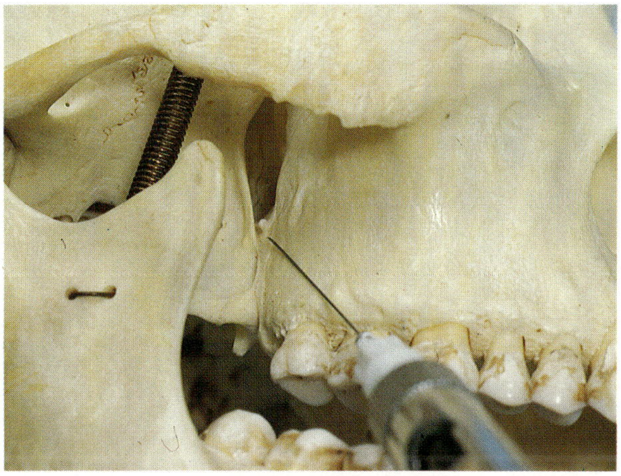

56

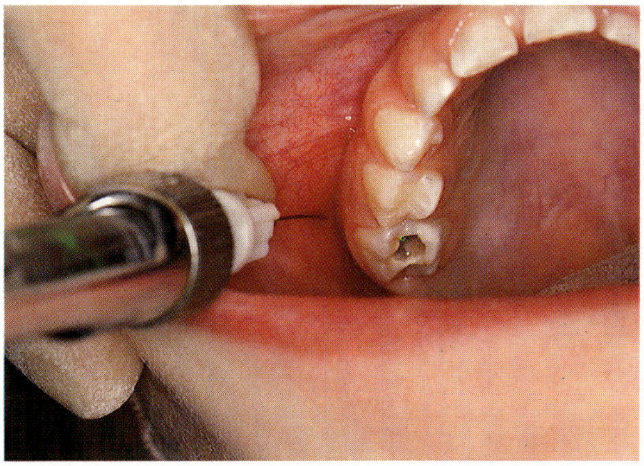

57

56 and 57 Analgesia of the posterior superior alveolar nerve

THE MAXILLA: MIDDLE SUPERIOR ALVEOLAR NERVE BLOCK

The mesio-buccal root of the first molar, together with the roots of both premolars – and the mucosa and periosteum associated with them – is supplied by the middle superior alveolar nerve. Analgesia of this nerve is achieved by the deposition of 1ml of solution deep in the sulcus, between the mesio-buccal root of the first molar and the root of the second premolar (**58** and **59**).

58

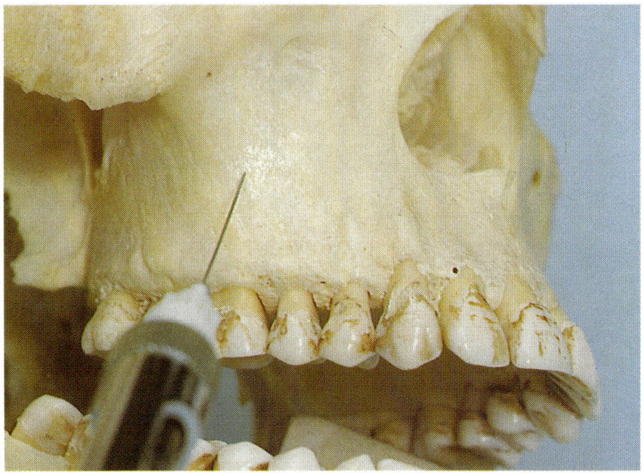

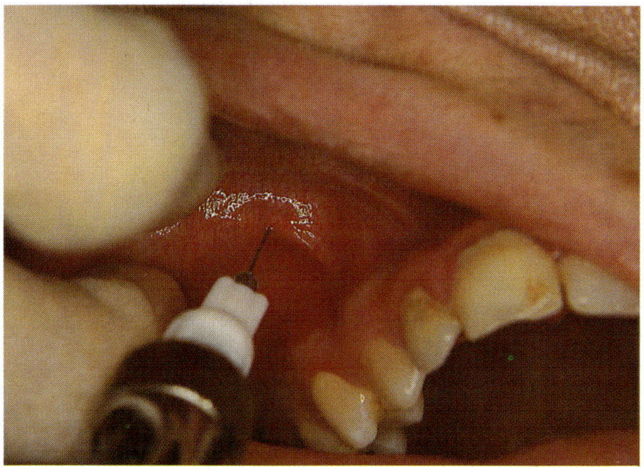

59

58 and 59 Analgesia of the middle superior alveolar nerve

THE MAXILLA: ANTERIOR SUPERIOR ALVEOLAR NERVE BLOCK

The anterior superior alveolar nerve supplies the upper canine, lateral incisor and central incisor. It can be blocked by infiltrating 1–1.5ml of solution deep in the sulcus below the level of the infra-orbital formation (**60**).

60

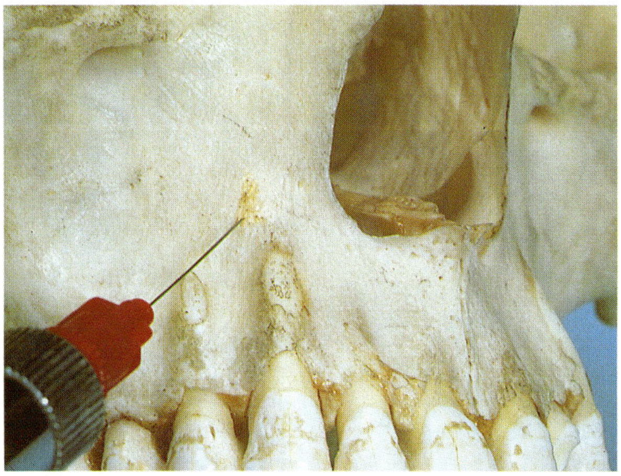

60 Analgesia of the anterior superior alveolar nerve

THE MAXILLA: INFRA-ORBITAL NERVE BLOCK

Extensive analgesia of the anterior part of one side of the maxilla can be achieved by making the infra-orbital nerve analgesic. This is particularly useful where infection precludes the use of infiltration techniques. The technique relies on the fact that analgesic solution deposited at the entrance to the infra-orbital foramen passes along the infra-orbital canal to involve both the anterior superior alveolar nerve and the middle superior alveolar nerve.

The intra-oral approach is most commonly used. The infra-orbital ridge is palpated and, using the tip of the first finger, the infra-orbital notch is identified. With the finger tip maintained in this position, the thumb is used to reflect the upper lip. The tip of the needle is inserted deep in the sulcus above the apex of the second premolar (**61**), and advanced in line with the long axis of the tooth until it is 1.5–2cm deep – when the analgesic solution is deposited. A swelling of tissue can be felt beneath the first finger when the tip of the needle is in the correct position. Allow approximately three minutes to elapse to ensure adequate analgesia.

61

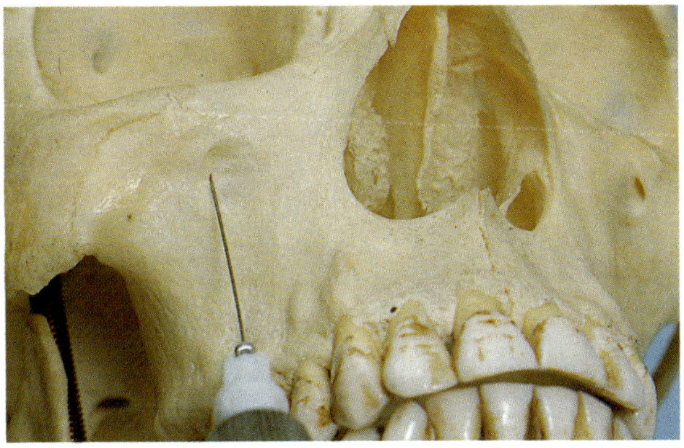

61 Analgesia of the infra-orbital nerve

THE MAXILLA: ANALGESIA OF THE PALATE

The whole of the palate is innervated by three nerve bundles (**62**). The paired greater palatine nerves supply the right and left sides as far forward as the canine, while anteriorly, the mucosa and periosteum palatal to the upper incisors and the mesial half of the canines are served by the nasopalatine nerve bundle.

Analgesia of the whole of the palate can be achieved by blocking these three nerves. Alternatively, part of the palate can be made analgesic by a local infiltration.

62

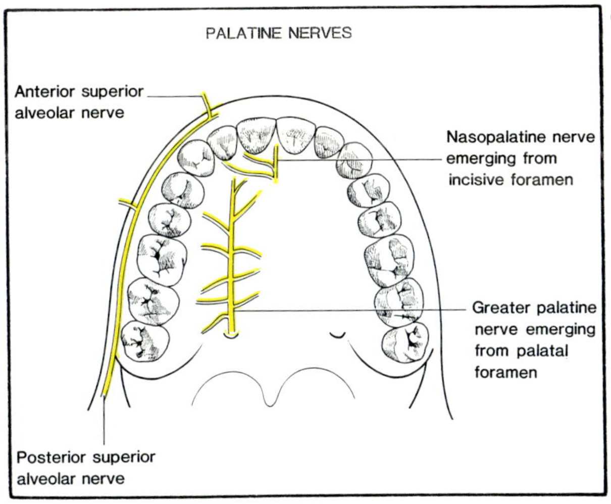

62 The nerves of the palate

THE MAXILLA: PALATINE NERVE BLOCK

Analgesia of the palate on one side as far forward as the canine can be achieved by depositing approximately 0.5–0.75ml of solution over the greater palatine nerves as they emerge from the greater palatine foramen.

In the skeletal photograph (**63**), the foramen can be seen opposite the distal surface of the second maxillary molar, at the junction between the hard palate and the alveolar process.

Clinically, the needle is inserted approximately 0.5cm (**64**). The injection is given slowly as the tissues are firmly bound down. The mucosa may blanch, and saliva from minor salivary glands may be extruded.

63

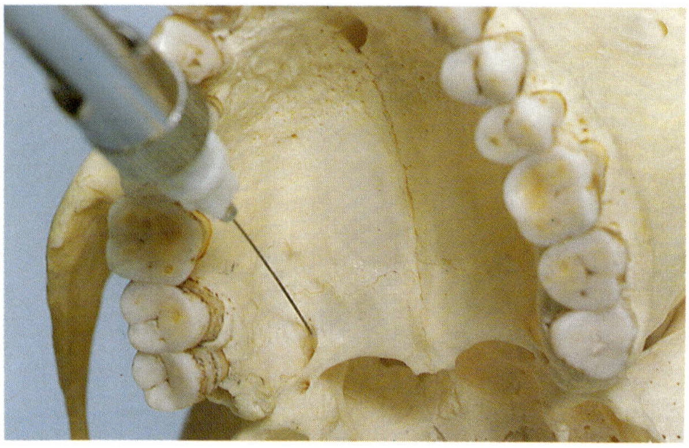

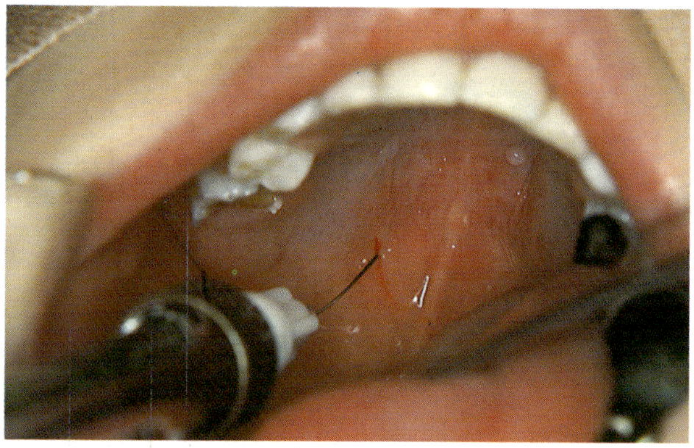

64

63 and **64** Analgesia of the palate

THE MAXILLA: NASOPALATINE NERVE BLOCK

The mucosa and periosteum in the anterior region of the hard palate are innervated by the nasopalatine nerve.

The tip of the needle is inserted through the nasopalatine papilla until it rests within the entrance to the incisal canal (**65**). If the bone is contacted the needle is withdrawn approximately 0.5–1mm. Approximately 0.1–0.2ml of solution is deposited (**66**); the solution must not be forced too rapidly as it will cause great discomfort. The tissue will blanch, and the onset of analgesia is rapid.

65

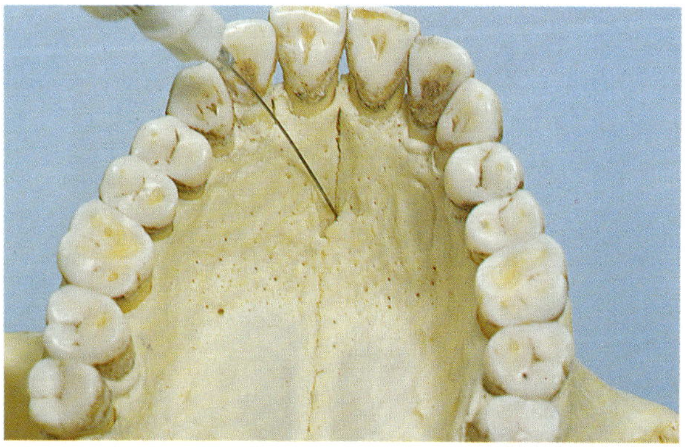

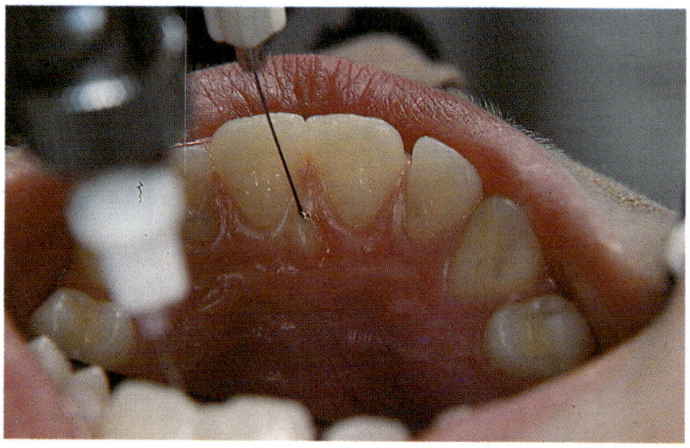

66

65 and **66** Analgesia of the nasopalatine nerve

The mandible: inferior alveolar nerve block

This nerve block technique is probably the single most important local analgesic injection in dental practice. Properly administered it provides, when combined with a lingual nerve block and long buccal nerve block, analgesia of the hard and soft tissues of one side of the mandible from the third molar to the central incisor. No other combination of injections achieves such widespread and profound analgesia. For the technique to be reliable, however, the dental surgeon must pay careful attention to the anatomical relationships of the inferior alveolar nerve.

ANATOMICAL CONSIDERATIONS

A few millimetres above the level of the occlusal plane, in the horizontal section, the inferior alveolar nerve lies against the medial surface of the ramus of the mandible in the pterygoid space. This space is bounded by the pterygo-mandibular raphe anteriorly. The fibres of the buccinator and superior pharyngeal constrictors are inserted into it. At the posterior is the parotid gland. The lateral wall is formed by the medial surface of the mandibular ramus, and the medial wall by the medial pterygoid muscle. The lingual nerve ascends diagonally backwards through the space until it joins the mandibular nerve superior to the mandibular foramen. There is a shallow bony depression just superior to the mandibular foramen into which local analgesic solution must be deposited to achieve profound analgesia of the inferior alveolar nerve (**67**).

The long buccal nerve is composed of a bundle of nerve fibres arising from the mandibular division of the trigeminal nerve. It is remote from the inferior alveolar nerve so a separate injection is necessary to achieve

67

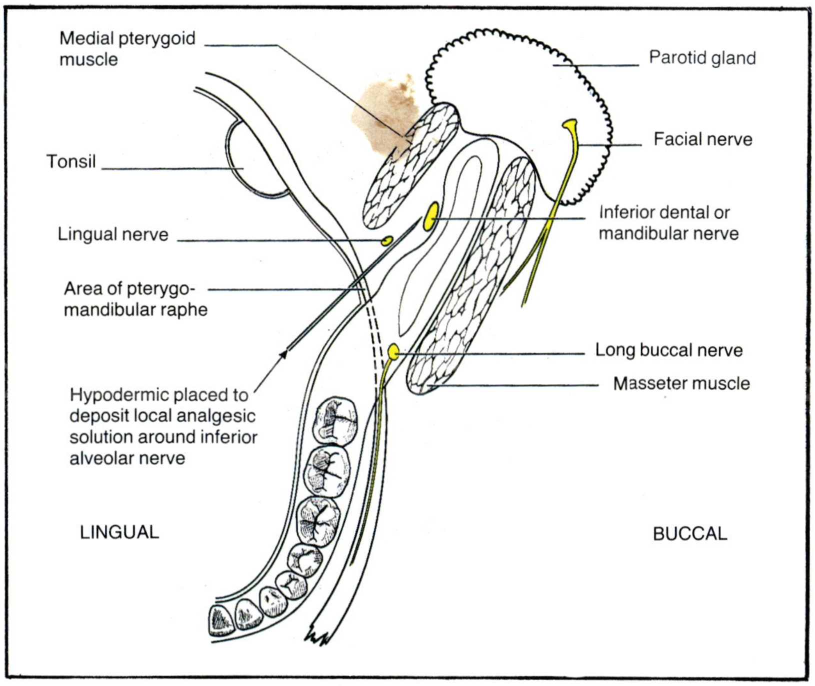

67 Inferior alveolar nerve block (horizontal section)

68 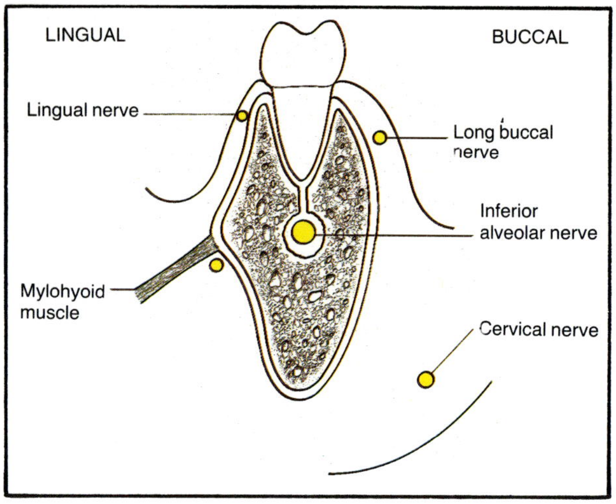

analgesia of the buccal mucosa and attached gingivae. At the level of the first permanent molar, in the coronal plane, these three nerves are in distinct bundles (**68**). The lingual nerve is beneath the mucosa in the lingual region. The inferior alveolar nerve is deep in the body of the mandible and gives off branches to the roots of individual teeth. The long buccal nerve lies in the tissues of the buccal mucosa.

68 Inferior alveolar nerve (coronal section in the first molar region)

OSTEOLOGY

69 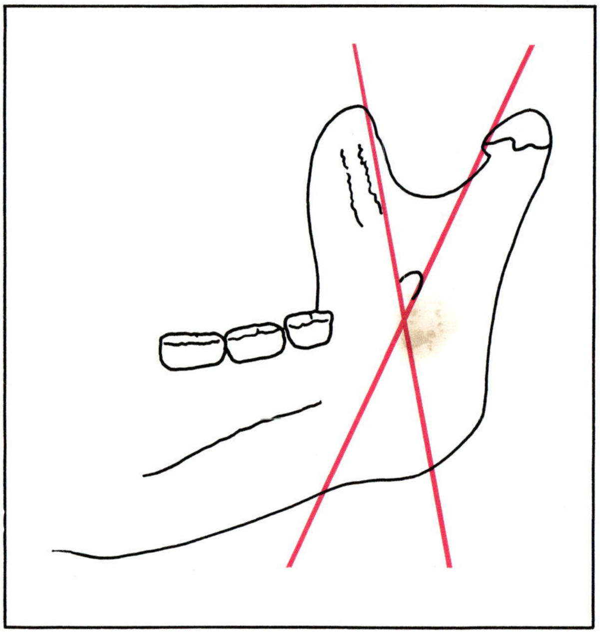

69 Locating the lingula

Notwithstanding the considerations of soft tissue anatomy given above, an important anatomical relationship when administering the inferior alveolar block clinically is the one existing between the lingula – and, therefore, the inferior alveolar foramen – and the coronoid process, mandibular condyle, mandibular notch and angle of the mandible.

The dental surgeon should imagine, in his mind's eye, a cross consisting of a line joining the coronoid process and the angle of the mandible intersecting with a line joining the mandibular condyle and the mandibular notch (**69**). The lingula is just superior to this notch. When administering an inferior alveolar block the dental surgeon should, by palpation, estimate the position of these bony landmarks and – coupled with the soft tissue landmarks – aim the tip of the needle to rest within 2–3mm of this point.

Clinical considerations

The success of the inferior alveolar nerve block technique depends upon the dental surgeon depositing approximately 2ml of local analgesic solution around the lingula where the inferior alveolar nerve enters the mandible.

The patient is seated and, after sufficient explanation and reassurance, the dental chair is laid flat to reduce the risk of a faint. The dental surgeon, too, should be seated, likewise the dental surgery assistant. The latter takes the local analgesic assembly and passes it behind the patient's head into the right hand of the dental surgeon. At the same time the needle guard, or plastic container, is held by the assistant so that when the dental surgeon grasps the syringe the needle guard is removed.

The patient is asked to open his mouth, so that the dental surgeon can inspect the retromolar area. It is usually possible to identify the ridge of mucous membrane, overlying the pterygomandibular raphe (**70**). The thumb is used to retract the cheek and simultaneously to delineate the apex of the buccal pad of fat. As the thumb is moved further back into the mouth the external oblique ridge is felt. The tip of the thumb is then moved medially to lie in the retromolar fossa: the mid point of the nail can now be used as a guide for insertion of the needle. In addition, the dental surgeon should use osteological landmarks to help direct the needle to the lingula. The horizontal angle of approach is estimated by holding the barrel of the syringe parallel to the occlusal plane, the oblique angle by placing the barrel of the syringe over the premolar teeth of the opposite side (**71**).

The needle is then inserted about 0.5cm and a few drops (0.1–0.2ml) deposited to anaesthetize the lingual nerve (the lingual nerve block). The needle should be advanced gently for a further 1.5–2cm until its tip lightly touches the bone above the mandibular foramen. It is then withdrawn slightly and aspirated. If there is no withdrawal of blood 1.5ml of solution is deposited (**72B**). The needle is then gently withdrawn. This is known as the direct method. The speed of onset is variable, but after three or four minutes the patient should experience pins-and-needles or a swollen feeling; surgical analgesia will be sufficiently profound within another two or three minutes.

The achievement of analgesia is assessed by the onset of pins-and-needles in the patient's lip. This can be verified, if necessary, by inserting a probe 2–3mm into the gingivae of the interdental space of any of the molar teeth.

70

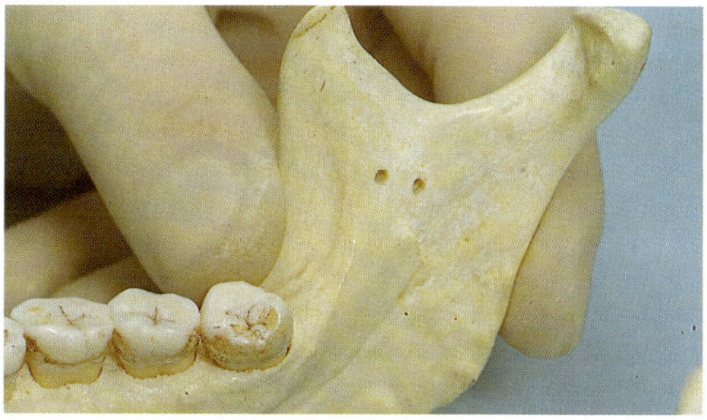

70 The ridge of mucous membrane, overlying the pterygomandibular raphe

71

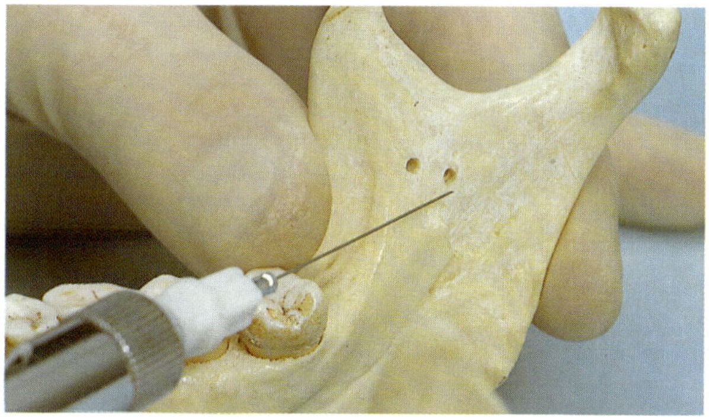

71 The oblique angle of approach is estimated by placing the barrel of the syringe over the premolar teeth of the opposite side

72A

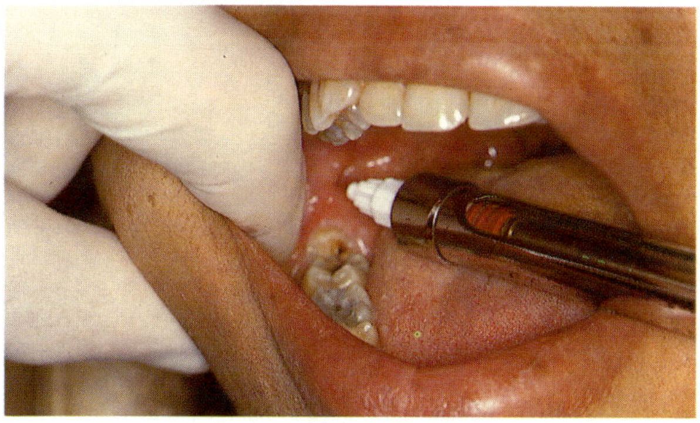

72A Positioning of syringe and needle, in order to administer an inferior alveolar nerve block.

72B

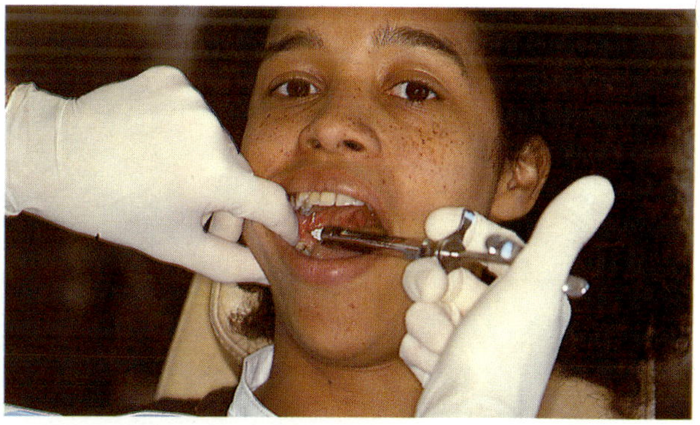

72B The needle lightly touches the bone above the mandibular foramen, and then is withdrawn and aspirated; if there is no withdrawal of blood, 1.5ml of solution is deposited

OLDER PATIENTS

If the patient has a lot of molar teeth missing and there is gross alveolar resorption, the relationship of the lingula to the occlusal plane is lost. The dental surgeon must then resort to using the osteological landmarks (**73** and **74**) as the principal guide to administering the inferior alveolar block.

74

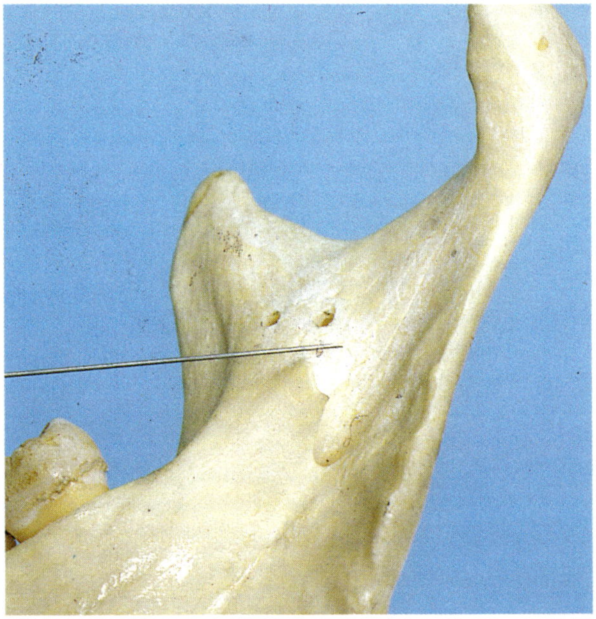

73

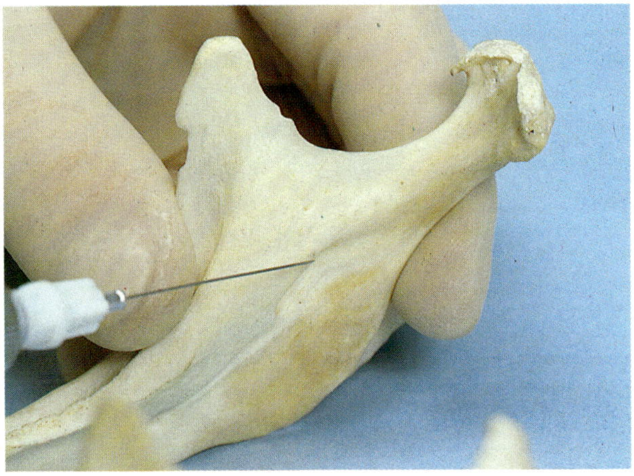

73 and 74 Using osteological landmarks to administer the inferior alveolar block

CHILD PATIENTS

Because of the relatively smaller distance from the anterior border of the ramus, only a short (20mm) needle is required. In addition, in young patients, the inferior alveolar foramen is placed below the occlusal plane. For this reason, in children up to the age of six or seven years, the needle should be angled downwards, so that the tip is brought to the lingula at approximately the level of the gingival margin (**75**).

75

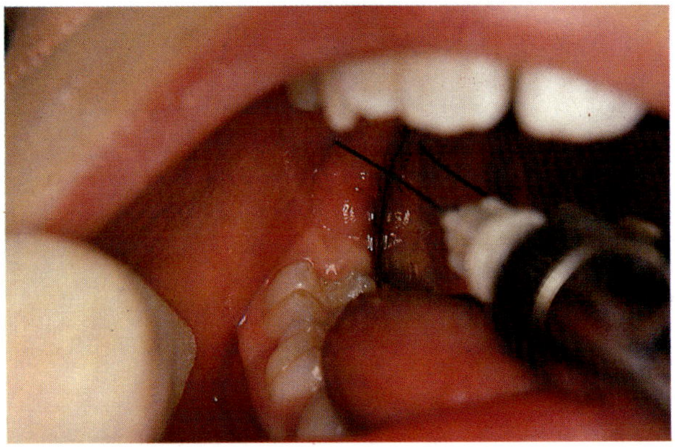

75 In children of six or seven, the needle is angled downwards, so that the tip is brought to the lingula at approximately the level of the gingival margin

EXTRA-ORAL APPROACH

Occasionally, severe trismus means that the patient is unable to open his mouth wide enough to allow the dental surgeon to insert the syringe. In this rare circumstance, an extra-oral approach can be used.

Using the osteological landmarks, particularly the angle of the mandible, the needle is inserted inferiorly for about 2.5cm (**76**). Once analgesia has been achieved, the mouth can usually be opened sufficiently wide to enable operative procedures to be carried out. It should be emphasized again, however, that this procedure is very rarely necessary.

76

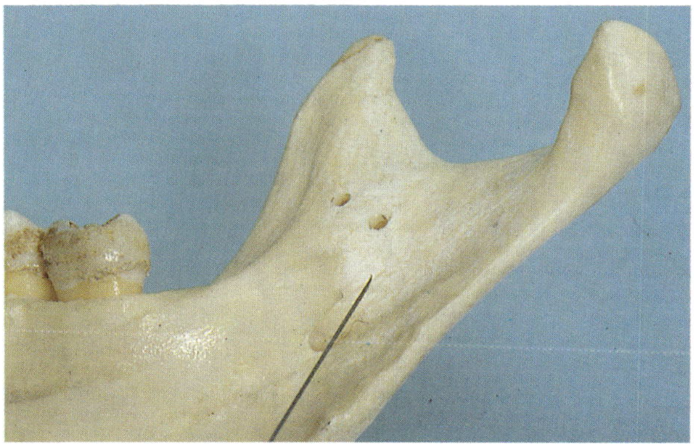

76 Extra-oral approach: using the osteological landmarks, particularly the angle of the mandible, the needle is inserted inferiorly for about 2.5cm

GOW-GATES TECHNIQUE

An alternative method of achieving analgesia of the inferior alveolar nerve is the Gow-Gates technique. The tip of the needle is placed at the neck of the mandibular condyle in the vicinity of the early path of the mandibular branch of the trigeminal nerve (**77** and **78**).

The mucosa is punctured higher than the conventional site for a block of the inferior alveolar nerve. The dental surgeon uses palpation of the mandibular condyle extra-orally as a guide when inserting the needle about 1.5–2cm. The whole of a 2.2ml cartridge should be deposited at this site.

The Gow-Gates technique has the advantage that it blocks the inferior alveolar nerve, the long buccal nerve and the lingual nerve with a single injection. A recent study showed, however, that it was less successful than the standard inferior alveolar block.

77

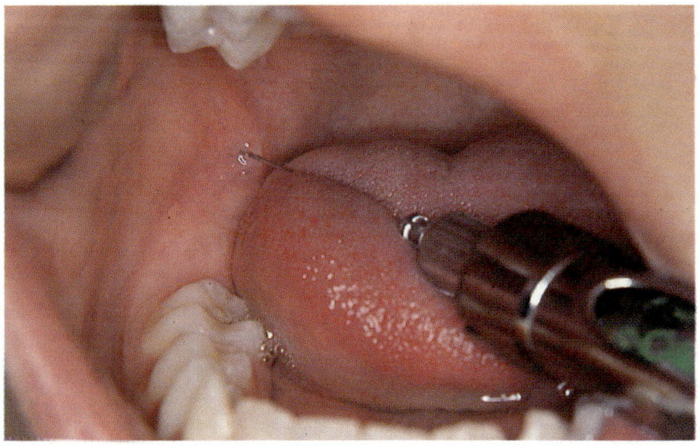

78

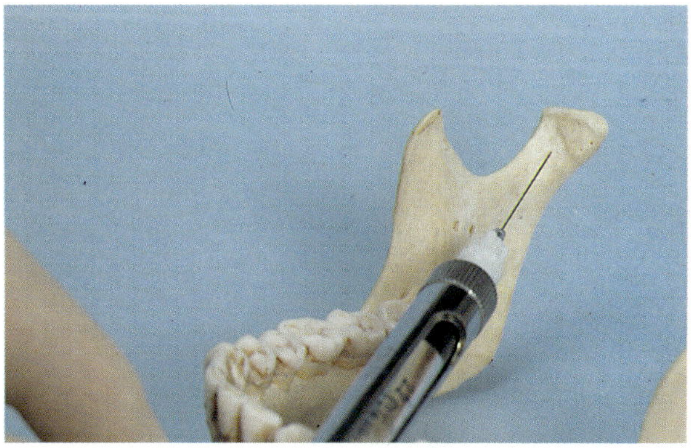

77 and 78 Gow-Gates technique: the tip of the needle is placed at the neck of the mandibular condyle in the vicinity of the early path of the mandibular branch of the trigeminal nerve

The mandible: lingual nerve block

This procedure is usually carried out in conjunction with an inferior alveolar nerve block. It is achieved by injecting 0.1–0.2ml of local analgesic solution at the level of the alveolar crest distal to the second or third molar (79). This can be done either as the needle is inserted, or as it is withdrawn after administering an inferior alveolar nerve block. The solution is deposited approximately 0.5cm mesially and inferiorly to the lingula (80).

79

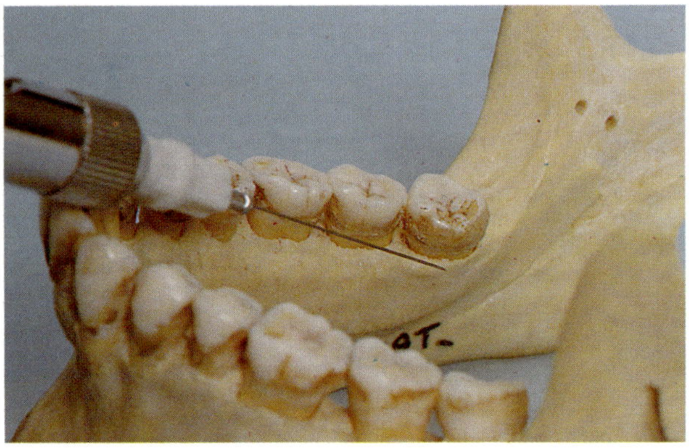

80

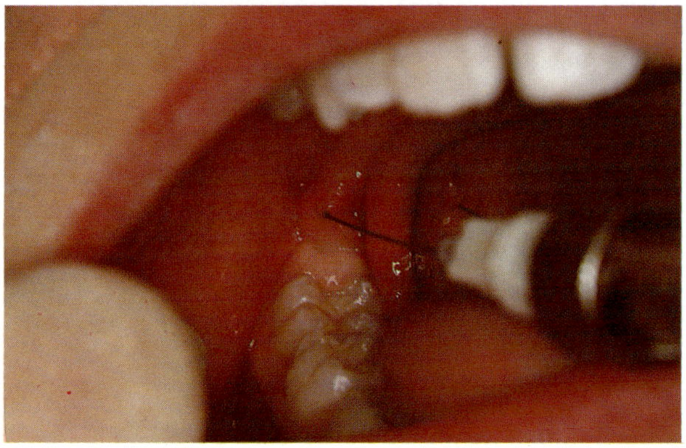

79 and **80** Lingual nerve block: 0.1–0.2ml of local analgesic solution is injected at the level of the alveolar crest distal to the second or third molar (**79**). The solution is deposited approximately 0.5cm mesially and inferiorly to the lingula (**80**)

The mandible: long buccal nerve block

The buccal nerve is a branch of the mandibular division of the trigeminal which courses from the region of the condylar neck on the medial side of the mandible. The terminal branches emerge from the buccinator muscle and innervate the buccal mucosa and the buccal gingiva in the molar region.

Analgesia of the buccal nerve is achieved by puncturing the mucosa distal and buccal to the third molar, approximately 1cm from the disto-buccal aspect. Approximately 0.5ml of analgesic solution is injected (**81** and **82**).

81

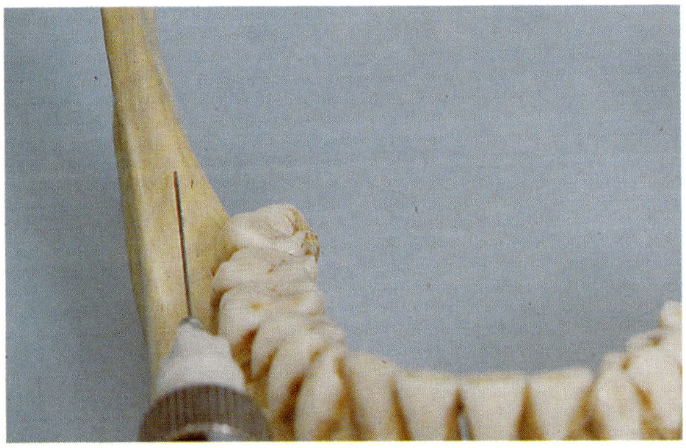

82

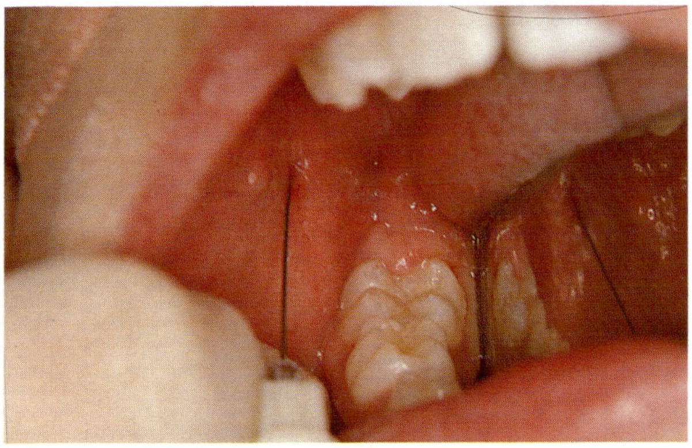

81 and **82** Long buccal nerve block: the mucosa is punctured distal and buccal to the third molar, approximately 1cm from the disto-buccal aspect (**81**). Approximately 0.5ml of analgesic solution is injected (**82**)

The mandible: mental nerve block

Local analgesic solution deposited near the mental foramen enters the inferior alveolar canal to produce analgesia of the premolars, canine and incisor teeth of that side. The mental foramen is usually situated between the apices of the premolar teeth at approximately the depth of the apex of these teeth (**83**).

Clinically, the cheek and lip are retracted and the tip of a short needle is placed deep into the sulcus: 1.5–2ml of solution is deposited (**84**).

The needle is not placed so deeply in younger patients, and only 0.75–1ml is deposited (**85** and **86**); in older patients, if there has been resorption of the alveolar ridge, the mental foramen is almost on the crest of the ridge (**87**). On the rare occasion when a mental nerve block is required in an edentulous ridge, the needle is inserted near the crest of the ridge and then 1–1.5ml of local analgesic solution is injected.

83

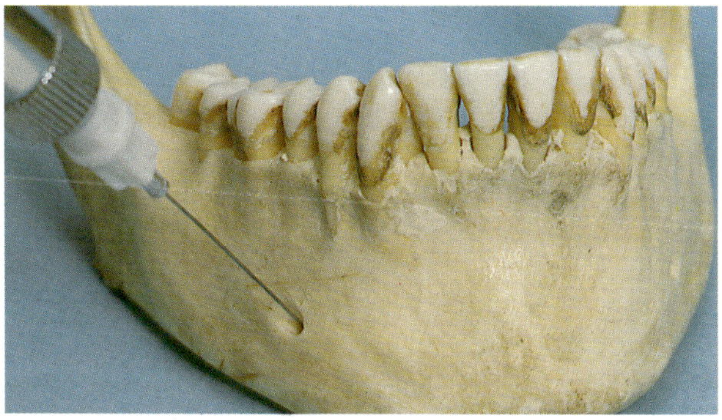

83 Local analgesic solution is deposited near the mental foramen

84

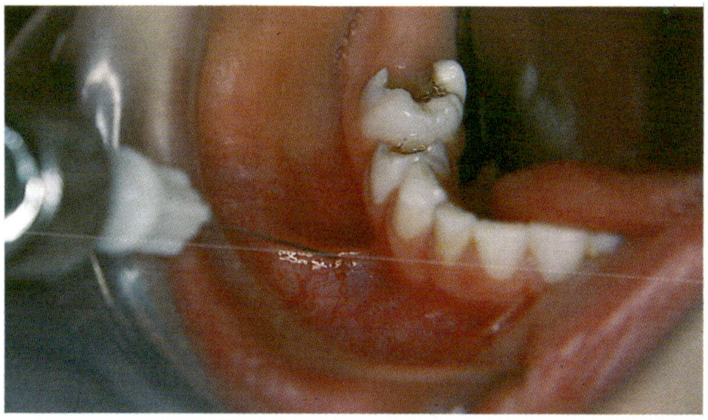

84 The tip of a short needle is placed deep into the sulcus: 1.5–2ml of solution is deposited

85

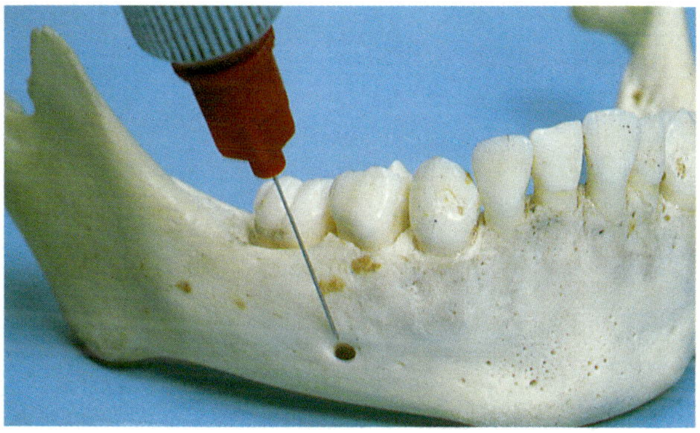

86

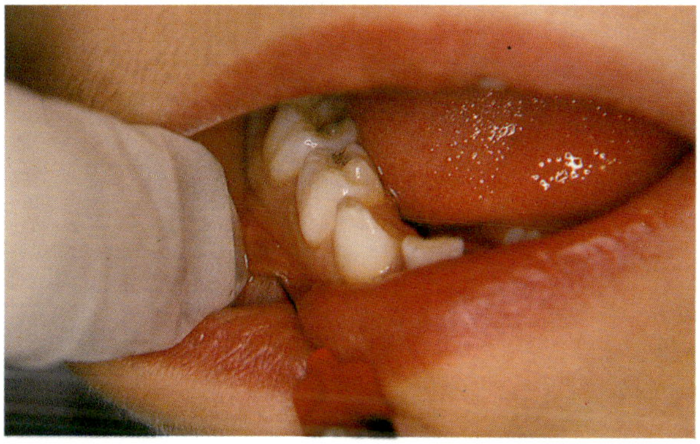

85 and 86 In the case of younger patients, the needle is placed less deeply and only 0.75–1ml of solution is deposited

87

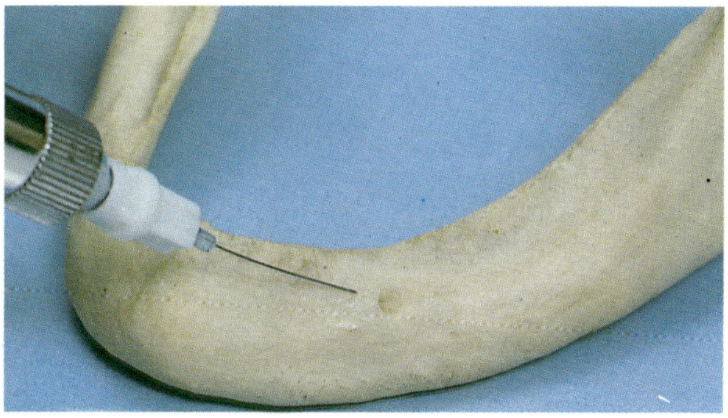

87 In older patients, where there has been resorption of the alveolar ridge, the mental foramen is almost on the crest of the ridge

Aspiration

Aspiration is the term used to describe the technique whereby negative pressure is applied to a local analgesic cartridge in a local analgesic assembly, to determine whether there is any fluid at the tip of the needle which can be drawn up into the syringe. In this way, if the tip of the needle is within the lumen of a blood vessel, blood will be drawn into the cartridge near the hub of the syringe (**88** and **89**).

The main purpose of aspiration is to prevent accidental intra-vascular injection. The technique is an aid to, and not an absolute guarantee of, the prevention of intra-vascular injection. If blood has leaked out into the tissues, occasional false positives can be obtained – these are of little concern. False *negatives*, however, can be a problem, as they can lead to a false sense of security in the dental surgeon.

False negatives result when:

- Small calibre veins collapse with minimal aspirating force.
- Excessive aspirating force has led to the collapse of a normal vein.
- The lumen of the needle lies against the internal wall of a vessel and is thus obstructed.
- Insufficient aspirating force has been generated.

The majority of intra-vascular injections are into veins. Such injections cause cerebral irritation leading to verbosity, respiratory depression, and a general feeling of unease. Reverse flow in arteries can cause visual disturbance, temporary blindness, and even transient hemiparesis.

88

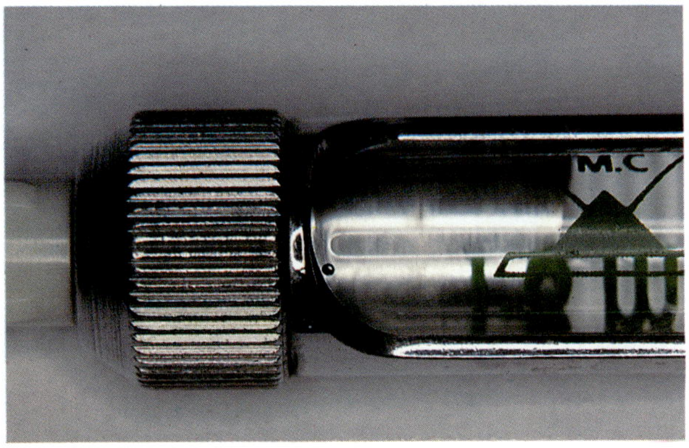

89

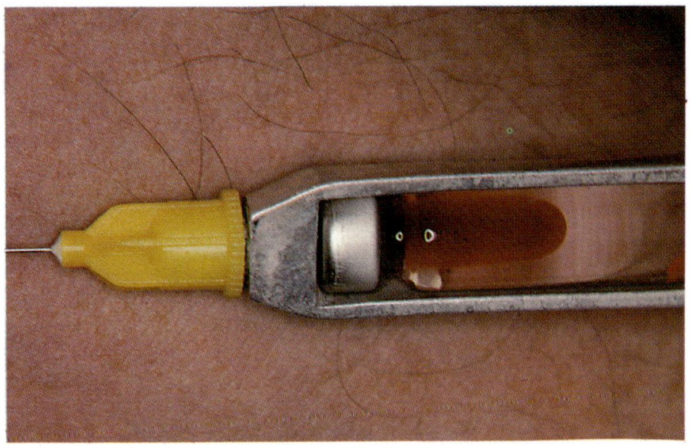

88 and **89** If the tip of the needle is within the lumen of a blood vessel, blood will be drawn into the cartridge near the hub of the syringe

The risk of intra-vascular injection

The reported incidence of positive aspiration varies from 0.65 per cent to 19 per cent and depends on the injection system used, the dental surgeon's technique, the age of the patient, and the type of injection being attempted. For example, 8.6 per cent of inferior alveolar block injections gave a positive aspiration against only 2.8 per cent of upper incisor infiltrations.

Several different aspirating systems are available, one of which is illustrated in the equipment section (page 28).

CONCLUSIONS

The use of an aspirating technique seems clearly advisable when administering nerve block analgesia, if less important in the case of infiltration analgesics. It is not possible to aspirate when administering intra-ligamental analgesics.

Latency of onset and failure

For a local analgesic injection to be successful it is essential that the solution is deposited around the target nerve. Placement of the needle tip in the tissues followed by depression of the plunger results in a pool of local analgesic solution being deposited in the tissues. Once the bolus of fluid has been injected, it takes a finite length of time before it diffuses around the neurovascular bundle; in the case of nerve blocks, the fluid diffuses into the nerve bundle itself and achieves analgesia of each of the individual nerve trunks.

If the bolus is deposited too far from the nerve sheath, the solution will not diffuse into the nerve bundle to cause analgesia (**90**). This is probably the most common cause of failure in nerve block analgesia.

When an inferior dental nerve block is given accurately the patient is aware of an 'electric shock' as the needle touches the nerve within the neurovascular bundle. In this event symptoms of local analgesia appear within 30 seconds or so. There is, however, a further 'latency of onset' due to the time taken for the solution to diffuse into the centre of the nerve bundle.

90

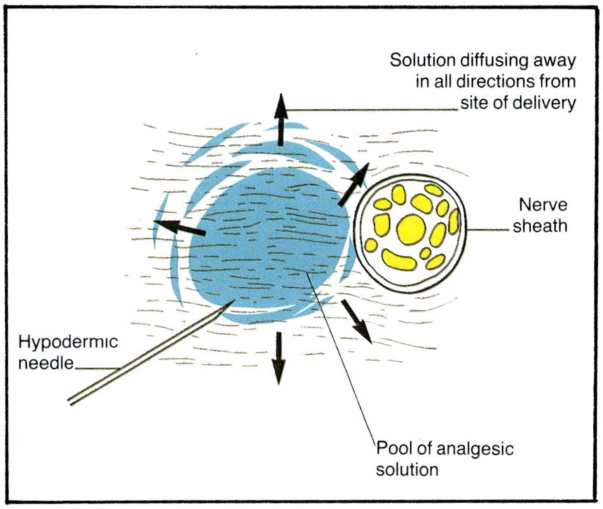

90 Latency of onset and cause of failure of nerve block analgesia

Failures with infiltration analgesia are rare because the nerves involved are extremely small and are easily surrounded by fluid deposited in the tissues.

Dosage of local analgesics

It is essential that a sufficient volume of solution is given at the site of the injection to ensure adequate analgesia. If the dosage is inadequate then analgesia itself will be inadequate. Throughout the text the optimum dosage volumes of 2 per cent lignocaine have been given. It is apparent that an inferior alveolar nerve block requires the greatest volume and an intra-ligamental injection the smallest.

The following example illustrates how the dosage of local analgesic administered can be calculated:

In the case of 2 per cent lignocaine in 1:80,000 adrenaline

2 per cent = 2 grams per 100ml	= 1 gram in 80,000ml
= 2000mg per 100ml	= 1000mg in 80,000ml
= 20mg per ml	= 0.1mg in 8ml
	= 0.0125mg in 1ml
i.e. approx. 40mg per cartridge	i.e. approx. 0.025mg per cartridge

(Cartridges range from 1.8–2.2ml.)

Using the above formula, the maximum dosages of local analgesic injections to remain within therapeutic guidelines are:

lignocaine 2 per cent	200mg = 5 cartridges
lignocaine 2 per cent + 1:80,000 adrenaline	500mg = 12 cartridges
prilocaine 3 per cent	400mg = 6 cartridges
prilocaine 3 per cent + 0.03 IU felypressin/ml	600mg = 10 cartridges

It can be seen from the above figures that there is a considerable safety margin between the maximum number of cartridges permissible (up to ten with a vasoconstrictor) and the recommended number of cartridges for therapeutic effect (usually two or possibly three are the maximum needed).

Local analgesia is so reliable and effective that if the dental surgeon considers that more than three cartridges are necessary then he should reconsider the local analgesic technique being used and perhaps use an alternative, e.g. an inferior alveolar block instead of an infiltration or an intra-ligamental analgesia instead of a nerve block.

Maximum dosage in children

The very wide safety dosages in adults are not applicable to children. Because of their very much smaller lean body mass the maximum dosages are a third or less than those for adults (**91**).

91

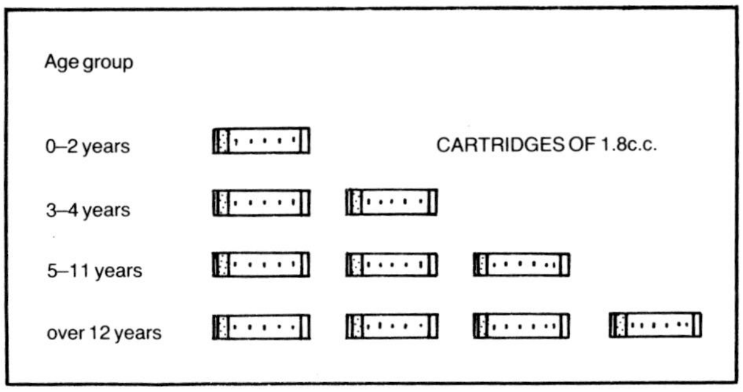

91 Upper dosage limit for solutions containing vasoconstrictor

Intra-ligamental analgesia

Introduction

The technique of intra-ligamental injection of local analgesic solutions is sometimes hailed as revolutionary but, as has recently been pointed out by Sowray (1988), it has been used for many years. What is new is the use of fine-gauge 30 needles which can gain ingress directly to the periodontal ligament. The other technical innovation comes in the shape of syringes which can achieve the high pressures necessary to force the local analgesic solution to the apex of the tooth, a ratchet mechanism preventing back pressure forcing the plunger back in the syringe. Of the two main types of syringe, the pistol-grip (**31** and **32**) features a trigger which is used to depress the plunger, while the pen-grip (**33** and **34**) uses a lever for this task. Both syringes have a plastic sleeve which protects the patient in the event of breakage of the cartridge glass when the high pressure for this injection technique is generated.

The technique

The 30-gauge needle is inserted, via the gingival sulcus, into the periodontal ligament. This is achieved by angling the needle at about 30° to the long axis of the tooth (**92**). The needle is pushed approximately 2mm into the periodontal ligament parallel to the root surface. Continuous and firm pressure is applied to the syringe lever over a period of 20–30 seconds. The dental surgeon should be able to 'feel' the very strong resistance to injection: if there is no resistance, it is likely that the needle is not properly inserted into the periodontal ligament. A relatively long time is necessary to ensure hydrofluid movement of the local analgesic solution to the apex of the tooth. Between 0.05ml and 0.1ml of solution is injected at each of the four 'corners' of a single rooted tooth, giving a maximum of 0.4ml of solution. The injection is given at each of the four corners of multirooted teeth, too – although here, the maximum volume of solution can be as much as 0.8ml.

Once the lever is depressed, the needle is held within the periodontal ligament for 5–10 seconds to allow the pressure generated within the cartridge to be dissipated. It is usual for the dental surgeon to start almost immediately as analgesia becomes profound very quickly.

Dental surgeons may initially have some difficulty in obtaining satisfactory results with the technique, but with a little practice a high degree of success can be expected.

ADVANTAGES

It is a simple technique.
It reduces unnecessary soft tissue numbness associated with other techniques.
It produces almost instantaneous analgesia.
It is especially suitable for patients with a bleeding disorder such as haemophilia.
The total volume of local analgesic solution required is very low.
It avoids complications associated with other techniques, e.g. lip biting, haematoma.

DISADVANTAGES

When conservative dentistry is carried out, patients complain of postoperative sensitivity. This is due to the tooth being slightly 'high' on the bite.

INDICATIONS

Any local analgesic where isolated teeth need to be anaesthetized.
Haemorrhagic disorders such as haemophilia or telangectasia.
Anxious patients, for whom an inferior alveolar block may be difficult to tolerate.

92

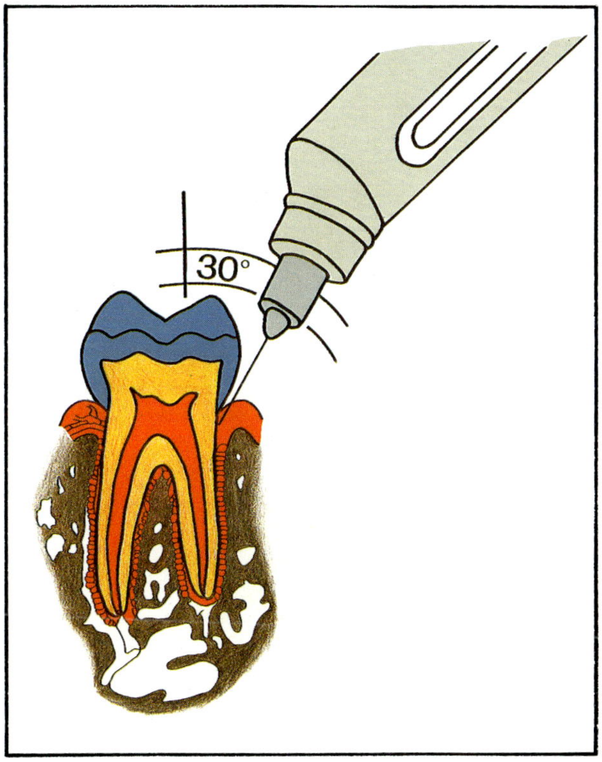

92 Intra-ligamental analgesia: inserting the needle into the periodontal ligament

CONTRAINDICATIONS

Presence of acute gingival or periodontal infection.
Note: A partially used cartridge must *never* be reused on another patient.

The maxilla

CENTRAL AND LATERAL INCISORS

The technique is basically the same for every tooth made analgesic by the intra-ligamental technique. The classical technique of intra-ligamental analgesia is to administer one injection in the mesial periodontal ligament and one in the distal periodontal ligament. In the author's experience, however, a higher success rate is achieved by administering four separate intra-ligamental injections, at the mesio-buccal, disto-buccal, disto-lingual and mesio-lingual corners, respectively, of the tooth to be made analgesic.

PREMOLARS AND MOLARS

The 30-gauge needle is angled appropriately to the mesio-buccal surface of 6/ and 0.05–0.1ml of solution is injected over 20 seconds (**93** and **94**). To make the disto-buccal corner of the 6/ analgesic the intra-ligamental syringe is rotated through 180° to enable the needle to be inserted at 30° into the periodontal ligament (**95** and **96**).

The angulation of the intra-ligamental syringe is maintained to enable the dental surgeon to insert the needle at 30° into the disto-lingual periodontal ligament of $\underline{6}$/ (**97** and **98**).

To inject into the mesio-lingual periodontal ligament of the $\underline{6}$/ the intra-ligamental syringe is rotated through 90° to enable the needle to be inserted at 30° to the long axis of the tooth (**99** and **100**).

93
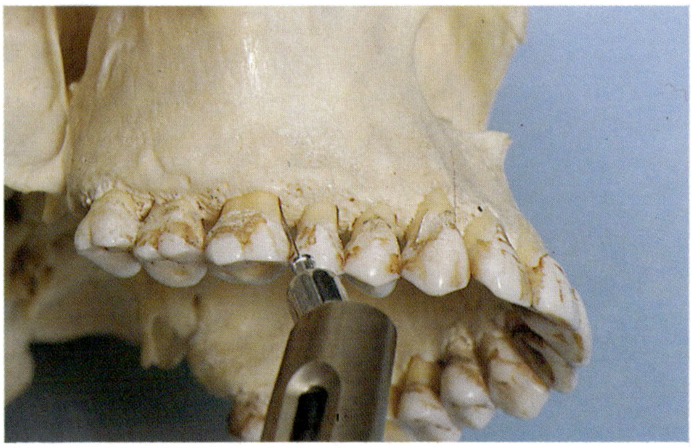

94
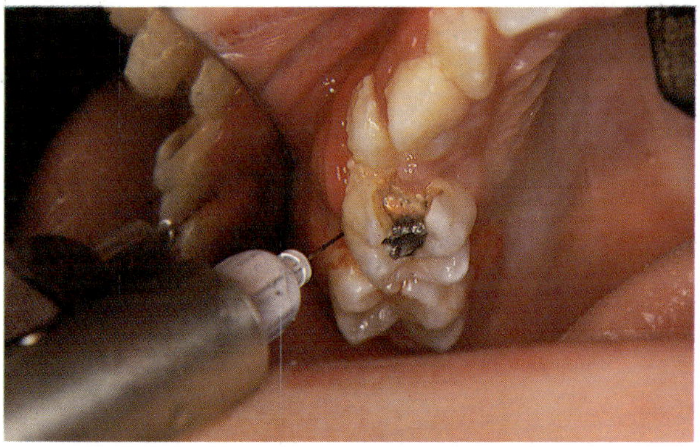

93 and **94** The mesio-buccal corner of the tooth is injected . . .

95
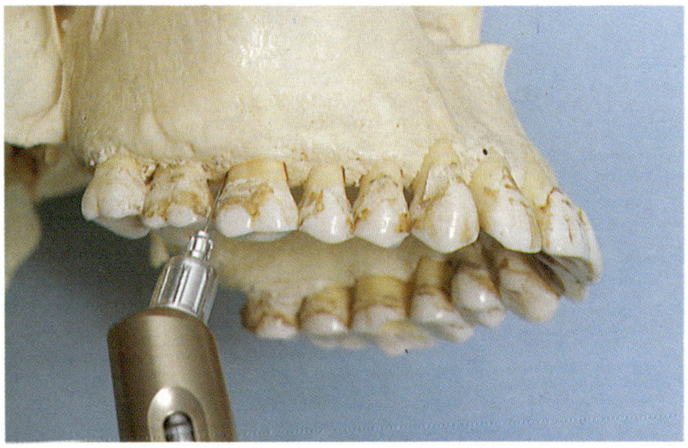

96
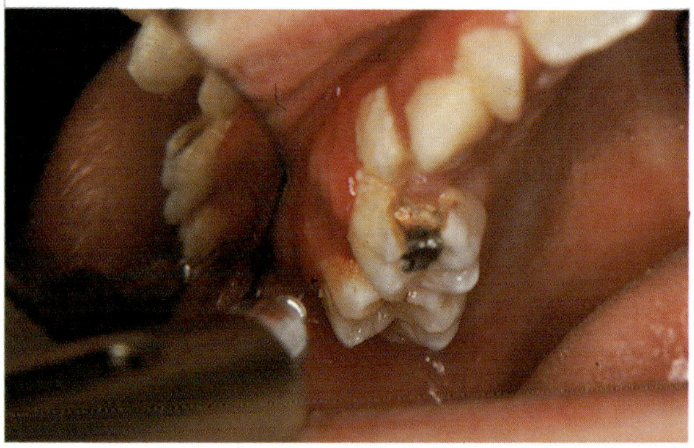

95 and **96** The disto-buccal corner is injected . . .

97
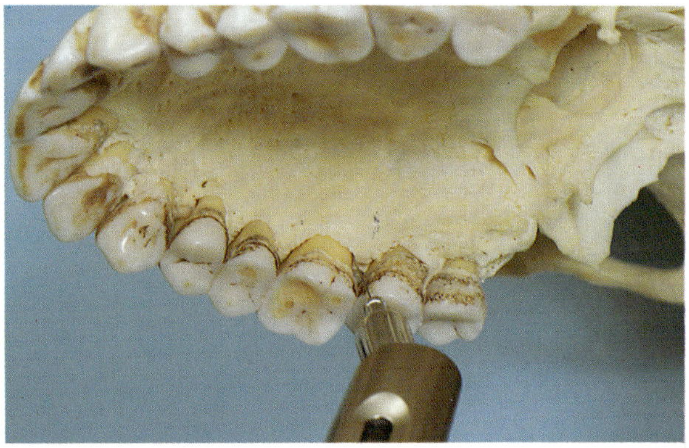

98
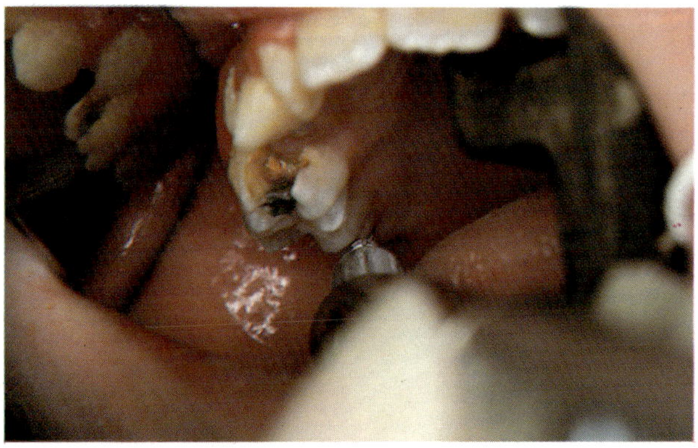

97 and **98** The disto-lingual corner is injected . . .

99 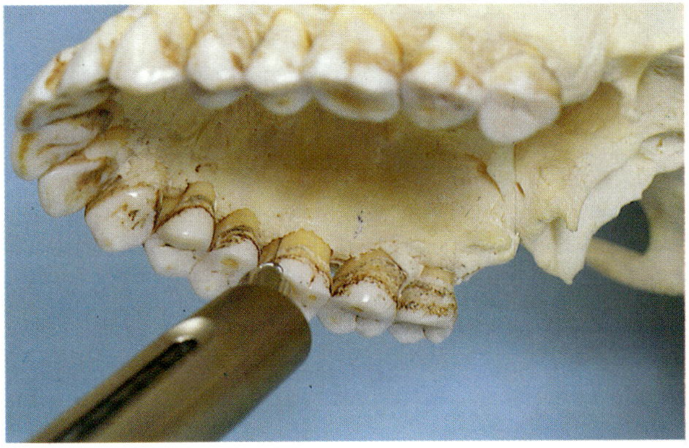 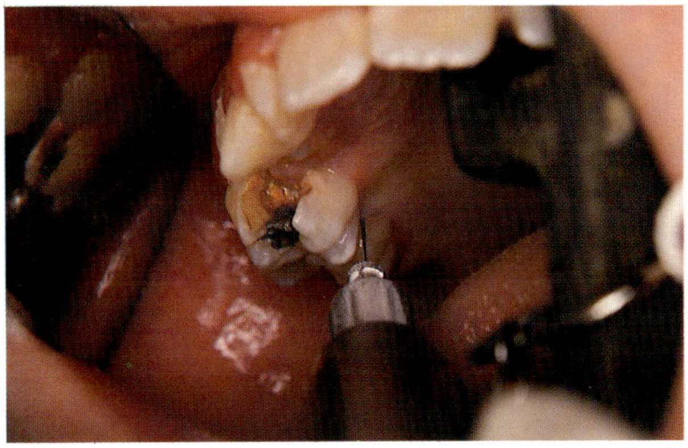 100

99 and 100 The mesio-lingual corner is injected

INCISORS AND CANINES

To make any of the upper incisor or canine teeth analgesic the needle is inserted into the periodontal ligament at 30° to the long axis at the mesio-labial (**101** and **102**), disto-labial (**103** and **104**), disto-palatal (**105** and **106**), and mesio-palatal (**107** and **108**) aspects of the tooth. In the example illustrated, an upper lateral incisor due for a crown preparation has been made analgesic in the upper central incisor position.

101 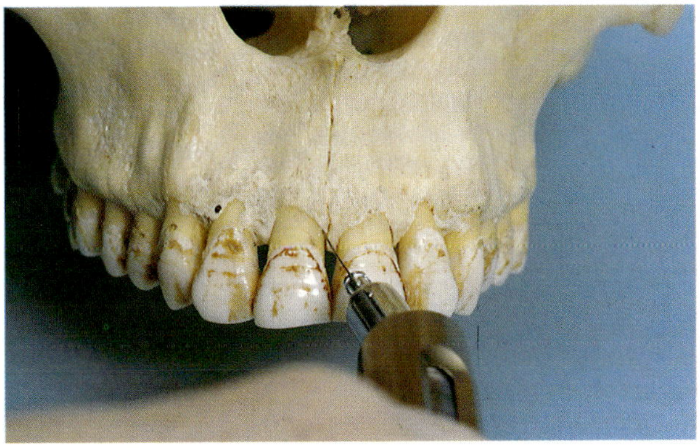 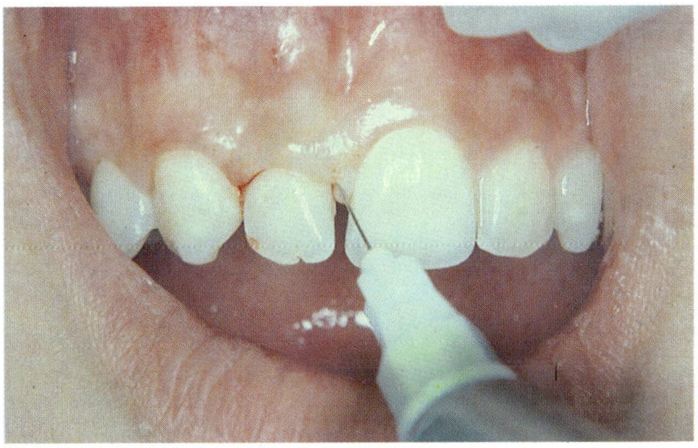 102

101 and **102** The needle is inserted into the periodontal ligament at the mesio-labial aspect of the tooth . . .

103 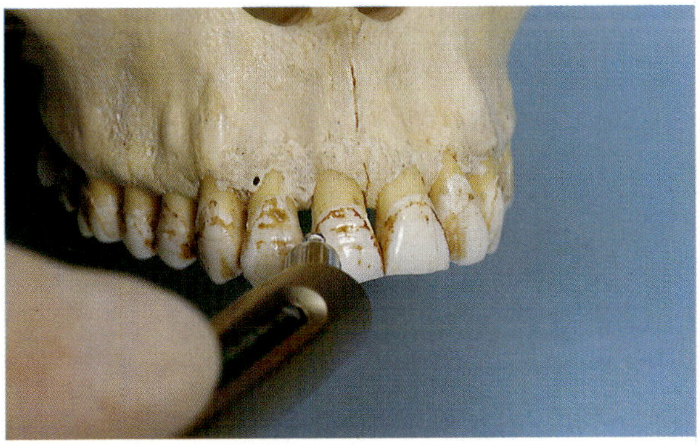 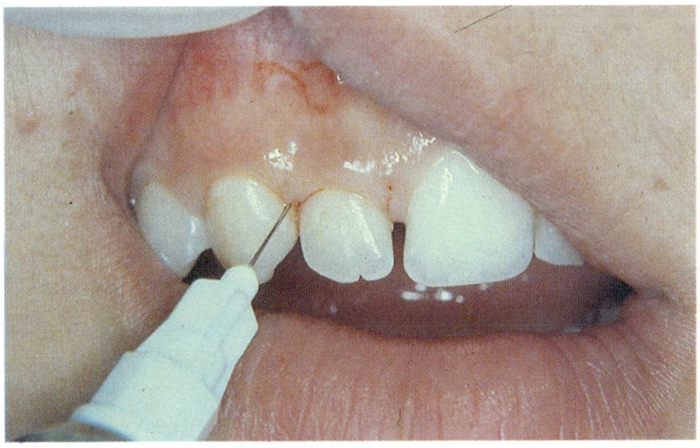 104

103 and **104** At the disto-labial aspect . . .

105 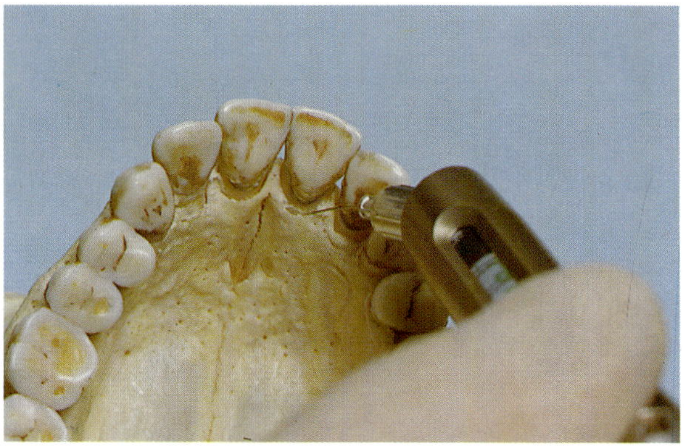 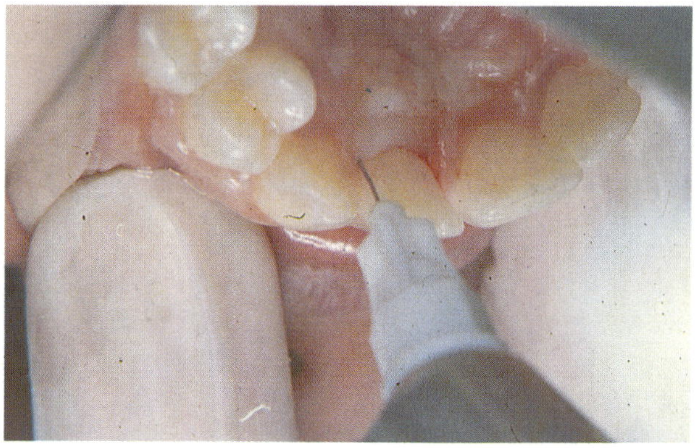 106

105 and 106 At the disto-palatal aspect . . .

107 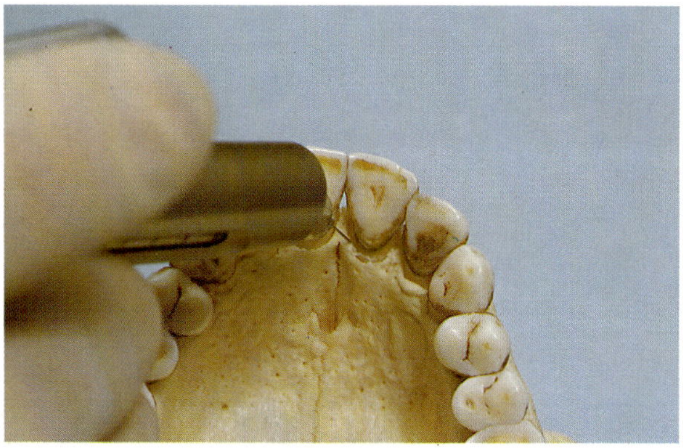 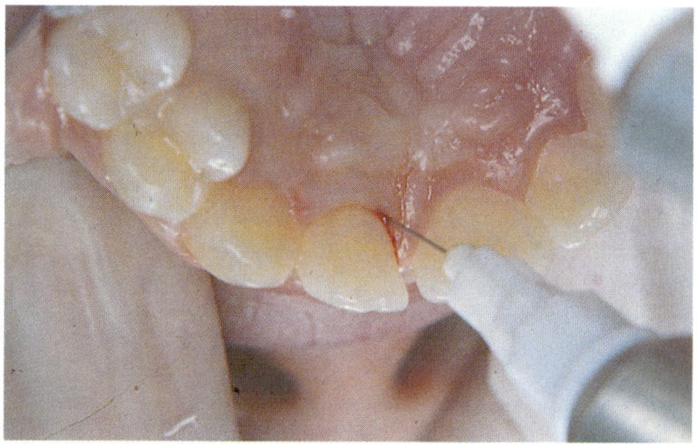 108

107 and 108 At the mesio-palatal aspect

The mandible

PREMOLARS AND MOLARS

Access to the back of the mouth is sometimes a problem. However, if this can be gained satisfactorily the needle is inserted, usually at 30°, into the periodontal ligament on the mesio-buccal (**109**), disto-buccal (**110**), disto-lingual (**111**) and mesio-lingual (**112**) corners.

Difficulty in obtaining access to orientate the syringe in the back of the mouth accounts for a significant proportion of failures. This is particularly the case with third molars, where trouble may be encountered in engaging the periodontal ligament on the distal aspect of the tooth.

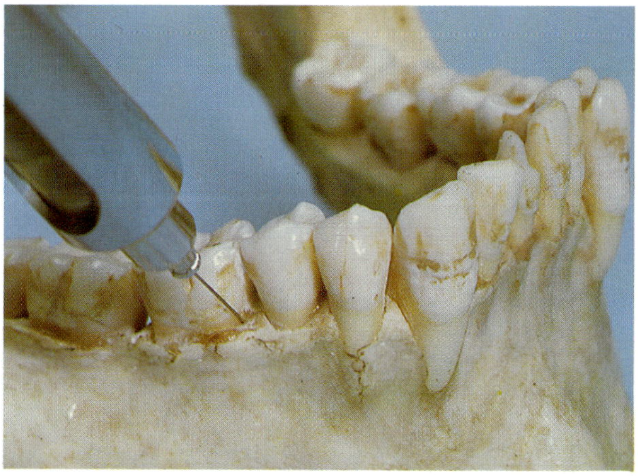 109

109 The needle is inserted into the periodontal ligament on the mesio-buccal corner . . .

110 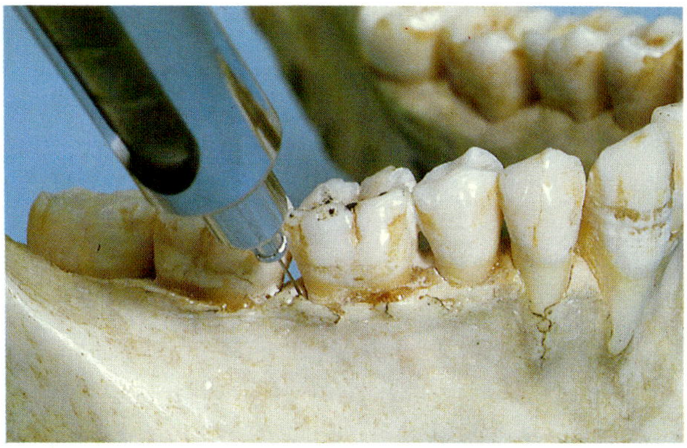

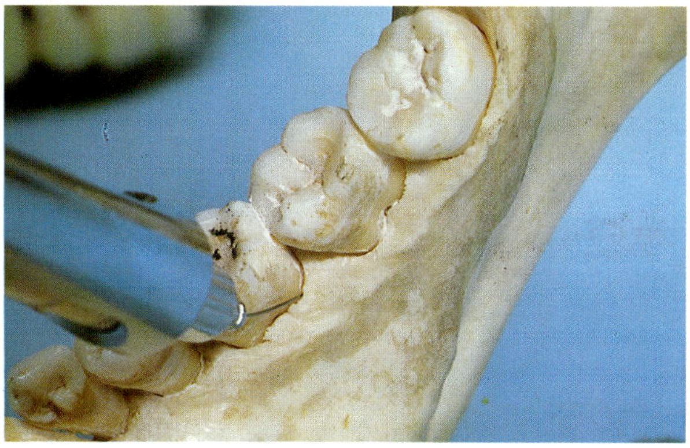 111

110 On the disto-buccal corner . . .

111 On the disto-lingual corner . . .

112 On the mesio-lingual corner

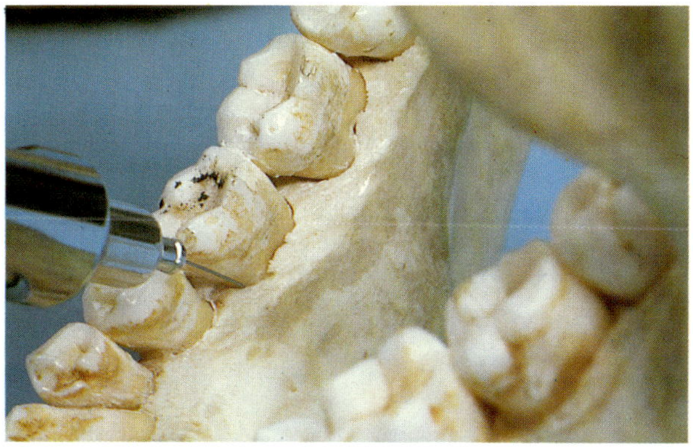 112

INCISORS AND CANINES

Intra-ligamental analgesia of the mandibular incisors is made a little more difficult than is the case with other teeth by the anatomical configuration of the alveolar crest – which in this region is thin and sweeps down labially. On the lingual side there is usually a noticeable shelf of bone which makes identification of the periodontal ligament easy.

To make any of the mandibular incisors and canines analgesic, the intra-ligamental syringe is angulated to enable the needle to be inserted at 30° or less into the periodontal ligament on the mesio-labial (**113**) and disto-labial (**114**) corners.

The angulation is changed to inject in the disto-lingual and mesio-lingual corners (**115** and **116**).

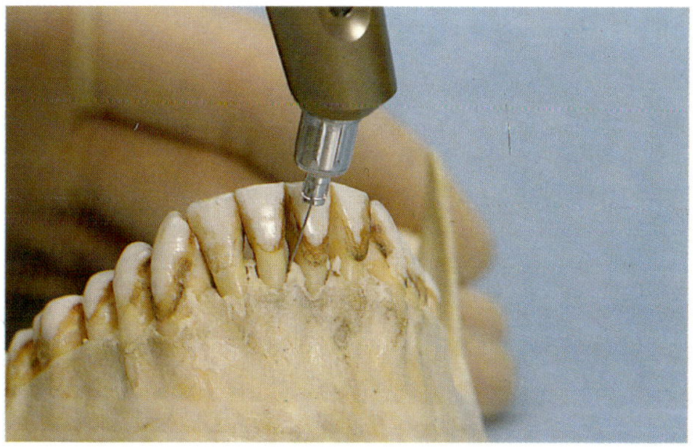 113

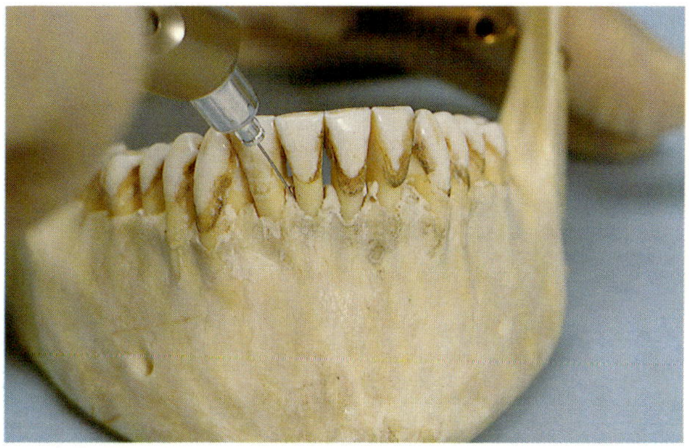 114

113 and **114** The intra-ligamental syringe is angulated to enable the needle to be inserted into the periodontal ligament on the mesio-labial (**113**) and disto-labial (**114**) corners

115 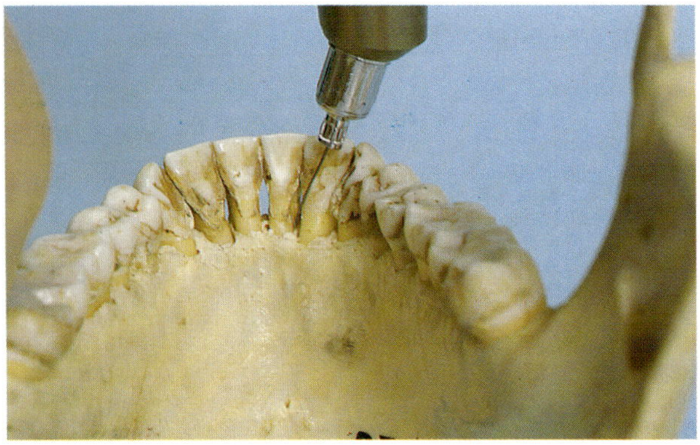 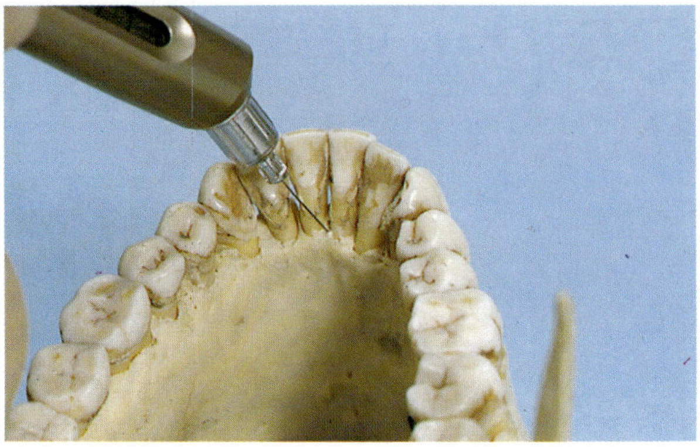 116

115 and **116** The angulation of the syringe is changed, to enable the needle to be inserted into the disto-lingual (**115**) and mesio-lingual (**116**) corners

Problems with the intra-ligamental technique

The technique of intra-ligamental analgesia has many advantages, not least being the very small volumes of solution needed to achieve analgesia. This means that systemic effects from the local analgesic solution are almost non-existent. However, in common with all techniques, there are problems which can only be overcome by careful application.

The greatest difficulty appears to be encountered in engaging the periodontal ligament with the tip of the needle whilst simultaneously applying sufficient pressure along the long axis of the needle to prevent analgesic solution flowing back up its sides as the ratchet mechanism is activated: very high pressures are needed to force the solution down the periodontal ligament, and the needle can very easily become bent in the process (**117**). With practice and increasing skill, this becomes less of a problem, but if it does occur it is best to discard the needle in the Sharpsafe box and use a new one.

Another possible consequence of the high pressures generated is that the glass of the local analgesic cartridge may shatter. If this does happen, the old cartridge must be carefully removed and discarded in a Sharpsafe box, and a new one substituted. The plastic sleeve surrounding the cartridge will prevent shards of glass falling into the mouth. As with bent needles, though, this problem occurs less often with mounting experience.

Of the few post-operative problems, the one which seems to cause the greatest distress occurs where intra-ligamental analgesia is used to make analgesic a tooth which has a restoration placed in it. After the restoration the tooth is 'high' on the bite and – because it is in premature contact – there is acute discomfort. However, the patient can be reassured that this will last for only 12–24 hours.

117 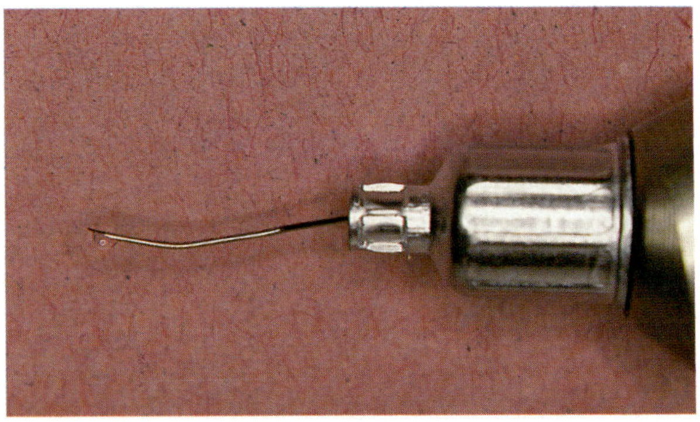

117 Very high pressures are needed to force analgesic solution down the periodontal ligament, and the needle can easily become bent as a result

Additional uses of intra-ligamental analgesia

It should not be forgotten that the intra-ligamental technique has other uses. First, it can be employed to give infiltration analgesia for simple procedures such as a frenectomy (**118**) and the removal of a small cyst (**119**).

Another valuable application is to provide supplementary analgesia where an infiltration technique is inadequate. This is particularly beneficial when the patient has a rubber dam on the tooth to be operated upon. In **120**, /3̲ is being given a supplementary injection whilst the rubber dam is left *in situ*.

118

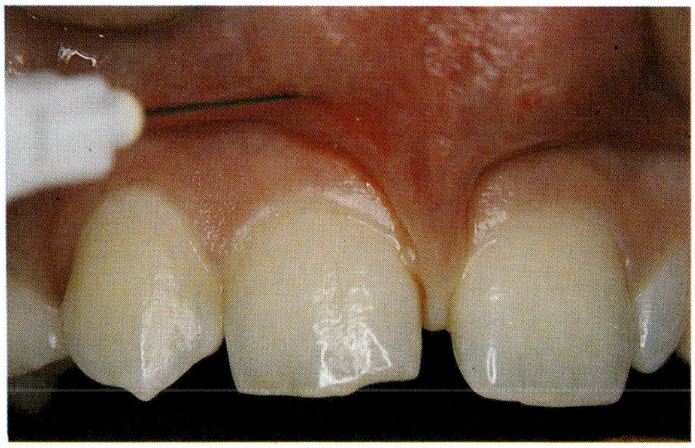

119

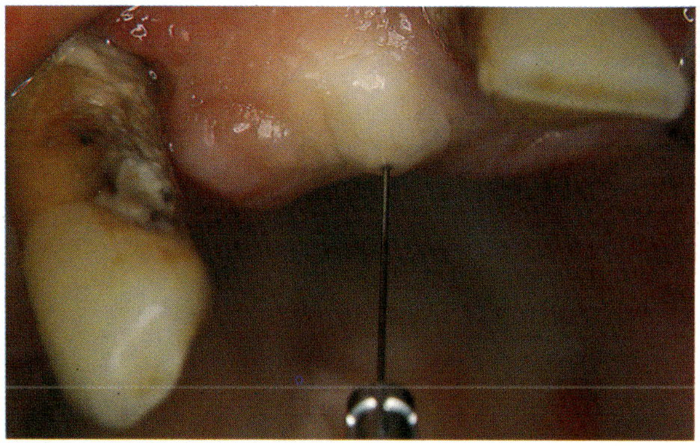

118 and 119 Intra-ligamental analgesia can be used for a frenectomy (**118**), and for removal of a small cyst (**119**)

120

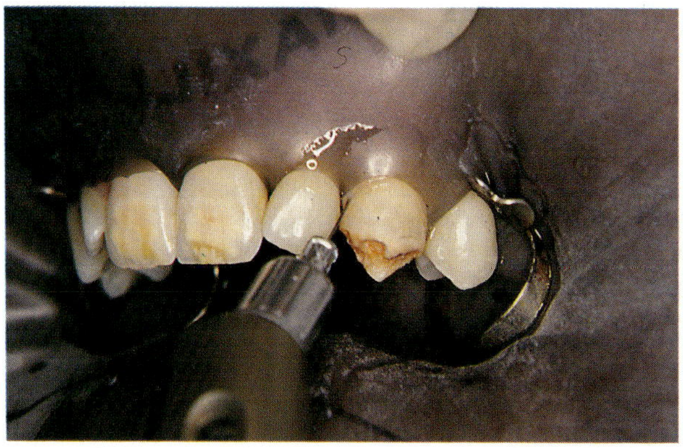

120 Intra-ligamental analgesia can be used to augment an inadequate infiltration technique – here, while a rubber dam remains in place on the tooth to be operated on

An appraisal of intra-ligamental analgesia

The technique of intra-ligamental analgesia seems to have been slow in finding acceptance by the dental profession. An active scepticism coupled with a few early failures has led many dental surgeons to dismiss it as ineffective. However, several excellent papers have addressed themselves to the use of the technique in general dental practice (Grundy, 1984).

The success rates quoted for the technique range from as low as 65 per cent to as high as 96 per cent. The multi-surgeon trial reported an overall rate of 70 per cent complete success with a further 20 per cent partially successful (**121**). This paper also showed differences between experienced and inexperienced dental surgeons. An important finding was the fact that over 92 per cent of patients expressed a preference for the intra-ligamental injection when compared to the inferior alveolar block.

Thus, in conclusion, the intra-ligamental technique has a high success rate (between 70 and 96 per cent) with a high proportion of patients preferring it to inferior alveolar block analgesia. There is no doubt that, judiciously used, it has an important role to play in pain control in clinical dental practice.

121

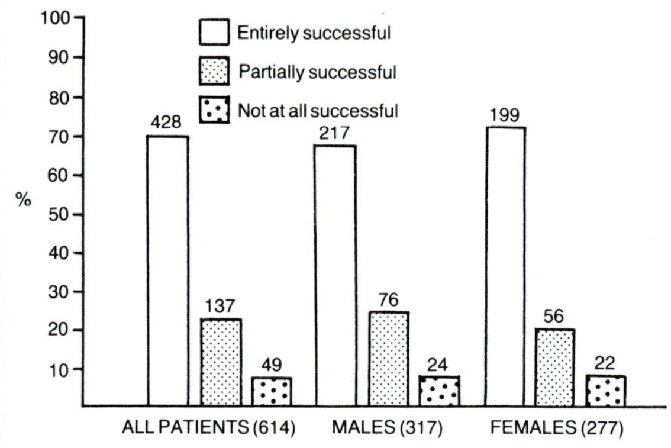

121 Success rates for intra-ligamental analgesia

Intra-osseous analgesia

This technique has been employed in the past to achieve analgesia of a tooth or group of teeth where a nerve block or infiltration analgesic has proved to be inadequate. A sterile 1 or 2 round bur – assisted by a copious supply of water – is used to drill through the mucosa, the cortical bone and some medullary bone. The local analgesic needle is then inserted into the bony medulla of the jaw and approximately 1–2ml of solution is deposited around the apex of the tooth to be made analgesic.

Although there is no doubting the profound analgesia this brings about, a serious disadvantage of the technique is that solution is deposited into a very vascular area and blood levels of the local analgesic solution rise dramatically. The technique is therefore not recommended for clinical use – indeed, with the advent of intra-ligamental analgesia, it has been rendered obsolete.

A typical local analgesic appointment

A dental surgeon may be excellent at giving individual local analgesic injections but this will mean very little to a patient if the whole analgesic appointment is not conducted in a sympathetic and efficient manner.

First, then, the dental surgeon should read the notes carefully. This is to ensure that there is no relevant medical history; to check the treatment that is to be carried out; to see if there were any special difficulties on previous visits; and to verify the precise type of local anaesthetic procedure to be used. The last matter should be discussed with the dental surgery assistant, so that she can be properly prepared.

The dental surgery assistant lays out all the relevant equipment and drugs on the work surface (**122**). Donning a pair of sterile rubber gloves, she then breaks open the sealed pack of cartridges, removes one, and – holding it close to her gloved hand – carefully checks the expiry date printed on the outside.

122

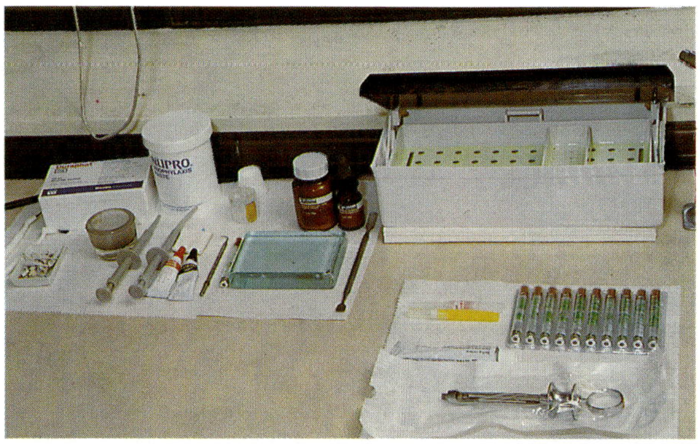

122 All relevant equipment and drugs for use in the local analgesic appointment are laid out on the work surface by the dental surgery assistant. In the foreground are the local analgesic syringe, the hypodermic, and a sealed pack of local analgesic cartridges

If the syringe is in a sterilized pack this is broken open and the syringe placed on a sterile towel on the work top. The seal on the hypodermic needle plastic container is checked to see that it is intact. It is then broken and the cap set aside for later reuse.

The hypodermic, still within the plastic container, is carefully screwed onto the end of the syringe (**123**). It is important that the end of the needle which should pierce the rubber diaphragm when the local analgesic cartridge is inserted is not bent: care must be taken to see that the whole needle is straight. The plastic cover or sheath is left in place to prevent inadvertent contamination of the needle and to ensure that neither the dental surgeon nor his assistant suffers 'needle-stick' injuries. The syringe is then extended and the plunger spring held back, so that the handle of the syringe can be disengaged from the barrel (**124**).

Next, the local analgesic cartridge is picked up from the work top and carefully inserted into the barrel of the syringe (**125**). Special care must be taken, when the cartridge is pushed the final few millimetres, to ensure that as its rubber diaphragm touches the short end of the needle it does not displace and bend it. As the initial resistance to penetration of the diaphragm occurs, a gentle push will ensure that the hypodermic pierces the rubber diaphragm.

The dental surgery assistant then straightens the syringe assembly, removes the plastic sheath, and tests the patency of the hypodermic by depressing the plunger a couple of millimetres: a few drops of local analgesic solution should be expressed. This check is important because, if for some reason the dental surgery assistant has not assembled the syringe properly, the dental surgeon will find himself giving an injection which will fail to deposit any local analgesic solution. And remember: with a very nervous patient, the dental surgeon may get only one chance to carry out an injection . . .

The dental surgery assistant replaces the plastic sheath using a Sharpsafe technique – being careful to avoid a 'needle-stick' injury (**126**).

After checking with the dental surgeon that he is ready, the dental surgery assistant goes out to the waiting room and, with a reassuring, welcoming and warm smile, brings the patient into the surgery.

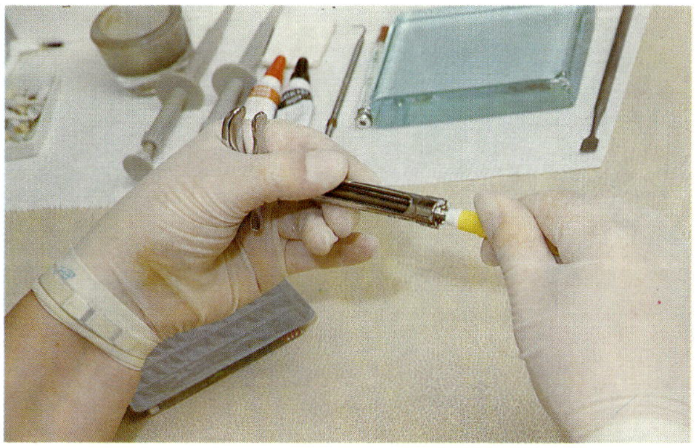 **123**

123 When screwing the hypodermic (which is still within the plastic container) onto the end of the syringe, it is important to check that the needle is straight – otherwise, the end which should pierce the rubber diaphragm when the local analgesic cartridge is inserted may be bent

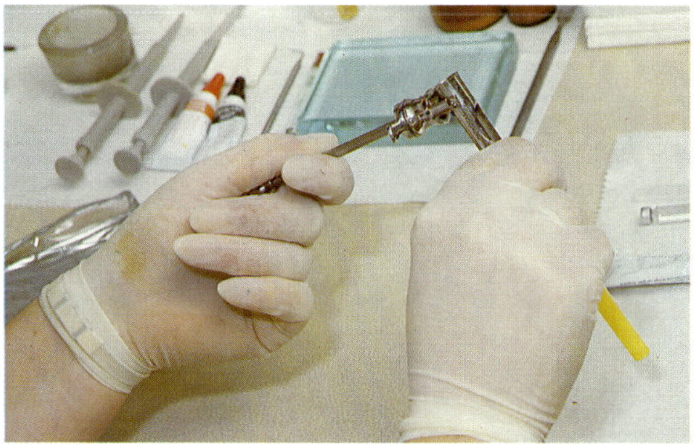 **124**

124 The syringe is extended and the plunger spring held back, so that the handle of the syringe can be disengaged from the barrel

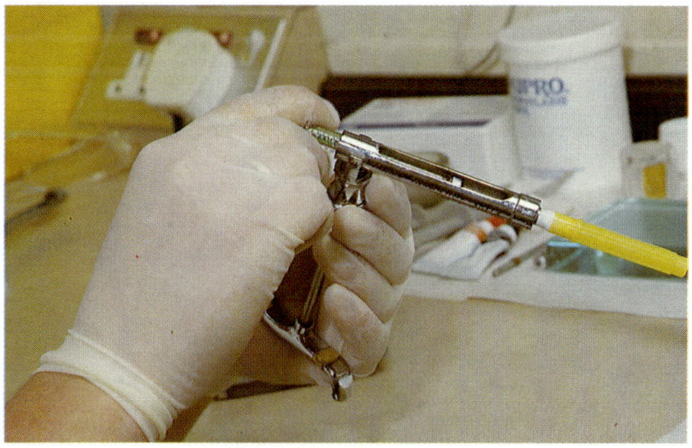 **125**

125 The local analgesic cartridge is carefully inserted into the barrel of the syringe

While the dental surgery assistant makes the final detailed preparations the dental surgeon welcomes and reassures the patient. Any important details of the patient's medical history are checked, and also any relevant fears, e.g. of the 'drill' or the 'needle', so that the dental surgeon can modify his approach to the patient accordingly.

Being sure first to tell the patient exactly when it is to happen, the dental surgeon reclines the dental chair. The warning is especially important in the case of nervous patients and children, who may otherwise become very distressed when the back of the chair suddenly disappears from behind them! The dental surgeon might place a reassuring hand on the patient's shoulder as the chair is reclined.

Now that the patient is supine it is important to protect his eyes by providing protective spectacles or eyeshields where necessary. If the patient is already wearing corrective spectacles it is probably better to leave him with these, as he will feel more comfortable and at ease this way. The dental surgery assistant, meanwhile, squeezes a pea-sized quantity of topical analgesic ointment onto a cotton roll – ready for the dental surgeon to place it in the patient's mouth, on the site of the proposed mucosal puncture by the hypodermic (**127**).

Next, the dental surgery assistant loosens the sheath on the local analgesic assembly and hands it to the dental surgeon behind the patient's back, i.e. out of his field of vision (**128**). This is important since many patients become extremely apprehensive at the sight of the needle, or what they imagine to be the needle. With appropriate reassurance and explanation, combined with counter pressure on the patient's cheek – and by keeping the syringe to the right and below the line of vision – the needle is placed in the correct alignment for the local analgesic injection (**129**).

The dental surgery assistant, meanwhile, takes the patient's left hand and holds it in a gesture of comfort: **this is an extremely important manoeuvre as it achieves the double objective of reassuring the patient and restraining the patient's hands.** The latter can be very important in nervous patients and children because if they suddenly lose courage and put up their hand to grasp the syringe or the dental surgeon's hand, they could knock the syringe up into their own face.

At the critical moment the dental surgeon says something to distract the patient, e.g. 'turn your eyes towards me', as he penetrates the mucosa and moves the needle forward in the tissues until the tip is at the injection site (**130**). If there is no sign of blood in the local analgesic cartridge after aspiration, the dental surgeon can proceed slowly with the injection until it is complete.

126

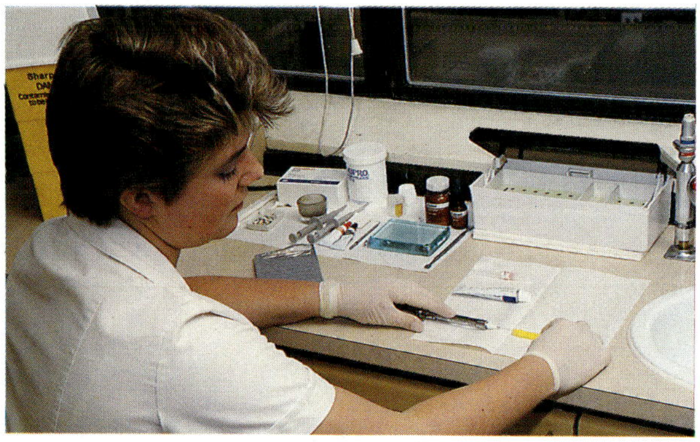

127

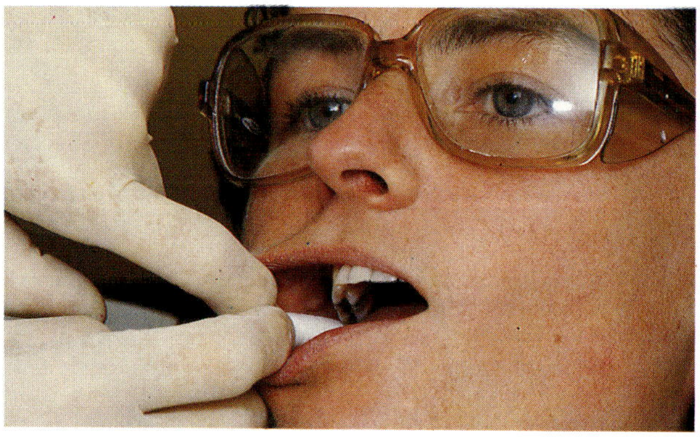

126 After testing the patency of the hypodermic, the dental surgery assistant replaces the syringe in its plastic sheath

127 The dental surgeon places the cotton roll – complete with blob of topical analgesic – in the patient's mouth, on the site of the proposed mucosal puncture

The dental surgeon then removes the syringe from the patient's mouth and transfers it to his left hand, grasping the barrel with his thumb and forefingers (**131**). This is in preparation for handing it to the dental surgery assistant, which he does with the needle pointing *away* from her. This is another aspect of the Sharpsafe technique which needs to be carefully executed by the dental surgeon and dental surgery assistant together.

128

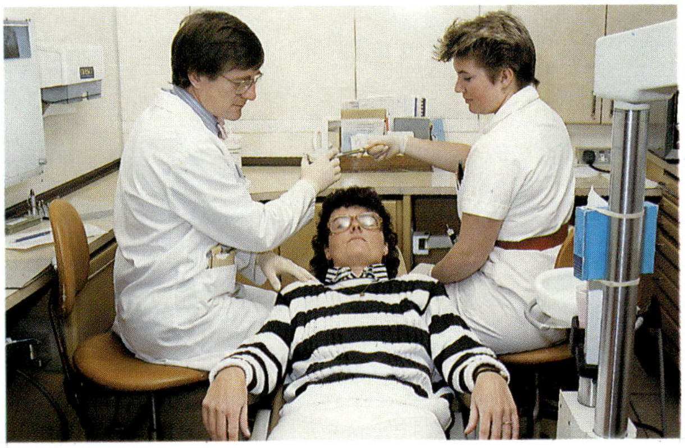

129

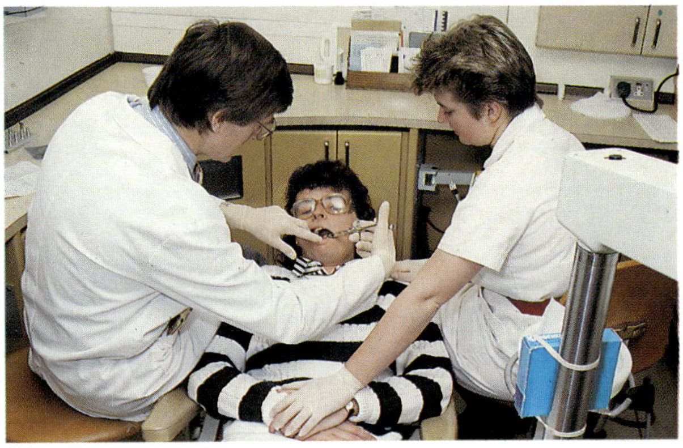

128 It is important to keep the needle out of sight of the patient. Here, the dental surgery assistant, having loosened the sheath on the local analgesic assembly, hands the assembly to the dental surgeon

129 Keeping the syringe to the right of the patient and below her level of vision, the dental surgeon aligns the needle for an inferior alveolar nerve block

130

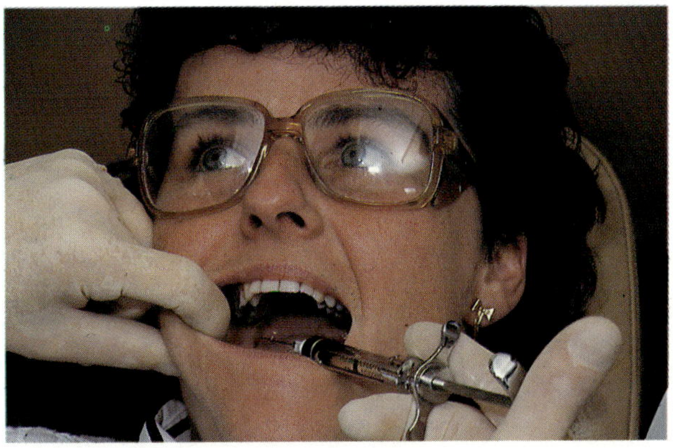

130 Having penetrated the mucosa with the needle, the dental surgeon moves it forward in the tissues until the tip is at the injection site

131

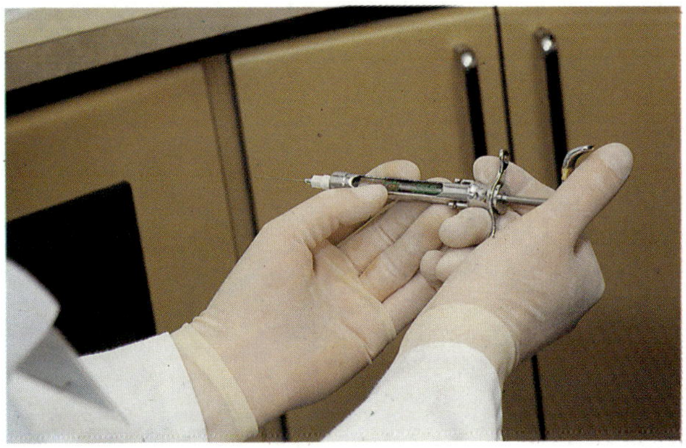

131 The injection complete, the dental surgeon removes the syringe from the patient's mouth and switches it to his left hand, grasping the barrel with his thumb and forefingers

Once again the dental surgery assistant places the syringe on the clean work top and, holding it firmly with the left hand, moves the plastic sheath carefully over the needle until it can be pushed firmly onto the hub (**132**).

After three to five minutes the dental surgeon checks that symptoms of adequate local analgesia are present and then tentatively starts drilling the tooth (**133**). Once operative dentistry has started, it is important that all three participants in the procedure – the dental surgeon, the patient, and the dental surgery assistant – are wearing either prescription spectacles or eye protectors.

At the completion of the appointment the dental surgery assistant removes the hypodermic from the syringe and bends the short end of the needle (**134**), making it impossible for it to be reused in error. It also thwarts any attempt at theft by drug abusers. The cap is then replaced on the hypodermic.

The partially used cartridge and the needle are then dropped into the Sharpsafe box, which is used as a holding point for all contaminated or disposable glass and needles. Each dental surgery has a routine by which Sharpsafe boxes are collected and the contents rendered safe by incineration.

When the appointment is over, the dental surgery assistant accompanies the patient out to the waiting room to make a new appointment. Where appropriate, the patient is given written post-operative instructions.

132

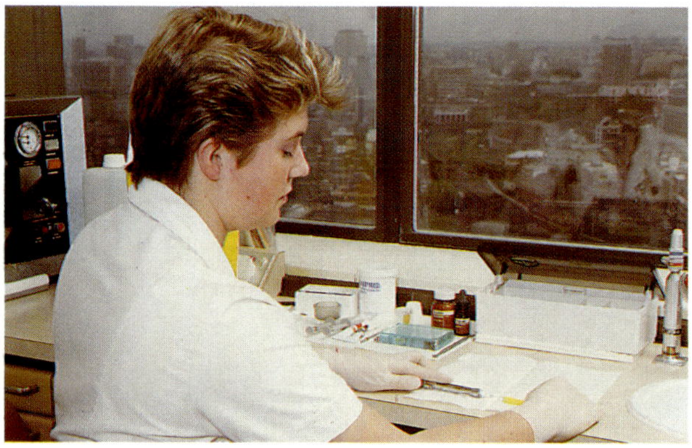

132 Once the dental surgeon has returned the syringe, the dental surgery assistant places it on the clean work top and, holding it firmly in her left hand, carefully replaces the plastic sheath

133

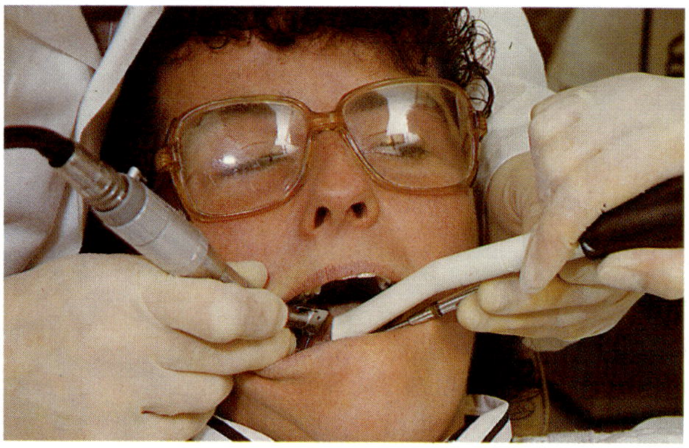

133 Having checked that adequate local analgesia is present, the dental surgeon starts drilling the tooth

134

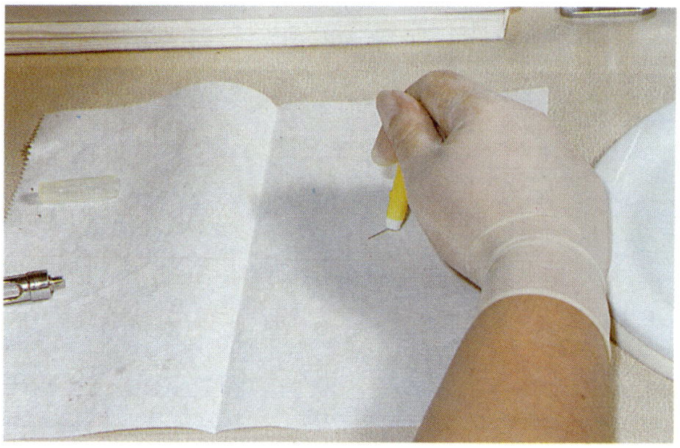

134 On completion of the appointment, the dental surgery assistant bends the short end of the needle to prevent it being reused by mistake

Combinations of local analgesic techniques for specific operative procedures

Over the years, the experienced dental surgeon will have developed specific local analgesic procedures to anaesthetize the teeth, soft tissues and bony tissues for given operative procedures. While this Atlas describes a large variety of specific techniques, it cannot give precise guidance on a local analgesic regimen suitable for *every* procedure. However, in general terms, the intra-ligamental technique is recommended for those procedures requiring highly localized analgesia. It can be used when conservative or surgical work is necessary in all four quadrants in one visit.

For profound analgesia of the mandible, a combination of inferior alveolar, long buccal and lingual nerve block is advised, while for other procedures a suitable combination of infiltration techniques may be appropriate.

It is important that the dental surgeon, when prescribing a plan of treatment for a patient, keeps an open mind. He must be willing to try different techniques to achieve the best results and provide the most effective pain control.

4 COMPLICATIONS OF LOCAL ANALGESIA

Introduction

Carefully and competently administered local analgesia with 2 per cent lignocaine and 1:80,000 adrenaline, or 3 per cent prilocaine with 0.03 international units of felypressin, is safe and effective. Nevertheless, the dental surgeon must be aware of the possible complications so that, if and when they do occur, early diagnosis and suitable treatment can be carried out.

It is convenient to divide potential complications into Local and General.

Local complications

Failure to obtain analgesia

This is experienced by every dental surgeon, although with decreasing frequency as he becomes more experienced. Failure to obtain analgesia is usually due to faulty technique. If analgesia is inadequate it is best to repeat the procedure, paying particular attention to anatomical landmarks and the details of the technique.

Another common reason for failure is the presence of infection: the local analgesic must be given in a site remote from the infection. In these situations nerve block analgesia has particular applications.

Pain during injection

Some patients will overreact to even mild discomfort, although a number do experience quite marked discomfort. This is usually due to a poor technique. The dental surgeon should take care to be gentle and inject slowly. Warming the local analgesic cartridge just before injecting it will also reduce the discomfort.

Rarely, during the administration of a nerve block, there is a sharp 'electric shock' pain along the distribution of the nerve being blocked. This symptom indicates that the nerve sheath has been penetrated and the needle should be withdrawn.

Haematoma formation

Some areas of abundant nerve supply to the orofacial tissues are extremely vascular. When giving a nerve block, particularly the posterior superior alveolar block, blood vessels can be punctured. This is followed by bleeding into the tissues and leads to the development of a haematoma. Antibiotic therapy should be instituted as a prophylactic measure, as there is the possibility that the haematoma will become infected. The patient should be reassured and advised that the haematoma will dissipate 'like a bruise' over a period of a week to ten days. The patient should be reviewed after two weeks.

Intra-vascular injection

This can be prevented by using an aspirating syringe (see page 28). There are no local effects except the risk of a small haematoma.

Blanching

Occurring at the site of the injection, this is due to the combined effect of the hydrostatic pressure of the local anaesthetic solution and the vasoconstrictor. Occurring remote from the site of the injection, blanching is due either to an inadvertant intravascular injection or to interference with the automatic nerve supply of the blood vessels affected by the local analgesic (**135**).

Blanching covers a variable area of the face, and lasts from 30 seconds to 30 minutes – after which it disappears without any trace. No treatment is required other than reassurance.

135

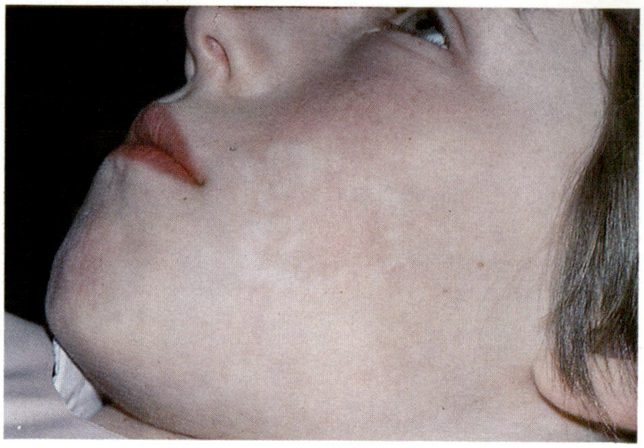

135 Blanching, following a local analgesic

Trismus

This is a muscle spasm which makes it difficult to open the jaws. It results when an injection into the medial pterygoid causes a tearing of the muscle fibres and a haematoma. Onset of the trismus is often more than 24 hours after the injection, but it usually resolves spontaneously.

Paralysis

Unilateral paralysis of the facial muscles is an uncommon complication and when it does happen it usually follows an inferior alveolar injection. It occurs because the tip of the needle is positioned too far back in relation to the mandible and enters the parotid gland, where it makes the branches of the facial nerve analgesic, causing paralysis of the muscles they supply – leading to paralysis of most of the side of the face (**136**). The patient is unable to activate either the orbicularis or the orbicularis oculi. Because the parotid gland is surrounded by fascia there is also a failure of the inferior alveolar nerve block. The complication is alarming to the patient and dental treatment should be abandoned until it resolves following dissipation of the local analgesic solution. The patient should be reassured; he should also be advised to protect the conjunctiva from dust and avoid scratching since the eyelid, too, will be affected.

136

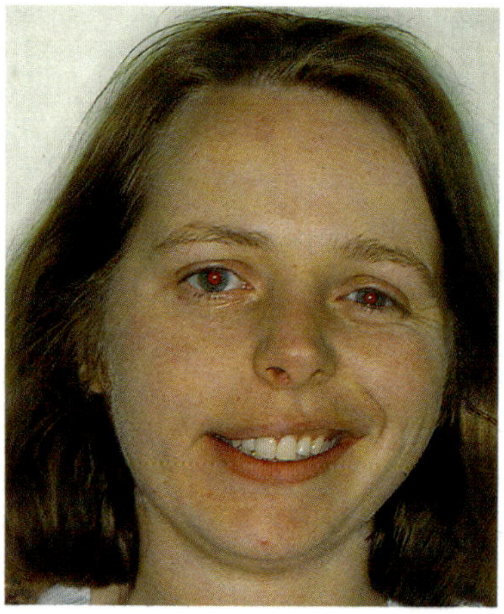

136 Paralysis of the facial muscles, following an inferior alveolar injection

Prolonged impairment of sensation

This is caused by direct damage from the needle or a small haematoma resulting from the injection. Following a local analgesic with failure of the return of normal sensation, the patient should be monitored at weekly intervals and the paraesthesia on the face 'mapped' by testing sensation. Recovery should be complete within three months.

Lip trauma

This usually occurs in children who have had an inferior alveolar nerve block. As sensation starts to return, but while the lip is still numb and rubbery, some children are inclined to bite their lip to test its 'feeling' – unaware that this can cause severe trauma (**137**). Untreated, a bite will develop a fibrin slough. Prevention being better than cure, the best 'treatment' is to advise the parents (or whoever is responsible for the child) to discourage the patient from biting his lip in the first place!

If lip trauma *does* occur, the wound should be kept moist by smearing a thin layer of sterile Vaseline over it every few hours. The traumatic ulcer usually heals without scarring.

Occasionally, an infiltration area is scratched by the patient, which leads to an ulcer (**138**). Necrosis at the injection site is a rare complication, possibly emanating from a local infection or subconscious trauma caused by the patient rubbing the site of analgesia.

137

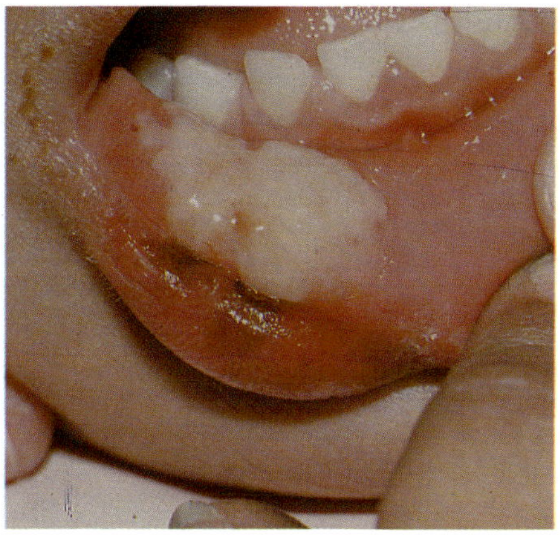

137 Severe lip trauma, the result of the patient biting the lip immediately after local analgesic

138

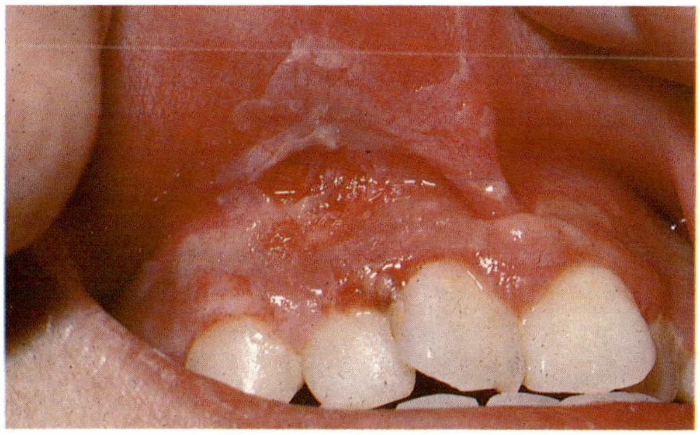

138 An ulcer can occasionally result if the patient scratches the infiltration area

Visual disturbances

Another rarity. Unilateral disturbance of vision is probably due to vascular spasm or intra-arterial injection. Normal vision usually returns within 30 minutes. The patient should be reassured but not discharged until vision has returned to normal.

General complications

Fainting or vasovagal attack

The most frequently encountered general complication of local analgesia is the common faint or vasovagal attack. Emotional disturbance leading up to the administration of the local analgesic predisposes to a faint: the patient appears to tense himself up to cope with the injection. Immediately afterwards, the strain of his exertions seems to overwhelm him – with the massive vagal discharge plus the arteriolar dilatation leading to a reduction in the blood returning to the heart, which in turn results in a gross reduction in cardiac output. The consequence of this is a sudden loss of consciousness, the patient appearing to collapse within a few seconds.

It is important to note that the majority of faints can be prevented by ensuring that the patient is laid fully supine *before* the local analgesia is administered. An upright posture is still the most common preventable contributory factor.

SIGNS AND SYMPTOMS

The patient becomes pale, suffers nausea and dizziness, and breaks out in a cold sweat. His skin feels cold and clammy, and – if nothing is done – he will lose consciousness and his pupils will become dilated. His pulse will feel weak and thready, and may for a short while appear to be absent altogether.

TREATMENT

If the dental surgeon has failed to place the patient in a supine position before the commencement of operative procedures, this must be done immediately. If the dental chair will allow it, the patient's feet should be placed higher than his head, to encourage the return of blood to the heart – which in turn will stimulate cardiac output. The airway should be checked and, if necessary, the jaw drawn gently forward; any tight clothing should be loosened.

Most patients will respond and recover within two or three minutes. However, a few take several minutes longer and seem to be confused for some considerable time.

An apparently simple faint represents a severe disturbance of the cardio-vascular and central nervous systems, and should not be taken lightly. Unless it is essential or extremely important to complete the dental procedure during that appointment it should be abandoned for the day, the patient allowed to recover, and treatment rescheduled.

Other causes of collapse

Special precautions may be necessary before treatment can be undertaken in the case of patients with an equivocal medical history, e.g. where diabetes, epilepsy, or familial dysautonomia has occurred. Clearly, special emergency drugs should be on hand to enable effective treatment of such complications.

SYSTEMIC TOXICITY

Despite the fact that local analgesic solutions are concentrated and injected into very vascular areas, toxic reactions are exceedingly rare. When they do occur (possibly due to an intra-vascular reaction) there may be convulsions, respiratory depression, or even circulatory collapse. Fortunately these symptoms pass relatively quickly. Indeed, they may be of such short duration that they are not even observed. It is possibly for this reason that the author cannot recall a patient suffering from acute toxicity in 15 years' experience.

DRUG INTERACTIONS

This is a potential problem when any patient is taking systemic medication. In general terms, drug interactions with local analgesics are extremely rare. However, local analgesic solutions containing noradrenaline can potentiate the blood pressure response in patients receiving tricyclic antidepressants (e.g. mitriptyline). For this reason, noradrenaline is not recommended for use in dental local analgesics. Solutions containing adrenaline (as recommended here) potentiate the blood pressure response to a small degree only.

It should be emphasized that, whilst any untoward effect could be due to drug interaction, it is more likely to be a simple faint.

ALLERGY

A steady trickle of patients attending dentists say that they are 'allergic to the local'. The dental surgeon is thus faced with the problem of how to effect pain control in a patient who believes that he cannot accept the local analgesic drug. In the author's experience, however, such patients have usually been given misinformation based on mistaken diagnoses. It is important, therefore, to establish whether or not a given patient really is allergic – and this is done by means of a small subcutaneous injection. Provided there is no skin erythema, the patient can then be given a local analgesic without worry.

On the rare occasion when a patient does appear to be allergic, this should be investigated systematically using the individual constituents of the local analgesic solution. Occasionally, the preservative (methylparaben) will be the substance causing the allergic reaction.

IDIOSYNCRASY

There are systemic complications that result in an individualized reaction in the patient; they are rarely predictable and do not fall into the pattern of known complications. Psychogenic factors play an important role in this type of reaction. An example is toxic symptoms reported by the patient when the dose is well below the maximum allowable. Apparent idiosyncrasy should not be ignored as it may well be the early or minimal signs of a more serious reaction. A heightened awareness of problems should be engendered.

Treatment of collapse

This is covered in detail in Part 2 of the atlas, on Intravenous Sedation.

5 RELATIVE ANALGESIA: INHALATION SEDATION WITH OXYGEN AND NITROUS OXIDE

The technique of inhalation sedation and analgesia with oxygen: nitrous oxide gas mixtures (relative analgesia) is aimed at alleviating fear, reducing pain, and improving patient cooperation. The principal objective is to achieve sedation. The general analgesia, when inadequate for a given operative procedure, is supplemented with local analgesia.

The technique is particularly suited for use by the dental surgeon/sedationist – that is, a dental surgeon performing the dual role of sedating the patient *and* carrying out the operative treatment. However, he can perform this role safely only when the dental surgery assistant, too, has had adequate training in the techniques of inhalation sedation, resuscitation and monitoring, to the extent that she qualifies as the 'second appropriate person'.

Relative analgesia consists of a triad of interrelated elements:

1. The administration of low to moderate concentrations of nitrous oxide in oxygen (**139**).
2. The use of a machine designed specifically for relative analgesia; it cannot administer less than 30 per cent oxygen and it has a fail-safe device that cuts off the supply of nitrous oxide if the oxygen supply runs low.
3. The accompaniment of a steady flow of reassuring and encouraging talk to the patient. (The importance of this form of semihypnotic suggestion should not be underestimated.)

139

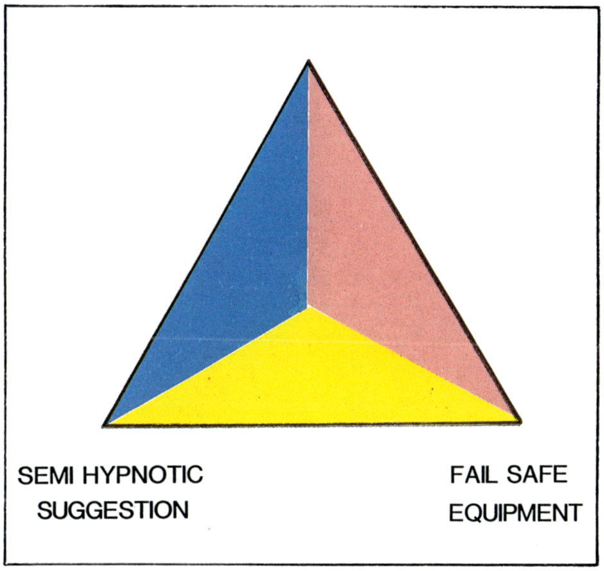

139 Relative analgesia – oxygen: nitrous oxide mixtures

Over the years, relative analgesia has been established as a safe and effective procedure for the dental surgeon to use as part of the overall strategy of managing oro-dental pain and dentally instigated anxiety in children, adults and geriatric patients.

Note. Throughout this section the terms inhalation sedation, oxygen: nitrous oxide sedation, relative analgesia and inhalational psychosedation are all used interchangeably.

Historical note

Joseph Priestley discovered oxygen in 1771 and nitrous oxide in 1772. However, it was not until 1798 that the analgesic properties of nitrous oxide were discovered by Humphrey Davy (later knighted) when carrying out experiments to determine the effects of inhaling the gas. Coincidentally, Davy was suffering from the pain of a wisdom tooth, and when the nitrous oxide was inhaled the pain from the pericoronitis was relieved. In 1800 Davy wrote:

'As nitrous oxide in its extensive operations appears capable of destroying physical pain it may probably be used with advantage during surgical operations in which no great effusion of blood takes place'.

Horace Wells, an American dentist, demonstrated the value of nitrous oxide as an analgesic in 1844. In 1868 Edmund Andrews, a surgeon from Chicago, had the ingenious idea of administering the nitrous oxide with 20 per cent oxygen. In 1881 nitrous oxide in oxygen was used for obstetric analgesia in St. Petersburg, Russia. In 1889, at the University of Liverpool in the United Kingdom, nitrous oxide was used to provide analgesia for the preparation of cavities in teeth.

During the 20th century the technique has enjoyed varying degrees of popularity. It wasn't until the 1940s that Dr. Harry Langa, a dental surgeon working in New York State, developed and refined the technique of relative analgesia as it is now practised world-wide (Langa, 1976). With some minor modifications this is the technique that is described and recommended here.

The stages of analgesia

The technique of inhalation sedation (relative analgesia) can best be understood by considering it in relation to general anaesthesia. The classic signs of either in the unpremedicated patient have been described by Guedel (1953), who divided analgesia into four stages; the same stages occur with nitrous oxide. As the patient passes through the stages there is selective depression of the nervous system, probably in phylogenetic order.

140

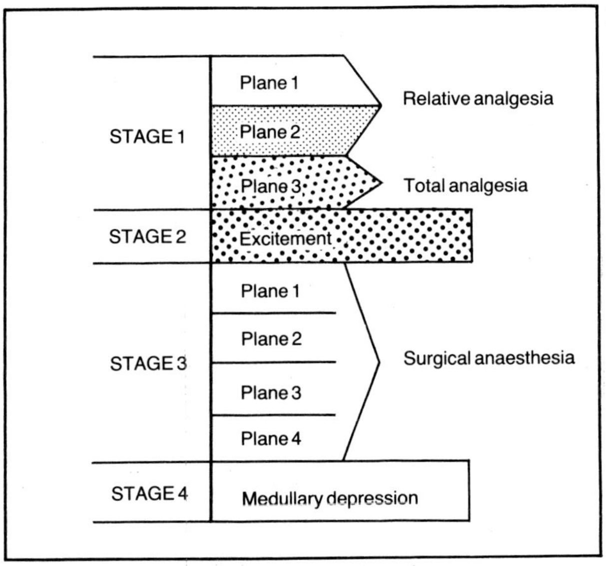

140 The stages of analgesia

Stage 1: Analgesia

There is loss of memory, psychomotor function, loss of sense of time, depression of intellect, and disorientation. The pain threshold is raised and the patient can tolerate minor surgical procedures. At first, the patient is awake and able to converse with the dental surgeon. As the concentration of nitrous oxide increases, however, he becomes increasingly disoriented and eventually starts to lose consciousness. This leads on to the second stage.

Stage 2: Excitement

During this stage breathing becomes irregular. In addition, any stimulation causes a violent reaction from the patient. Vomiting can occur because the laryngeal reflex is obtunded, and there is a significant risk of inhalation of gastric contents. For this reason analgesists attempt to pass patients through this phase as quickly as possible.

Stage 3: Surgical analgesia

This covers the period from the onset of a regular respiratory pattern to the cessation of respiration. The patient can withstand surgical or painful stimuli. This stage is divided into four planes, and leads into the fourth stage.

Stage 4: Respiratory paralysis

This is characterized by the onset of diaphragmatic paralysis, apnoea and death. It is a stage without any clinical use. The technique of relative analgesia is limited to the first, or analgesic, stage of anaesthesia.

The planes of analgesia

The principal changes that occur from inhalation of low to moderate concentrations of nitrous oxide in oxygen have been defined as a result of clinical work carried out at the Royal Dental Hospital and Guy's Dental Hospital, London. This extends the work of Langa (1976) and Parbrook (1967).

The planes of sedation and analgesia constitute the analgesic plane of anaesthesia, and they are usually represented by a schematic diagram (**140**). There is no clear-cut demarcation of the planes – in fact, they overlap to a considerable degree, merging imperceptibly. In practice it is often impossible to be sure which plane of sedation a patient is in at any given time.

An important feature of the third zone is that it acts as a buffer between the clinically useful planes one and two of sedation.

Plane 1: Moderate sedation and analgesia usually obtained on concentrations of 5–25 per cent N_2O (95–75 per cent O_2)

OBJECTIVE SIGNS (**141**)

The patient is wide awake and does not look particularly relaxed. There is a lessened reaction to painful stimuli with a slight reduction in spontaneous movements. Heart rate, blood pressure and respiratory rate are all normal. There is no change in pharyngeal and laryngeal reflexes, the mouth is easily maintained open and the patient is able to converse at will with the dental surgeon.

SUBJECTIVE SYMPTOMS (**142**)

The patient starts to feel some sense of relaxation and diminution of fear. There may be some symptoms of paraesthesia (pins and needles), and he begins to be indifferent to the surroundings. Altogether, the patient feels almost normal.

141

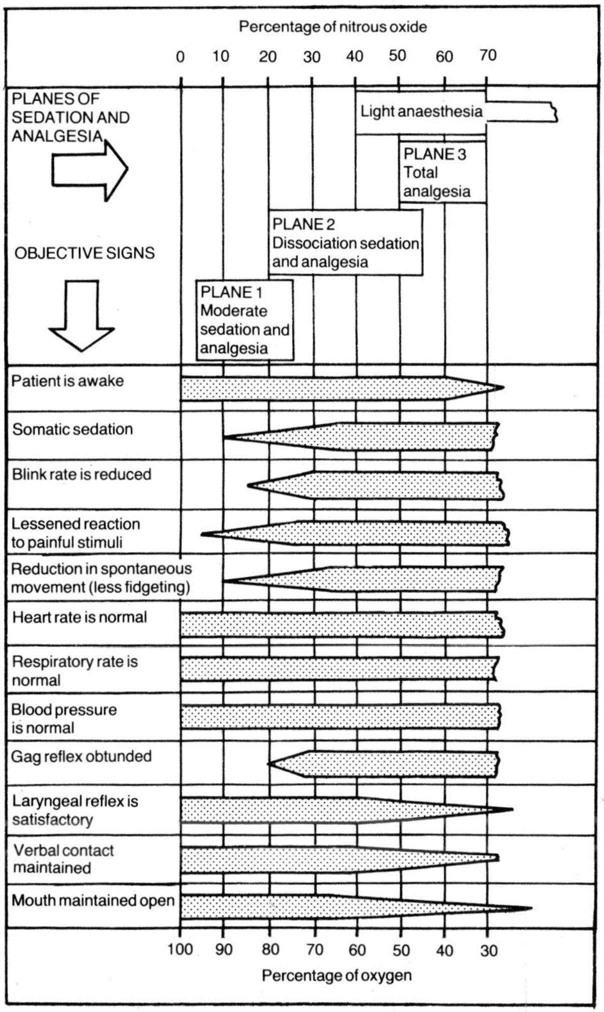

141 Objective signs of the planes of sedation and analgesia

Plane 2: Dissociation sedation and analgesia usually obtained on concentrations of 20–55 per cent N_2O (80–45 per cent O_2)

OBJECTIVE SIGNS (**141**)

In this plane the patient is also awake but may appear a little sleepy. There is a relaxed demeanour. One of the few tangible physical signs is a reduction in the blink rate. There is a significantly lessened reaction to painful stimuli and the patient exhibits somatic sedation (less fidgeting in small children). Heart rate, blood pressure and respiratory rate are all normal, and though there is a marked reduction in the gag reflex the laryngeal reflex functions normally. Verbal contact is maintained, although the response to any questions or commands may be delayed. The mouth is maintained open quite easily by the patient.

SUBJECTIVE SYMPTOMS (142)

The patient begins to experience psychological symptoms described as dissociation or detachment from the environment. The dissociation may be minimal or extremely profound. The patient may also feel widespread paraesthesia, usually most profound in the fingers and toes. It can occur quite markedly in the lips and tongue. Other senses become partially impaired, the patient reporting abnormal sensations of hearing, taste and visual disturbances. In addition, there are marked proprioceptive changes, which accounts for the patient feeling a dramatic floating sensation.

Further subjective symptoms are an apparent loss of memory and indifference to the passage of time. There is a tendency to dream; in some patients the results are very vivid, and occasionally they are unpleasant. In the latter case, simply reduce the nitrous oxide by 15 per cent. An additional symptom experienced by a small number of patients is that of nausea, but it is estimated that less than one in 300 patients undergoes this side effect.

142

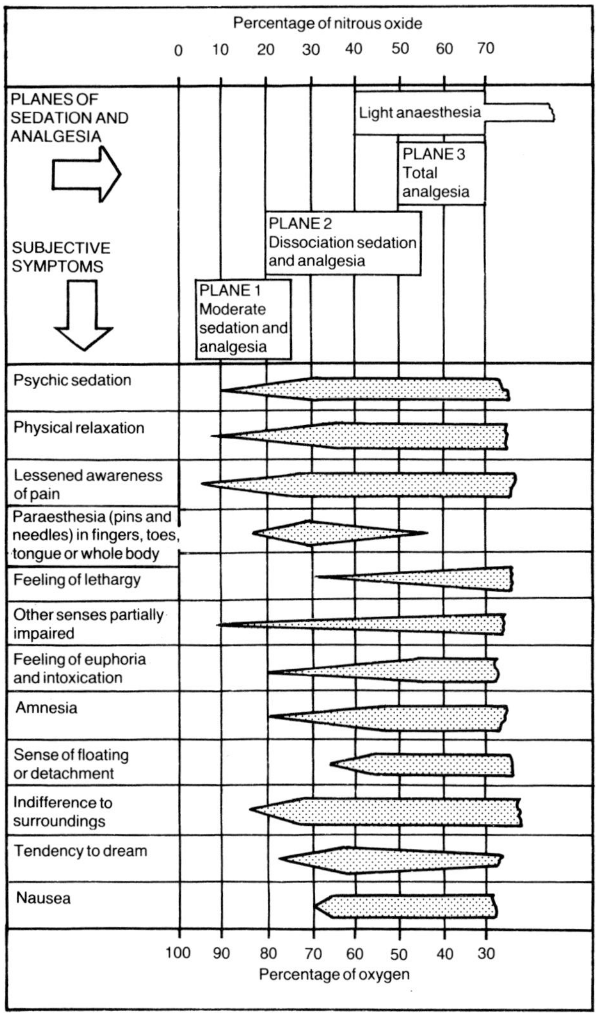

142 Subjective symptoms of the planes of sedation and analgesia

Plane 3: Total analgesia usually obtained on concentrations of 50–70 per cent N_2O (50–30 per cent O_2)

OBJECTIVE SIGNS (141)

In some patients, although analgesia is very nearly complete, it is not sufficiently profound to allow the extraction of teeth. The patient exhibits sleepiness, the gag reflex is reduced, and the laryngeal reflex – although reduced – still functions satisfactorily. Verbal contact is beginning to be lost. A further sign is that the patient exhibits a hard stare to the eyes. In the deeper level of this plane the ability of the patient to maintain the mouth wide open is lost. This loss of the ‘open mouth sign’ is an important guide to the dental surgeon, indicating that the patient is beginning to lose consciousness and therefore becoming too deeply sedated. The dental surgeon should thus reduce the concentration of nitrous oxide to a level where the patient is able to maintain an open mouth independently. **It is essential that a mouth prop is never used** to help a patient keep the mouth open, as this would obviously preclude this vital physical indication.

SUBJECTIVE SYMPTOMS (**142**)

In the lighter stages of this plane the patient is awake, but as the sedation deepens he begins to exhibit the signs of impending analgesia, i.e. closure of the eyes, loss of verbal contact, and sleepiness. The patient becomes almost unresponsive to painful stimuli. A further important sign that the patient is in the third plane of analgesia is a failure to respond to any questions or commands, i.e. verbal contact is lost. In addition, the patient's mouth closes despite any request to the contrary from the dental surgeon. These two signs together indicate that the patient is sedated too deeply and that analgesia is the next stage.

For the above reasons, the third plane of total analgesia is regarded as a buffer zone between the clinically useful planes of moderate sedation and analgesia and dissociation sedation and analgesia.

It bears repeating that a mouth prop is absolutely forbidden because it masks loss of the 'open mouth' sign.

Indications

Relative analgesia has application to almost all fields of dentistry and minor oral surgery where either psychic or somatic sedation is required to improve patient cooperation. The following conditions are regarded as benefiting considerably from the use of oxygen: nitrous oxide inhalation sedation.

1. Dental anxiety.
2. A marked gag reflex.
3. Exceptionally traumatic procedures, e.g. orthodontic extractions in a child who usually accepts conservation, or minor oral surgery in an adult.
4. Sickle cell trait and/or sickle cell anaemia.
5. Bleeding disorders, e.g. haemophilia.
6. Mental handicap.
7. Physical handicap.
8. Asthma.
9. Epilepsy.
10. Pregnancy (avoid sedation in the first three months, if possible).
11. Cardiac disorders.
12. Psychiatric disorders (with the physician's approval).

The vast majority of patients fall into the first three categories and can be treated in general dental practice. The remaining groups, if severe, may need to be availed of facilities and personnel normally only available in a hospital environment.

Contraindications

Although the use of the technique of relative analgesia is not limited by any absolute contraindications, any of the following would make for obvious difficulties.

1. The common cold.
2. Tonsillar and adenoidal enlargement.
3. Serious pulmonary conditions, e.g. bronchiectasis and emphysema.
4. Undergoing psychiatric treatment.
5. Multiple sclerosis.
6. Myasthema gravis.

The last four conditions preclude treatment in general practice, but such patients can be treated in hospital with the appropriate support of medical personnel.

Patient assessment

Before patients can be accepted for oxygen: nitrous oxide sedation, a preliminary attempt at 'routine' treatment should be made. If behaviour management techniques prove inadequate then a preliminary assessment of the patient is made to determine the need for inhalation or intravenous sedation. The preference of both the dental surgeon and the patient are important, here.

In addition, factors such as the amount of treatment and the degree of trauma involved in the surgery – together with any relevant details in the medical history – may tip the balance one way or the other. With increasing experience the dental surgeon becomes adept at assessing patients and choosing the most suitable method of sedation.

Uptake and elimination of nitrous oxide

At rest the normal adult breathes 12–15 times per minute. Such a breath is approximately 500ml (TV). So over a 60-second period approximately six to eight litres are inspired and expired – this is the so-called minute volume (**143**). At the start of a dental appointment the patient may be anxious, causing an increase in his minute volume. It is necessary, therefore, to establish an adequate flow rate on the relative analgesia machine, sufficient to match the patient's tidal or minute volume.

Nitrous oxide is carried in simple solution in the body and does not enter into any of the body's chemical processes. When a sparingly soluble gas such as nitrous oxide is inspired at a steady concentration, for example 25 per cent N_2O (75 per cent O_2), the uptake of gas into the blood proceeds rapidly. As equilibration of the gas occurs in the blood and tissues, the alveolar concentration rapidly approaches that of the inspired concentration (**144**).

The increase in alveolar tension is rapidly followed by an increase in the tension of the gas in the blood and the grey matter of the brain. The main reason for this is the poor solubility of nitrous oxide in blood and tissue (the blood/gas solubility coefficient is 0.47). This explains why induction of relative analgesia is usually so rapid, blood and tissue saturation being approximately 90 per cent of the inspired concentration within five minutes.

Over ten or 15 minutes, the blood level of nitrous oxide continues to rise, but very slowly, occasionally resulting in a deepening of sedation beyond that suitable for a given patient. The solution to this problem is to lighten the sedation by reducing the

143

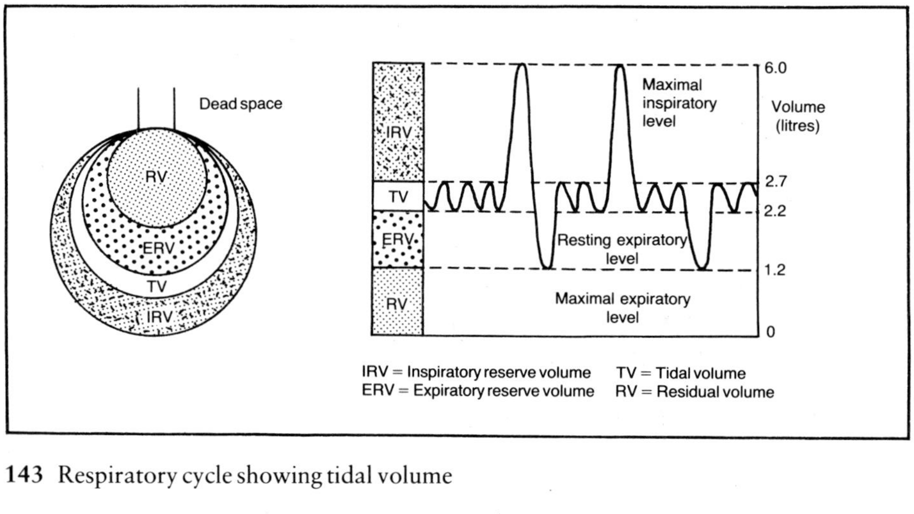

143 Respiratory cycle showing tidal volume

144

Alveolar and grey-matter tension during uptake of 25 per cent nitrous oxide
(After Mapleson 1963)

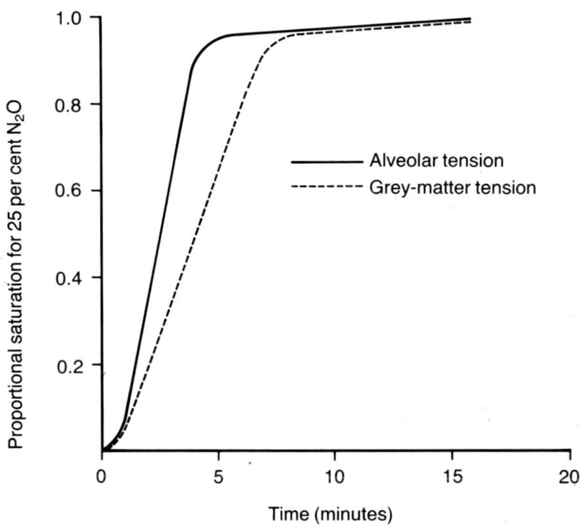

145

Rate of elimination of nitrous oxide following administration for 20 minutes and two hours, respectively
(After Mapleson 1964)

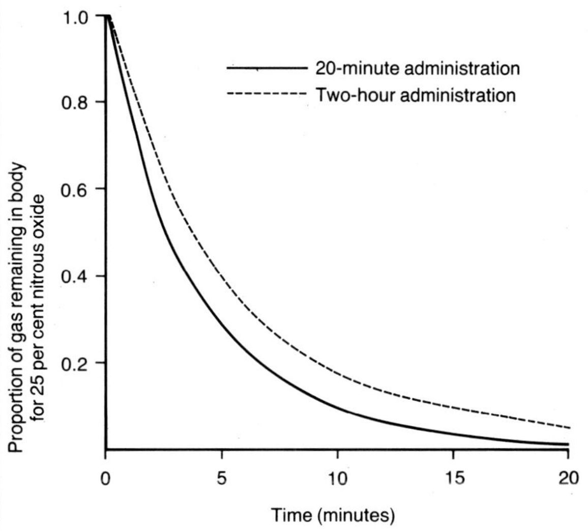

concentration of nitrous oxide by ten or 15 per cent.

The elimination of nitrous oxide from the body is very rapid, 95 per cent of the gas being eliminated within ten minutes following short administration (**145**). Even after administrations lasting two hours or more, 90 per cent of the nitrous oxide is eliminated within 15 minutes. During recovery, diffusion of nitrous oxide out of the blood and into the lung alveoli will occur so rapidly that it will dilute the inspired air and lead to a diffusion anoxia. This is probably of no consequence in fit and healthy patients, but in those with respiratory disease it may lead to a significant drop in oxygen arterial tension. This is the principal reason for oxygenating patients for two minutes at the end of treatment.

The technique of inhalation sedation (relative analgesia) using oxygen: nitrous oxide gas mixtures

The following technique, developed by the author and his colleagues, is the easiest and the most flexible of all those available.

Equipment

Apart from a conventional dental surgery, the only equipment needed is a flow control meter, a scavenging nasal hood, and a waste gas scavenger to direct waste gases away from the surgery environment.

FLOW CONTROL METER: QUANTIFLEX MDM (**146**)

This is inclined at 45° for easy reading. Both oxygen and nitrous oxide flow meters are calibrated up to 10l/min (10 litres per minute); their glass tubes are tapered, which means that the gradations between each one-litre mark are equidistant. This type of flow meter is the easiest to read accurately.

146

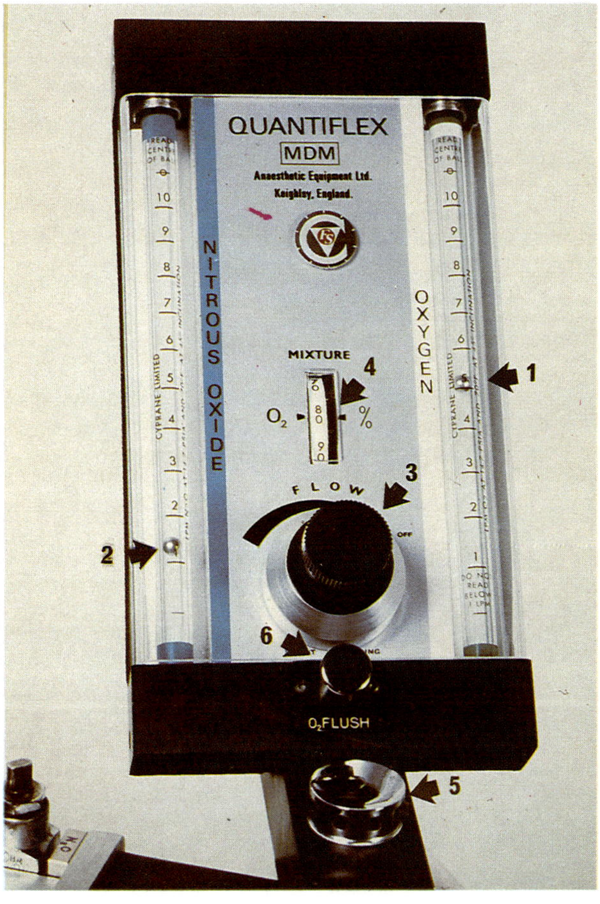

146 The ubiquitous Quantiflex MDM flow control meter. 1 indicates the oxygen meter, and 2 the nitrous oxide meter. The total flow of gases from the machine is regulated by turning the flow control knob (3), while the relative flow of gases in the oxygen and nitrous oxide flow meters is controlled by the mixture control dial (4). Other features are the air entrainment valve (5) and the oxygen flush button (6)

GAS DELIVERY HOSES AND NASAL HOOD

The whole of the inhalation assembly can be seen as an inter-connected unit (**147**). One corrugated hose, 2.5cm in diameter, brings fresh gases from the flow control meter to the specially designed nasal hood (**148**), which fits over the patient's nose. Another corrugated hose, also 2.5cm in diameter, leads on from the nasal hood to the scavenged exit (see 'Waste gas scavenger' below). To prevent the patient rebreathing expired gases, an expiratory valve has been built in to the exit port, next to the nasal hood (there used to be an expiratory valve together with an air-entrainment opening, situated in an aperture on the front of the nasal hood – but both were abandoned because of the leakage of nitrous oxide into the surgery atmosphere).

147

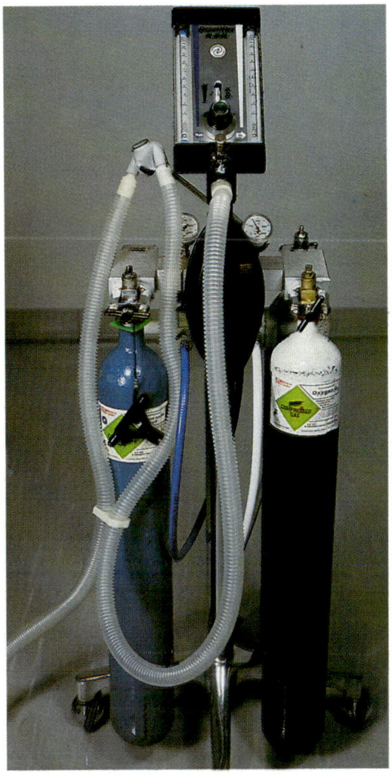

148

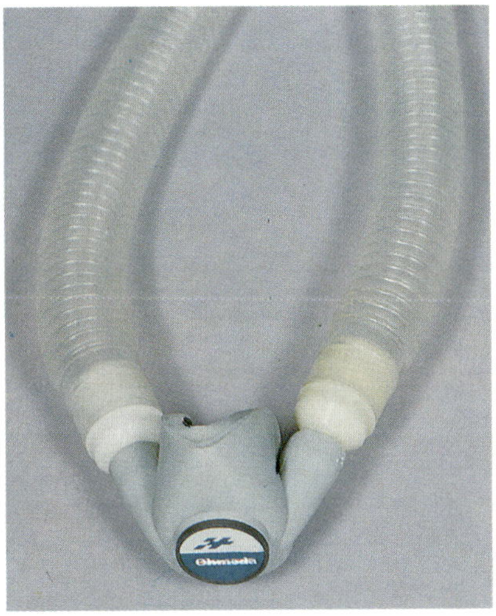

147 Flow control meter mounted in a four-cylinder stand, with corrugated hose, nasal hood, expiratory valve and scavenged gases exit port

148 Nasal hood. The blue-and-white disc on the front covers an aperture which formerly accommodated an expiratory valve and air-entrainment opening

WASTE GAS SCAVENGER

The corrugated hose carrying waste gases to the scavenging outlet, at 2.5cm in diameter, provides only minimal resistance to expiration. The hose is connected to a steel block, which is in turn connected to a 2.5cm copper pipe which vents gases to the outside atmosphere (**149**). This is by passive transfer from the patient's expired air pressure, or active transfer by a negative pressure of approximately 2cm of water.

149

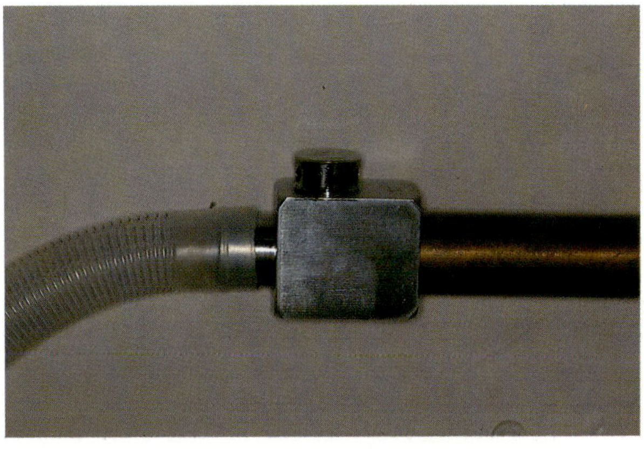

149 Waste gases are vented to the outside atmosphere via the copper pipe

A small valve incorporated in the steel block allows the entrainment of air should the pressure within the exit hose from the nasal mask fall too low. In this way negative pressure is not applied to the patient's lungs under any circumstances.

Procedure

1. At the beginning of each session the machinery is checked by the dental surgeon or dental surgery assistant to see that it is working properly. It is particularly important to make sure that there is a sufficient supply of oxygen for the forthcoming session. In addition, the safety 'cutout' on the machine must be checked to ensure that it is functioning correctly – if it is not, the machine must *not* be used.
2. The three sizes of nasal mask are examined so that the dental surgeon can choose the most appropriate one (**150**).
3. The nasal mask is connected to the 2.5cm-diameter corrugated hose so that it is ready for use. The expiratory valve is fixed open in the white plastic cylinder on the left, or exit, side of the nasal mask.
4. The mixture dial is set at 100 per cent oxygen and the patient is settled in the dental chair.
5. The flow control is turned to approximately 3l/min and the reservoir bag is allowed to fill with oxygen. The nasal mask is positioned gently and comfortably on the patient – frightened patients can be encouraged to hold it for themselves.
6. As the patient breathes in, the oxygen flow is increased – in this example, to 5l/min; in some cases, even further.
7. The reservoir bag is observed to flatten or deflate (**151**).
8. As the patient breathes out the reservoir bag expands again. This expansion is caused by the gases from the machine, which has a light non-return valve set into its outlet pipe.
9. The process is repeated: the patient breathes in again and the reservoir bag deflates again. The amount of expansion

150

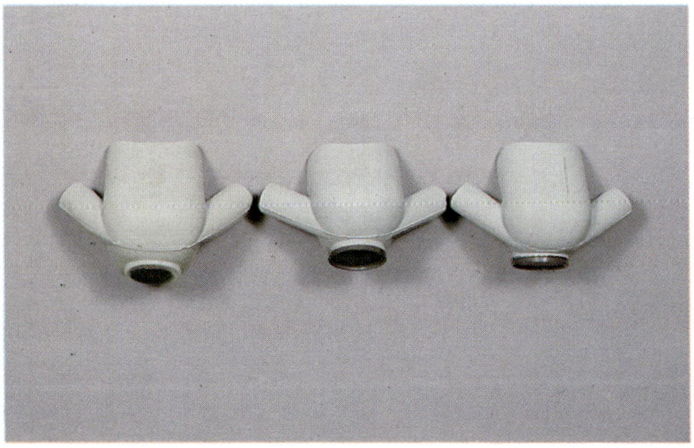

150 Nasal masks come in different sizes to suit the patient

151

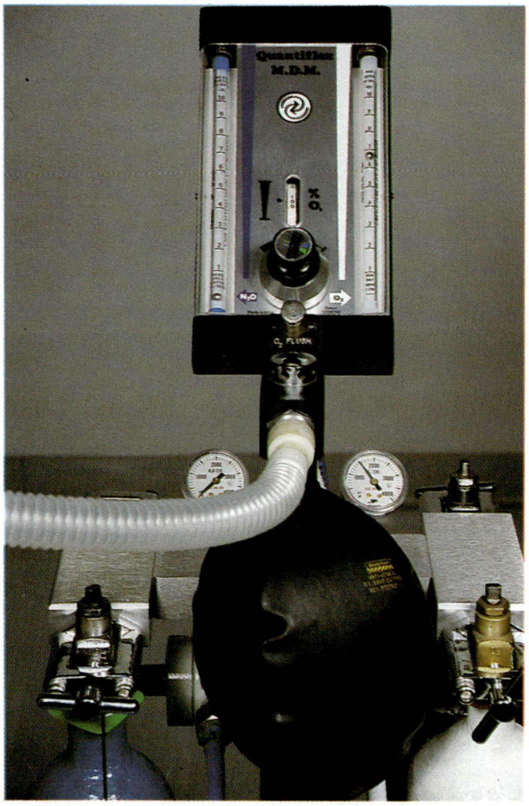

151 The reservoir bag expands and deflates as the patient breathes in and out

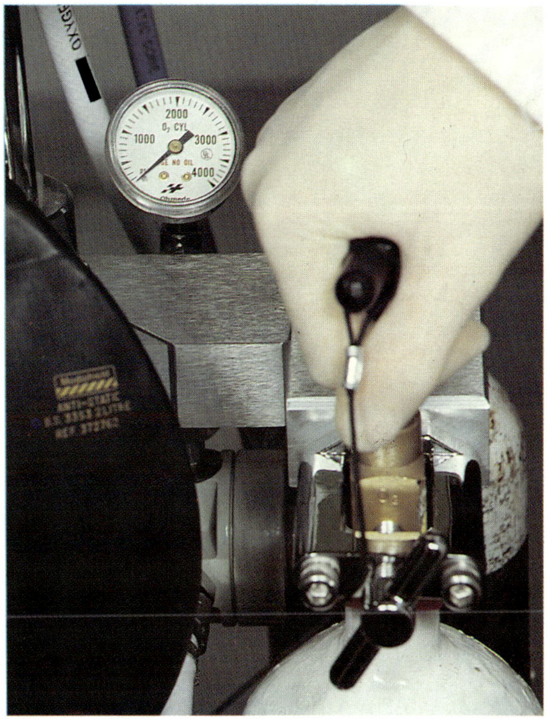

152

152 Turning off the oxygen cylinder, the procedure completed

and flattening is judged to be to the correct degree for satisfactory sedation, the flow from the machine in litres per minute having been matched to the patient's minute volume (here, of 7l/min). This process takes about 15–20 seconds.

10. The mixture dial is turned to 90 per cent oxygen, giving an increment of ten per cent nitrous oxide, and is timed carefully for a period of 60 seconds.
11. The flow meters are monitored by the dental surgeon or dental surgery assistant, to make sure that the settings are correct.
12. After 60 seconds has passed the mixture control dial is turned to 80 per cent oxygen, the balance being 20 per cent nitrous oxide. This is held for a further 60 seconds, during which time the dental surgeon continually reassures the patient, explaining what will happen and what will be felt.
13. On completion of the 60 seconds the mixture dial is turned to 70 per cent oxygen, the balance being 30 per cent nitrous oxide. This is held for a further 60 seconds. Usually by this time the patient is beginning to feel quite profound symptoms of sedation. However, the sedation can be deepened by increasing the flow of nitrous oxide by increments of five or ten per cent, as the dental surgeon considers appropriate. Once the optimum level of sedation has been achieved the dental surgeon can carry out treatment.
14. With the sedation completed, the patient can be recovered. This is achieved by turning the mixture dial to 100 per cent oxygen again. The flow meters read 7l/min for oxygen and 0l/min (that is, zero litres per minute) for nitrous oxide. This flow of 100 per cent oxygen is maintained for two minutes, for the purpose of:

    i. preventing a diffusion anoxia (caused by the very rapid elimination of nitrous oxide from the blood into the lung alveoli)
    ii. reducing the amount of pollution in the dental surgery (if the patient breathes out into the surgery it causes considerable atmospheric pollution)
    iii. speeding up the rate of recovery.

15. The machine is switched off and the oxygen cylinder is turned off completely (**152**).

The technique of sedation using the Quantiflex RA

This technique is included because there are still a large number of Quantiflex RAs (**153**) in circulation – and, indeed, being sold.

The controls are similar to those on the MDM but somewhat more basic in design. There is a simple on/off switch set in the middle of the front plate. The oxygen and nitrous oxide flow is controlled separately on this machine, by individual flow control knobs: that on the right, the white one under the oxygen flow meter, regulating the oxygen flow; that on the left, the blue one beneath the nitrous oxide flow meter, controlling the nitrous oxide flow.

Procedure

1. The preliminary steps are carried out as for the MDM (stages 1–4). As the patient starts breathing through the nasal head the oxygen flow meter is turned on to a flow of 3l/min to allow the reservoir bag to fill.
2. The oxygen flow is turned up as the reservoir bag responds to the patient's breathing, until the rate from the machine matches the patient's minute volume. At this point the technique differs markedly from that used with the Quantiflex MDM. Because there are separate controls for the oxygen and the nitrous oxide, the mixture of gases required has to be created by turning the oxygen and the nitrous oxide flow control knobs. The required mixtures and flow rates are tabulated below.

153

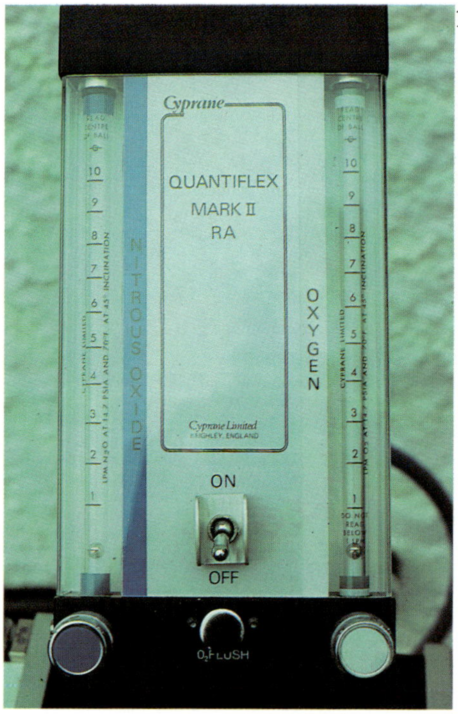

153 Quantiflex RA flow control meter

Flow rates for nitrous oxide and oxygen with a total flow of 9l/min

N_2O		O_2	
%	*l/min*	*l/min*	%
0	0.0	9.0	100
10	0.9	8.1	90
20	1.8	7.2	80
30	2.7	6.3	70
40	3.6	5.4	60
50	4.5	4.5	50
60	5.4	3.6	40
70	7.0	3.0	30

Similar tables can be constructed for each of the individual flow rates from 6l/min up to 12l/min. Note that at 30 per cent oxygen (70 per cent nitrous oxide) the flow rates for oxygen and nitrous oxide are altered to 3l/min and 7l/min, respectively, breaking the even steps of 0.9l/min increments. This is necessary because the Quantiflex RA and similar machines have a minimum flow of 3l/min.

3. To enable this to be done accurately the dental surgeon should visualize a percentage chart for the total flow. The table gives the flow of nitrous oxide (N_2O) and oxygen (O_2) for each ten per cent increment of nitrous oxide.
4. The first ten per cent is achieved by turning the nitrous oxide flow control to 0.9l/min and the oxygen flow down to 8.1l/min.
5. The second ten per cent, i.e. 20 per cent nitrous oxide, is achieved by turning the

nitrous oxide flow to 1.8l/min and the oxygen down further to 7.2l/min.

6. The third ten per cent, i.e. 30 per cent nitrous oxide, is achieved by turning the nitrous oxide flow to 2.7l/min and the oxygen down to 6.3l/min.
7. The fourth ten per cent, i.e. 40 per cent nitrous oxide, is achieved by turning the nitrous oxide flow to 3.6l/min and the oxygen down to 5.4l/min.

In this case, the patient was successfully treated on 40 per cent nitrous oxide, so no further increments were needed.

8. Once treatment is completed, the patient is recovered by administering 100 per cent oxygen for a period of two minutes. This speeds up the rate of recovery and prevents a diffusion on anoxia.

Signs and symptoms for both techniques

It is important that the dental surgeon should have a clear idea of the patient's state to ensure that all is well and that the patient is adequately sedated. To this end the following is a summary of the signs and symptoms encountered in both of the techniques of sedation described here:

Objective signs

1. The patient is awake.
2. The patient is relaxed and comfortable.
3. Pulse rate, blood pressure, respiration, skin colour and pupils are all normal.
4. The blink rate is markedly reduced.
5. Vital reflexes, particularly laryngeal, are all functioning normally.
6. The gag reflex is obtunded.
7. The mouth is maintained open on request.
8. Verbal contact is maintained.
9. Lessened reaction (sometimes absent) to painful stimuli.
10. A general reduction in spontaneous movements or fidgeting (particularly in small children).

Subjective symptoms

1. Psychic and somatic sedation.
2. Mental and physical relaxation.
3. Lessened awareness of pain.
4. Paraesthesia or tingling sensation in one or more of the following: lips, fingers, toes, legs, tongue – or over the whole body.
5. A feeling of lethargy or mild intoxication.
6. Euphoria.
7. A sense of detachment sometimes interpreted as a floating or drifting sensation.
8. A feeling of warmth.
9. Indifference to surroundings or the passage of time.
10. Dreaming.

Clinical status of a sedated patient

There are five clinical criteria by which a dental surgeon can determine a patient's level of sedation. If he is adequately – though not over- – sedated, the patient should still possess:

154

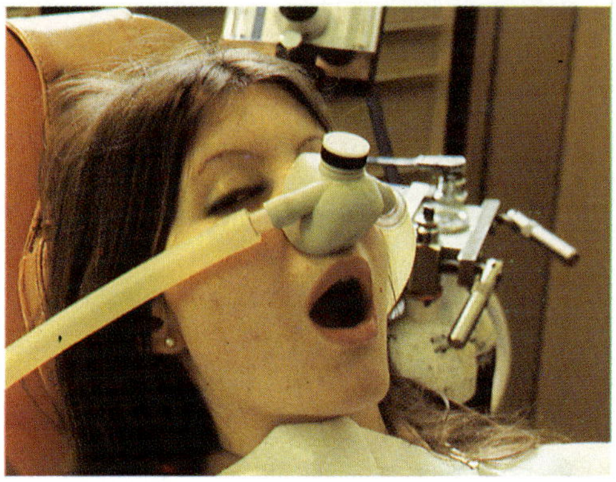

154 The ability to keep the mouth open – without any assistance – is one of the essential criteria by which adequate sedation is judged

1. *The ability to maintain a patent airway independently.* This can be tested by the dental surgeon flexing the head forward to cause the tongue to touch the back of the pharynx. In a properly sedated patient the suprahyoid and infrahyoid muscles change their posture to maintain a clear airway: the so-called 'head-flexure test'.
2. *The ability to maintain verbal contact.* This can be tested simply by asking the patient to give his name or the time he arrived at the surgery. A coherent and sensible reply immediately tells the dental surgeon that the patient is only lightly sedated.
3. *The ability to maintain an open mouth independently: the 'open-mouth sign' of Langa.* Patients in a suitable state of sedation are able to keep the mouth open independently (**154**). For this reason it is absolutely forbidden to use a mouth prop.
4. *The ability to maintain the eyes open.* Patients who are sedated can, if required, keep their eyes open. Some dental surgeons allow patients to go to sleep. However, the author prefers patients to keep their eyes open because then their status can be readily ascertained.
5. *The ability to swallow.* The patient maintains the normal swallowing function. This ensures that any fluid accumulating in the mouth will, when swallowed, pass down past the larynx into the oesophagus without causing any problems with normal laryngeal function.

Miscellaneous problems with relative analgesia

The technique of relative analgesia poses a number of special problems which do not fit easily into any of the other sections.

Fear of the mask

With the improvement in dental health that has occurred over the last ten years, far fewer general anaesthetics are now being given for the extraction of teeth. However, a small number of children and adults are still frightened of the mask. Fear is hardly a surprising response,

155

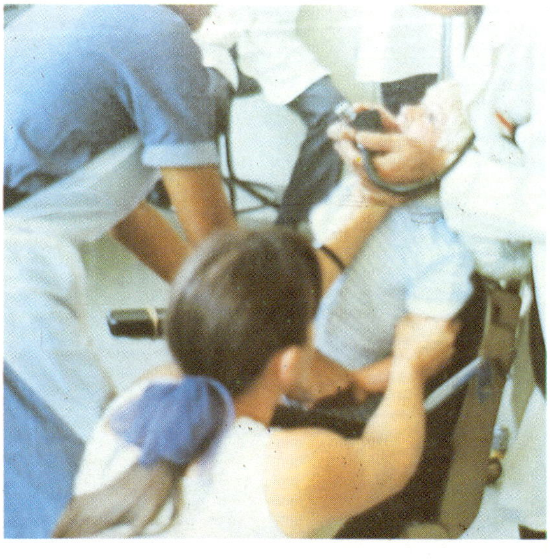

155 How *not* to go about relative analgesia . . . . Physical compulsion can have a traumatic effect on a child, instilling a deep-rooted fear of the mask

though, when a child has been forcibly restrained as in **155**.

The anaesthetist is gripping the girl's jaw whilst holding the mask forcibly against her face. Although the child has succeeded in pushing her head up and away in an attempt to escape, the mother has gripped her arm to counteract this and appears to be trying to hold her still by grasping her throat! The staff nurse is 'assisting' by holding the child's hands . . . .

The following, alternative, strategy is recommended to overcome fear of the mask:

1. The dental surgeon should explain in detail to the child (or adult) exactly what is expected, and do this beforehand.
2. He should promise the child that no one will force the mask onto his face or hold him down.
3. He should promise that no dental treatment will be carried out there and then: 'Today is only a trial run'.
4. At the same time, he should quietly insist that the child himself tries holding the mask over his nose.
5. He should insist, too (with the parents' agreement), where a child is concerned, that the child cannot go home until he has tried the 'happy air' or 'magic wind'.
6. He should encourage the child to hold the mask on his nose whilst he – the dental surgeon – counts to five; he should repeat the process until the child is cooperative, and then use a count of ten, and so on.
7. He should praise the child for his cooperative behaviour.

Following the above approach, the dental surgeon will still be able to impose his will on the patient – but *without* the use of force. With the dental surgeon's guarantee that there will be no pain, the patient's confidence can be gradually built up until adequate trust in the dental surgeon is achieved.

Advanced operative procedures

The most sophisticated operative dentistry and endodontics are undertaken using a rubber dam (**156**). Relative analgesia can be a great help in relaxing the patient sufficiently to enable the dental surgeon to carry out a high standard of work. The dam, once in place, can be a significant contributory factor in reducing atmospheric pollution because it cuts down leakage from the mouth.

This application emphasizes an important feature of relative analgesia: it allows the dental surgeon to perform clinical work of the highest quality.

156

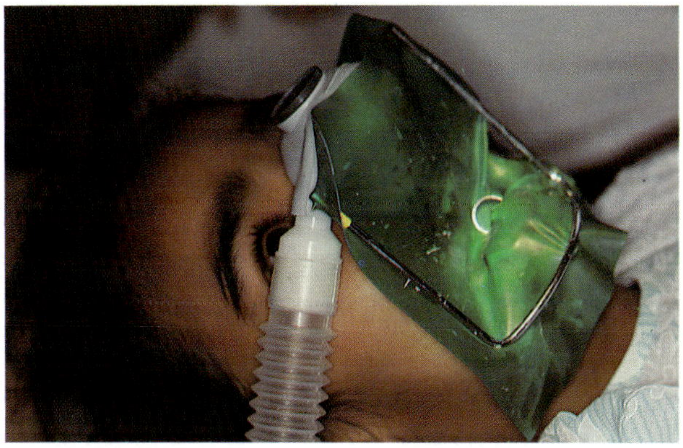

156 Use of a rubber dam facilitates effective operative dentistry

The reservoir bag

Many dental surgeons labour under the misapprehension that the two-litre reservoir bag on the machine (**151**) is for rebreathing. In fact, the bag is there solely as a **reservoir** of gases so that when the patient breathes in there is always an adequate supply of gas available to him. Rebreathing is prevented by the non-return valve set into the outlet pipe of the Quantiflex MDM flow control meter.

An unexplained leakage

When a dental surgery assistant replaces an E-sized cylinder on a sedation unit there is, occasionally, a significant and audible leak from the manifold when the cylinder is turned on. This is usually because the metal-and-rubber seal has stuck to the cylinder head as it is removed from the machine. Before replacing a cylinder, therefore, the dental surgery assistant should check to see that the bodock seal is still in place on the cylinder manifold (**157**).

157

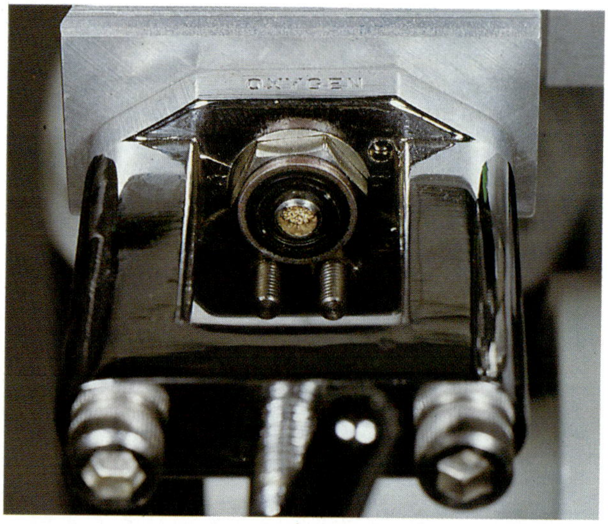

157 The bodock seal can stick to the cylinder head when a cylinder is replaced, leading to a leak. A check that the seal is still in place on the cylinder manifold is therefore essential

Limited access

Because the nasal hood covers the nose and upper lip it is difficult to obtain access to the upper incisor area when carrying out an apicectomy. This problem can be surmounted by holding the nasal hood in place with the palm of the hand and retracting the upper lip with the fore, middle, and ring fingers (**158**). A mucoperiosteal flap can then be lifted quite easily, although occasional readjustments to the mask are necessitated.

158

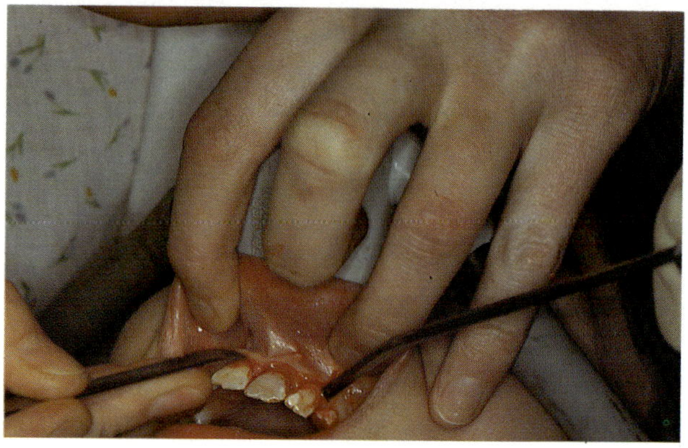

158 How to gain access to the upper incisor area when carrying out an apicectomy. (*Note:* this photograph was taken before the wearing of gloves became mandatory, and is used here solely to illustrate the technique involved. Gloves *must* be worn in all such cases.)

Handicapped patients

Handicapped patients can present particular problems. Often, the handicap itself can dominate the person's thinking, to the extent that dental matters are neglected. While if the handicapped person has considerable medical problems, it can be undesirable to administer a general anaesthetic. However, in a large number of cases, the need for general anaesthetics has been significantly reduced.

In fact, though, the dental requirements of the majority of handicapped patients can usually be met by the use of oxygen: nitrous oxide sedation. However, their response to sedation can be unpredictable: occasionally, the result is much more favourable than was anticipated; but other times, despite the dental surgeon's optimism, treatment can prove to be impossible. It is always worth giving it a try, though. The need for general anaesthetics in the case of a large number of handicapped patients has been significantly reduced, lessening the risk, the discomfort and the cost associated with treatment.

The dental surgery assistant as Second Appropriate Person

Before a dental surgeon can use sedation techniques – in this case, relative analgesia (oxygen: nitrous oxide sedation) – it is recognized that he should have undergone a suitable course in the subject. What is not always appreciated, however, is the extent to which the dental surgery assistant, too, can become involved in the provision of dental care to patients. In fact, a dental surgery assistant's general training should encompass all of the following:

1. The relevant anatomy and physiology of the cardiovascular system, including venous and arterial supply to the forearm.
2. The relevant anatomy and physiology of the respiratory system, including the importance of maintaining an unobstructed airway.
3. The pharmacology of the drugs used for the sedation of patients and of the techniques of: i. inhalation sedation; ii. intravenous sedation; and iii. resuscitation.
4. General pre- and post-operative instructions for patients receiving dental treatment.
5. The indications and contraindications of inhalation sedation and intravenous sedation.

In the specific area of relative analgesia, the dental surgery assistant should:

1. Know about oxygen: nitrous oxide sedation equipment such as the Quantiflex MDM flow control meter.
2. Be able to give adequate pre-operative instructions, such as: i. that the patient should eat a light meal only; ii. that extremely nervous patients should be accompanied; and iii. that children should be accompanied.
3. Be able to test the machine and cylinder manifold to verify the amount of oxygen and nitrous oxide remaining in the cylinders, and report to the dental surgeon.
4. Be able to test the flow meters to verify correct working of the fail-safe device should the oxygen supply inadvertently run out, and report to the dental surgeon.
5. Know about the clinical technique of relative analgesia.
6. Be able to alter machine settings, under the direction of the dental surgeon.
7. Be able to monitor and record the pulse rate.
8. Be able to monitor and record the respiratory rate.
9. Be able to take and record the systolic and diastolic blood pressures.
10. Be familiar with the open-mouth sign, verbal contact and open eyes, and their use in determining a patient's consciousness.
11. Be aware of the importance of not using a mouth prop.
12. Be aware of the importance to the patient of the 15-minute recovery period after nitrous oxide sedation.
13. Be able to give adequate post-sedation instructions to children or adults, viz. the need to be careful when driving or cycling following a relative analgesia appointment.

Once the dental surgery assistant has been trained in the above matters, she will qualify as a Second Appropriate Person, and the dental surgeon will be able to utilize her skills to the advantage of the patients.

Monitoring of patients undergoing oxygen: nitrous oxide sedation

During treatment the dental surgeon and the dental surgery assistant should keep a watchful eye on the patient to ensure that all is going well. The following should be monitored intermittently throughout the procedure:

1. The oxygen flow meter.
2. The nitrous oxide flow meter.
3. The reservoir bag (to ensure adequate inhalation of gases).
4. The general level of sedation of the patient.
5. Respiration (to ensure that the patient is breathing comfortably).

Pulse and blood pressure need to be monitored only where patients present a special risk by virtue of cardiac insufficiency or some other potentially serious complication.

Monitoring of oxygen saturation

This is achieved using a pulse oximeter (**159**). Recordings are gained by placing a simple, light-emitting probe on the finger (**160**) or ear (**161**).

With the advent of sophisticated oxygen monitors the dental profession needs to consider whether or not it is still necessary to carry out oxygen monitoring.

Preliminary studies with oxygen: nitrous oxide sedation show that blood/oxygen levels are 98 per cent or higher during induction and maintenance of sedation. During recovery, the phenomenon of diffusion anoxia causes the level of oxygen saturation to drop – though it still exceeds 95 per cent (**162**). These levels are well within the acceptable range for patients undergoing out-patient care. The author's view is that pulse oximetry is not necessary for patients treated under relative analgesia unless there are potentially serious medical problems which may justify the use of such close and careful monitoring.

159

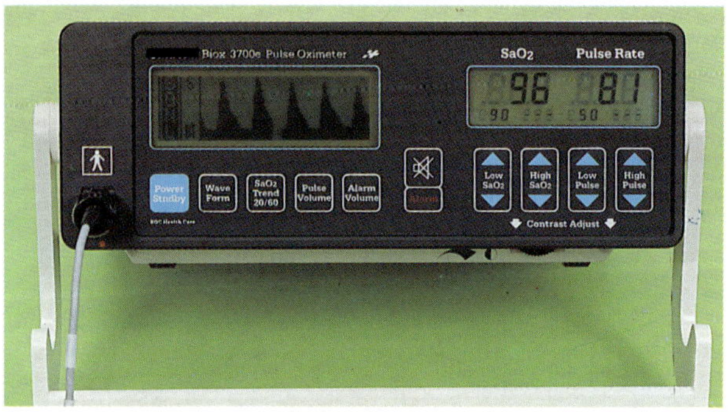

160

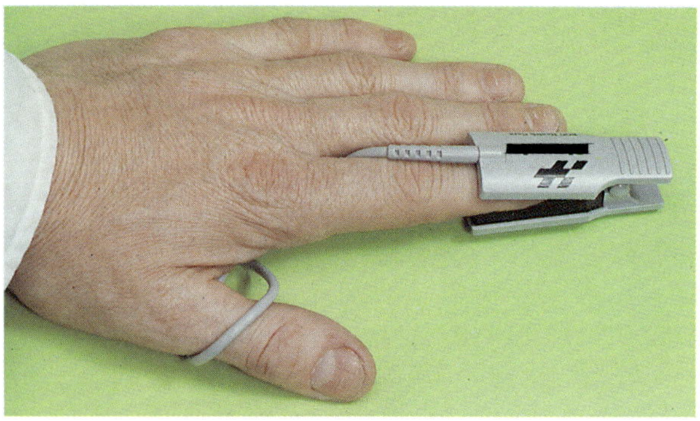

161

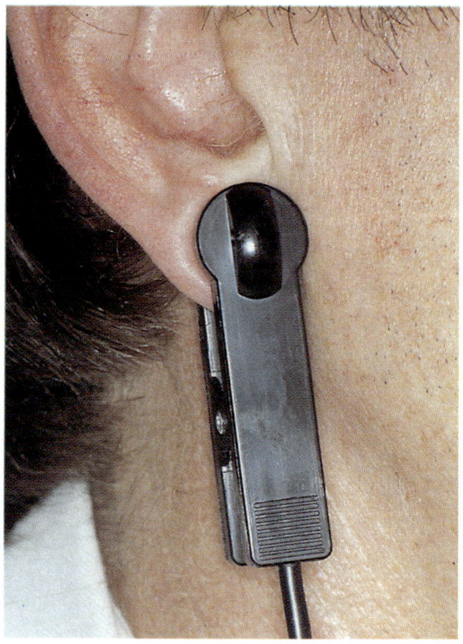

159 to **161** Pulse oximeter (**159**). Recordings are achieved via a probe placed on the finger (**160**) or ear (**161**)

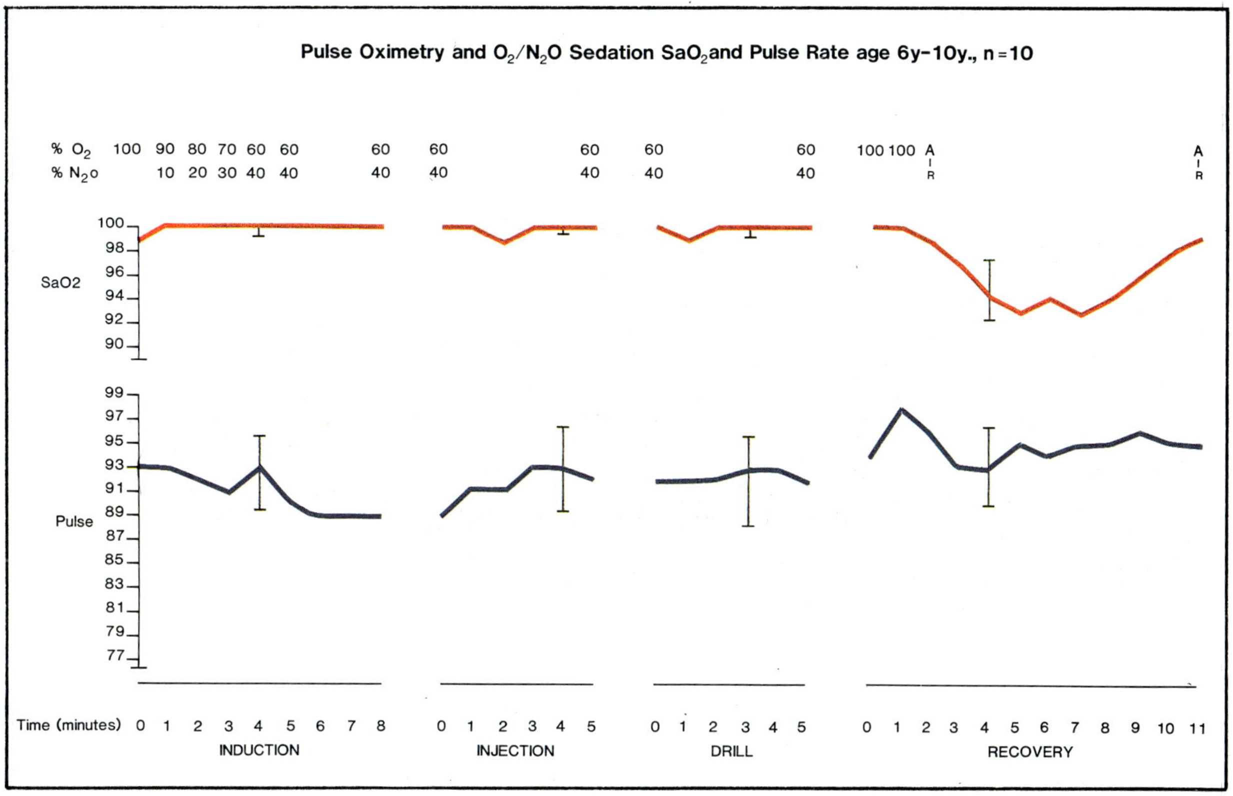

162

162 Pulse oximetry shows high O_2 saturation with relative analgesia. The small amount of diffusion anoxia at the end is within acceptable limits

The physiological status of patients during oxygen: nitrous oxide sedation

Five criteria, viz. blood pressure, heart rate, respiratory rate, psychomotor ability and laryngeal competence, are used to assess the degree of intrusion – if any – upon the patient's physiological state of inhalation sedation.

Blood pressure

At the commencement of treatment the systolic and diastolic blood pressures are slightly elevated because of the patient's high anxiety levels. Once a local analgesic is given there is a slight elevation of the systolic blood pressure (**163**), but as treatment proceeds the tendency is for it to drop a few millimetres – although intensive drilling brings a slight elevation. Towards the end of treatment there is another slight increase, but the systolic value does not approach the pre-treatment level. This is interpreted as a loss of anxiety once treatment is complete. The diastolic blood pressure shows minor fluctuations which are of no significance.

163 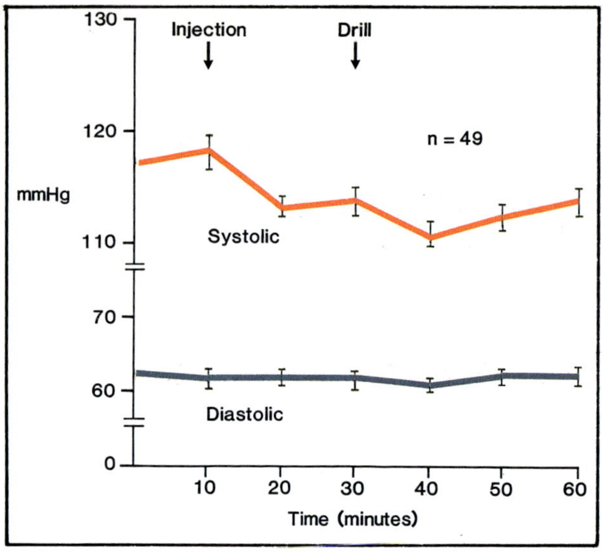

163 Mean systolic and diastolic blood pressures at ten-minute intervals throughout treatment (age six to 16 years)

164 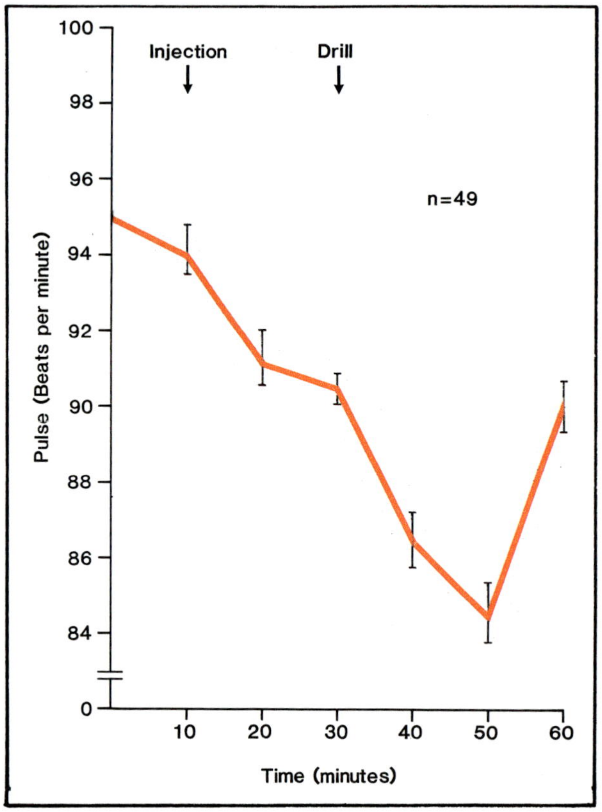

164 Mean pulse rate at ten-minute intervals throughout treatment (age six to 16 years)

Pulse rate

The trends shown with systolic blood pressure are repeated in the case of the pulse rate. That is to say, there is an elevated heart rate at the start of treatment. Then, as sedation takes effect, the rate begins to drop – although the drop slows with the increased anxiety associated with the administration of the local analgesic (**164**). As treatment proceeds the pulse rate drops further; intensive use of the drill, though, will cause this drop to slow down, as in the case of the injection. During packing and carving of the amalgam restorations, the pulse rate drops to what can be regarded as a basal level. It rises again after the nitrous oxide is turned off, but not as high as the pre-operative level.

Respiratory rate

Nervous children, when first attending the dental surgery, have a slightly elevated respiratory rate, presumably due to their heightened anxiety (**165**). During treatment the rate fluctuates by two or three breaths per minute, as a result of gasping or breath-holding by patients under stress. Come the end of treatment the respiratory rate is lower than at the start.

COMMENT

The most significant finding of these three vital parameters is the fact that all values recorded, and the slight changes that were observed, are well within the range of normal. This means that, as far as the cardiovascular and respiratory systems are concerned, the technique of oxygen: nitrous oxide sedation represents only a minimal intrusion into the patient's physiological state.

So beneficial are the effects on the cardiovascular system that an extensive study carried out on adults 'at risk' because of ischaemic heart disease showed that circulating levels of adrenaline and nonadrenaline were reduced when these patients received inhalation sedation. The conclusion is that oxygen and nitrous oxide at sub-anaesthetic levels are actually beneficial to patients with cardiac disorders. (Summers, 1981.)

165

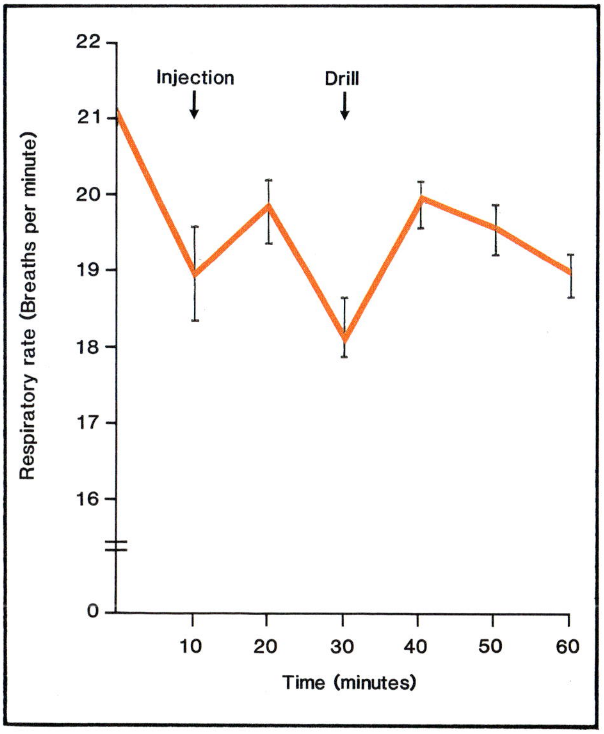

165 Mean respiratory rate at ten-minute intervals throughout treatment (age six to 16 years)

Psychomotor ability

A major advantage of inhalation sedation is the fact that patients remain conscious throughout the period of sedation. They are therefore able to perform a simple pencil-and-paper drawing test, via which their psychomotor ability can be assessed (Trieger *et al*, 1971).

At baseline, breathing 100 per cent oxygen, the patient (a 12-year-old child) is able to produce clear lines passing through the centre of most of the dots (**166**) – the object of the exercise; score, 49. Five or six minutes later, however, breathing 40 per cent nitrous oxide in oxygen, the performance has deteriorated: there is an increased number of missed dots and several lines have been drawn over (**167**); score, 86.

Following the completion of dental treatment, now breathing 50 per cent nitrous oxide in oxygen, the patient is slightly more heavily sedated (**168**); score, 92. After being given 100 per cent oxygen for two minutes to induce recovery, there is a dramatic improvement (**169**); score, 64. A further eight minutes breathing air, and the drawing test indicates that the patient's psychomotor ability has virtually returned to normal (**170**); score 51. Both the drawings (**166–170**) and the graph (**171**) illustrate two important points:

- Patients under the influence of low concentrations of nitrous oxide remain conscious.
- Recovery from oxygen: nitrous oxide sedation is rapid.

166

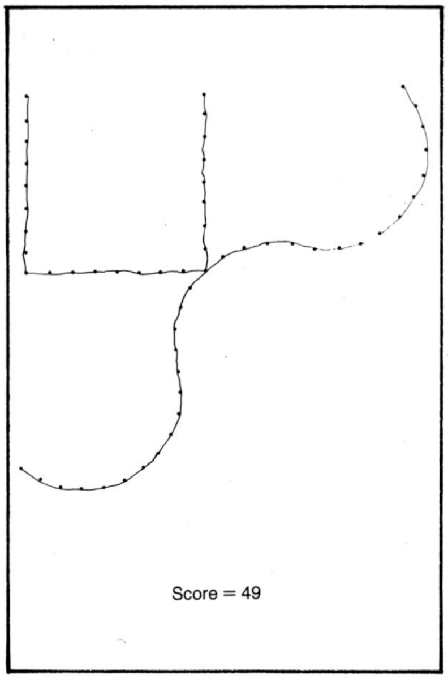

167

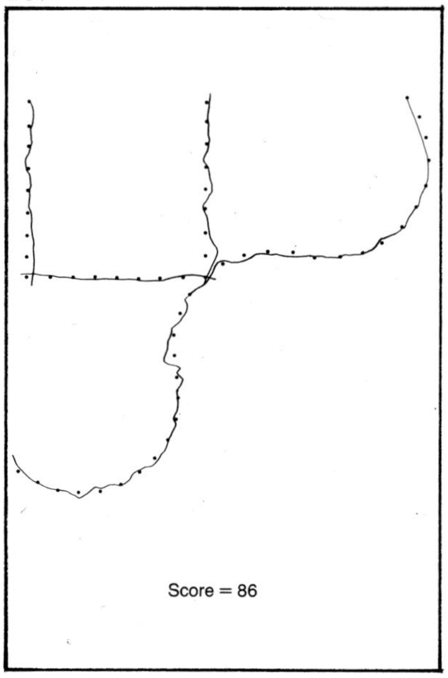

168

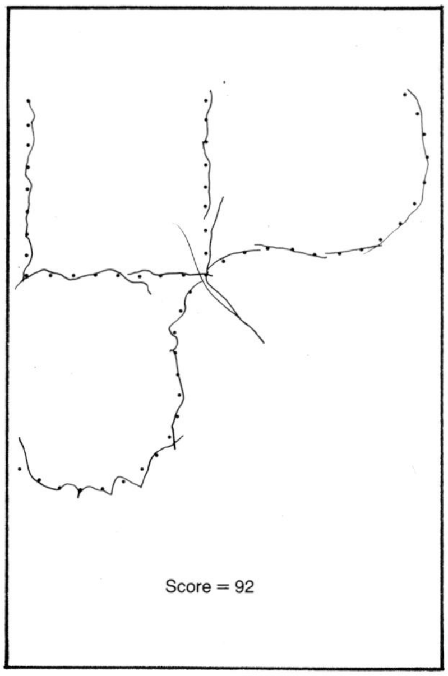

169

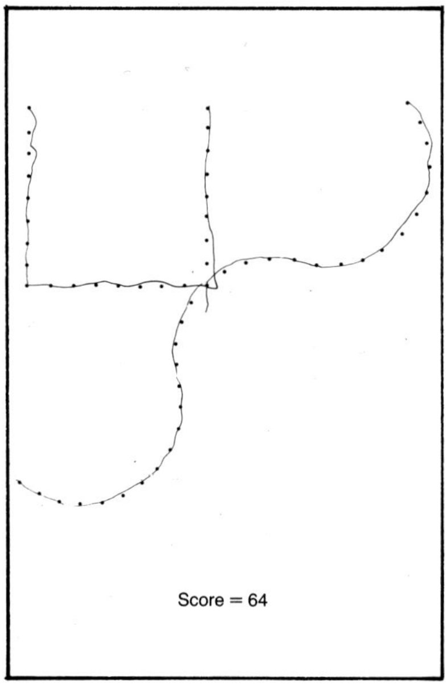

170

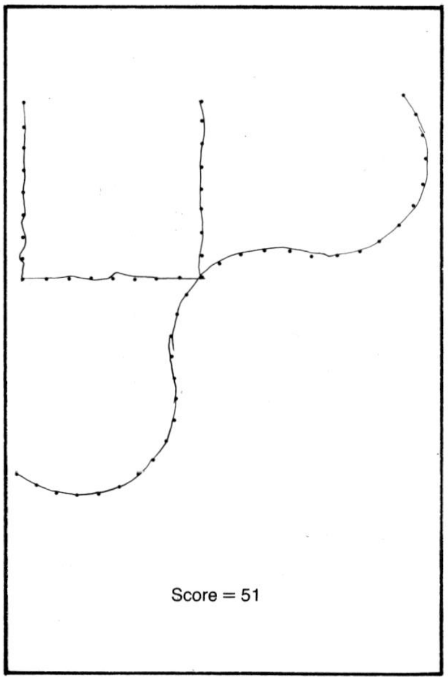

166–170 The simple drawing test used to assess a patient's psychomotor ability before, during and after inhalation sedation

171

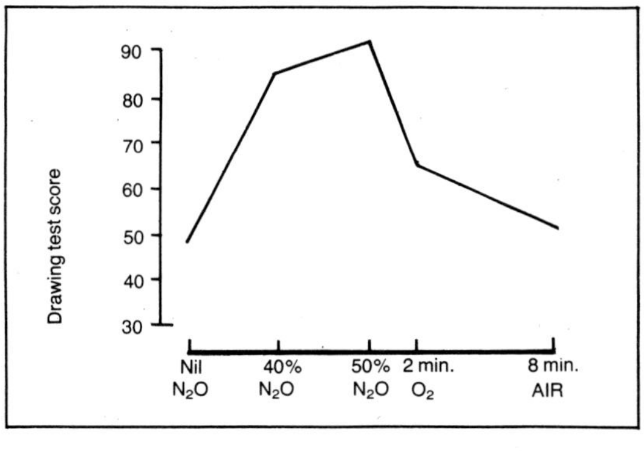

171 Graph with curve typical of a patient breathing nitrous oxide in oxygen and then being recovered on 100 per cent oxygen

Laryngeal competence

The effect of oxygen: nitrous oxide sedation is to achieve psychic and somatic sedation. This obtunds the gag reflex to an extent which allows patients who retch fiercely to accept dental treatment. However, concern has been expressed that other reflexes, particularly the laryngeal, may be depressed below a critical level. This possibility has been investigated by inducing patients to swallow a large or physiological bolus of radiopaque dye.

The results (**172** and **173**) demonstrate that when oxygen: nitrous oxide sedation is carried out using concentrations of gases titrated to the individual patient's needs, and with the open-mouth sign present, there is *no* risk of the aspiration of debris and material from the mouth as a result of laryngeal incompetence.

172

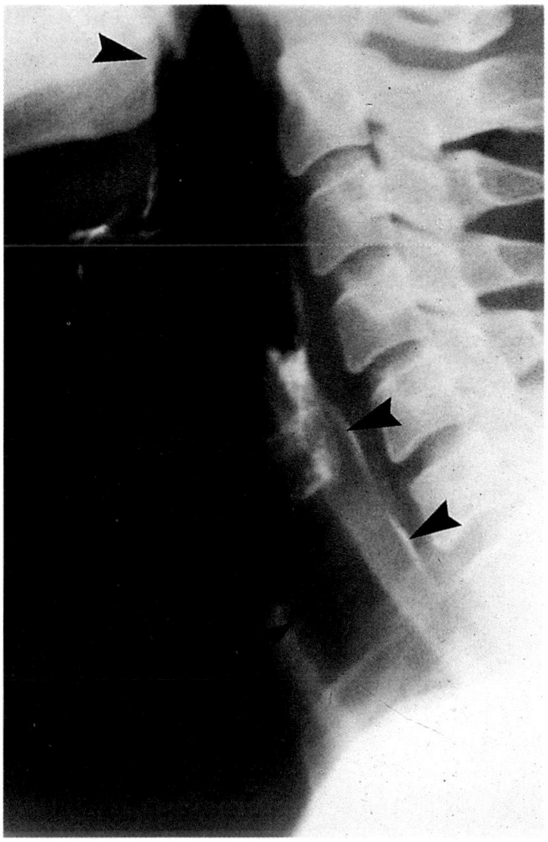

172 Lateral view of the throat, following ingestion by the patient of a large or physiological bolus of radiopaque dye. The three larger arrows indicate the dorsal surface of the tongue, the posterior wall of the pharynx, and the anterior and posterior walls of the oesophagus, all of which are coated with the dye; the two smaller arrows indicate the larynx and the upper trachea, both of which are completely clear of the dye

173

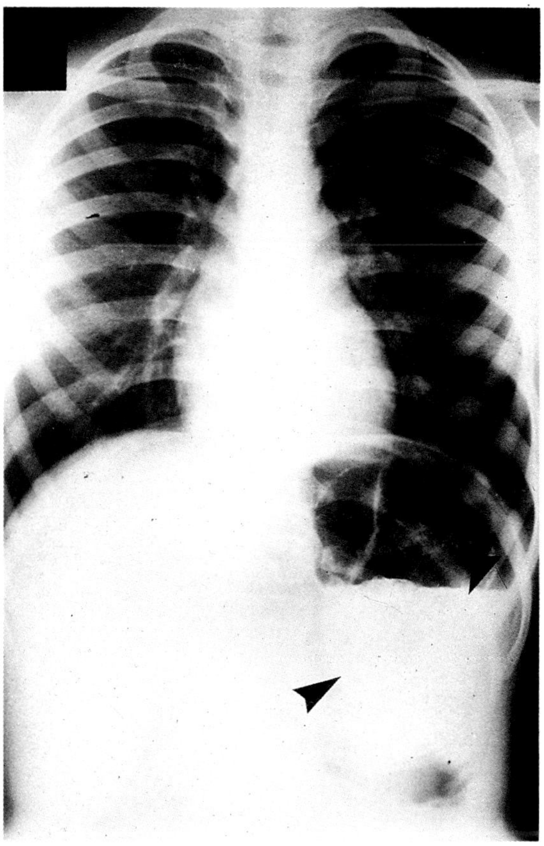

173 Postero-anterior view of the chest of the patient featured in **172**. Though the lungs are entirely free of the dye, the stomach – which is clearly outlined – is obviously not, a large amount of dye being discernible in the arrowed area

Behavioural changes during oxygen: nitrous oxide psychosedation

Little work has been undertaken on this topic. However, by compiling appropriate checklists, it is possible to monitor behavioural changes in both the patient (**174**) and the dental surgeon (**175**).

The first major finding, when comparing the use of relative analgesia with that of an air placebo, is that the time taken to complete similar amounts of dental treatment is approximately 40 per cent less when nitrous oxide is used (**176**).

The second important finding is that the total number of obstructive activities is considerably less (i.e. patients are more compliant) with relative analgesia than is the case with an air placebo (**177**).

Furthermore, patients require considerably less behaviour management when treated with oxygen: nitrous oxide gas mixtures than with air alone (**178**). The dental surgeon has to work appreciably less hard and his task is both simpler and safer.

174

Child's behaviour	1	2	3	4	5	6	7	8	9	10
Choking/coughing										
Verbal complaints										
Stops/won't allow treatment										
Cries out at injection										
Strikes out arms/legs										
Pushes away dentist										
Wants parent										
Restless										
Wants to see/asks about instruments										
Attempts to dislodge mask										
Other behaviour (weeping etc.)										
	1	2	3	4	5	6	7	8	9	10

(minutes)

175

Dentist's behaviour	1	2	3	4	5	6	7	8	9	10
Speaks very gently										
Entertains child										
Reprimands/is angry with child										
Reassures child (asks what's wrong, tells/suggests/shows what will happen, asks child how he feels)										
Praises										
	1	2	3	4	5	6	7	8	9	10

(minutes)

174 and 175 Changes in the behaviour of the patient (**174**) and the dental surgeon (**175**) occurring during oxygen: nitrous oxide psychosedation can be monitored by the use of suitable checklists

176

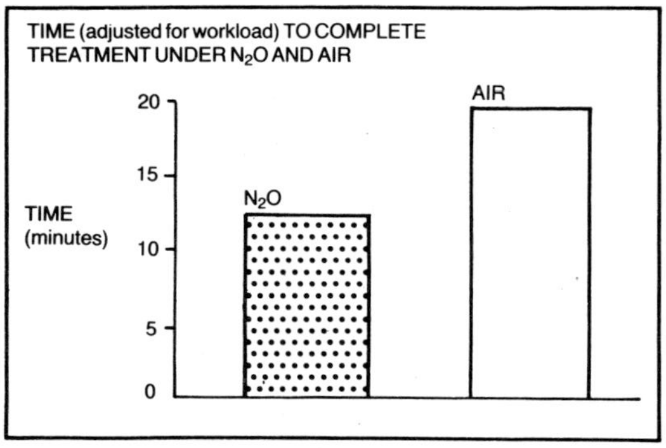

176 Relative analgesia *v.* air placebo: a comparison of the time taken in each case – adjusted for workload – to complete similar amounts of dental treatment

177 Relative analgesia *v.* air placebo: a comparison of the total number of instances of obstructive behaviour occurring in each case

178 Relative analgesia *v.* air placebo: a comparison of supporting activities undertaken by the dental surgeon in each case

177

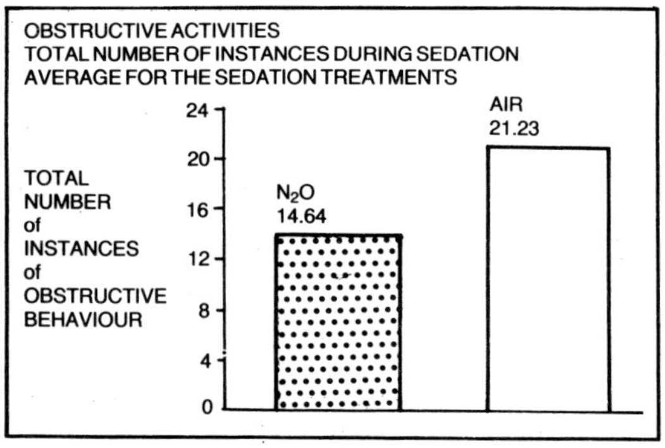

178

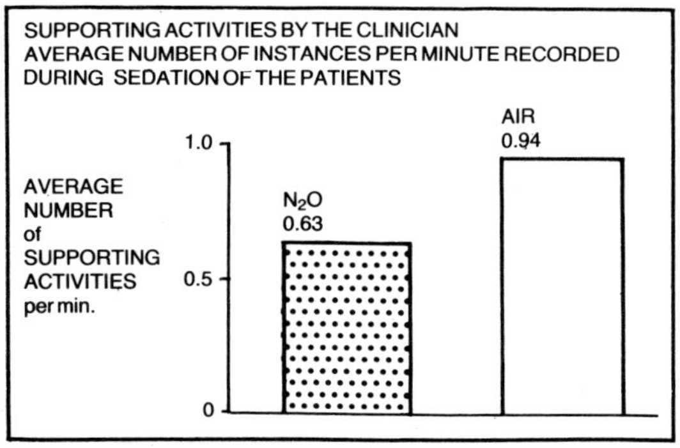

Anti-pollution system

Although the deleterious effects of chronic exposure to low levels of nitrous oxide in the operating room are now established, it is important to recognize that there is a threshold of about eight hours per week below which serious problems will not occur.

The use of a suitable passive scavenging system (**179**) will ensure that gases are vented away from the faces of the dental surgeon and the dental surgery assistant. A simple nasal hood with 2.5cm corrugated tubes is used (**147**). Note that the old expiratory valve port is blocked off, but that a new one is placed in the port, on the right, to prevent the patient rebreathing expired gases. This new expiratory valve is attached to a corrugated hose, which in turn is connected to an exit port with some negative pressure attached to it (**149**). This successfully directs any expired gases outside the building.

Other important prerequisites of scavenging are:

- A controlled background level of pollution, achieved by having satisfactory room ventilation.
- A good clinical technique, e.g. to prevent mouth breathing and ensure there are no leaks around the mask.

A short period of 100 per cent oxygen after completion of sedation is also required, to ensure that gases from the patient are expired via the scavenging system.

179

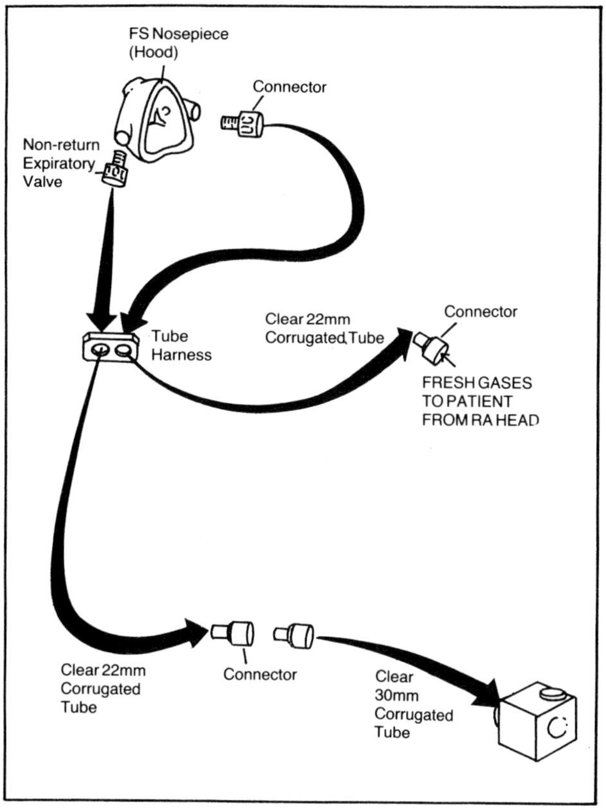

179 A passive scavenging system

By careful application of the scavenging system, levels of nitrous oxide can be kept below 50ppm (parts per million), which is the currently recommended level.

Oxygen: nitrous oxide sedation (relative analgesia) – a case record

The case record described here should assist understanding of the various aspects of relative analgesia covered in this chapter. The record is of a typical visit by a dentally anxious child – here known as 'Mark' – who requires a simple filling.

The dental surgeon and the dental surgery assistant, on being advised of Mark's arrival by the receptionist, review his patient records to verify the treatment plan, to check which tooth is to be filled, and to remind themselves of any special likes and/or dislikes that Mark may have.

The dental surgery assistant then makes a final check to ensure that the relative analgesia machinery is working properly, setting the flow control of the inhalation sedation control unit at 10l/min and the mixture control at 50 per cent (**180**). Both the oxygen and the nitrous oxide flow meters should read 5l/min.

The dental surgery assistant then collects Mark from the waiting area. She is initially a little surprised to see that he is accompanied by his father, since his mother brought him on his last visit. Then she remembers that Mark was very uncooperative on that occasion and that, as a result, his mother had said that she would try to get her husband to bring Mark next time, as her son would then be less likely to 'play you up'. The situation is therefore a new one, Mark's relationship with his father being an unknown quantity.

Mark is settled in the dental chair, with his father seated close by where Mark can see him. The dental surgeon then explains to Mark what is to be done today, being careful to avoid the use of any emotive words, and reassures him (**181**).

Next, he shows him the nasal hood, which he describes as a 'sky pilot's oxygen mask' or a 'spaceman's mask', making sure that Mark holds the hood himself. The atmosphere is relaxed and there is no attempt to rush the procedure. After some further explanation, Mark places the nasal hood onto his nose by himself. The dental surgeon supports the pipes, **but makes no attempt to force the mask onto Mark's face** – this is imperative if the dental surgeon is to gain his patient's confidence.

Under instruction from the dental surgeon, the dental surgery assistant turns up the flow control to ensure that the reservoir bag is sufficiently inflated. Mark is encouraged to breathe gently through his nose to check that there are no leaks due to mouth breathing. (It is helpful to count one . . . two . . . three . . . etc. at the speed that the patient should breathe.) He is very unsure of all this and frowns quite noticeably.

The oxygen is now flowing at approximately 6l/min, at which rate the reservoir bag is adequately expanded, showing that the flow rate from the machine is matching Mark's minute volume adequately. The dental surgeon, who has now donned a pair of rubber gloves, then starts his stop watch to enable him to time the 60-second intervals, and an increment of ten per cent nitrous oxide is introduced (**182**).

With further increments of the same, Mark becomes considerably more relaxed. The dental surgeon places a hand reassuringly on his

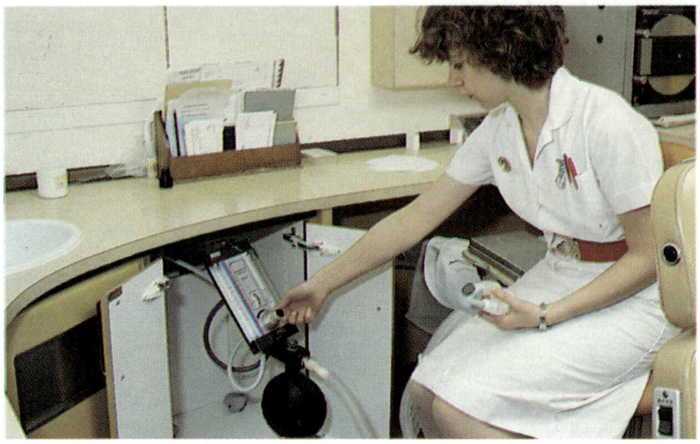

180 The dental surgery assistant makes a final check of the relative analgesia machinery, prior to collecting the patient from reception. She sets the flow control of the inhalation sedation control unit at 10l/min and the mixture control at 50 per cent. (Both the oxygen and the nitrous oxide flow meters should read 5l/min.)

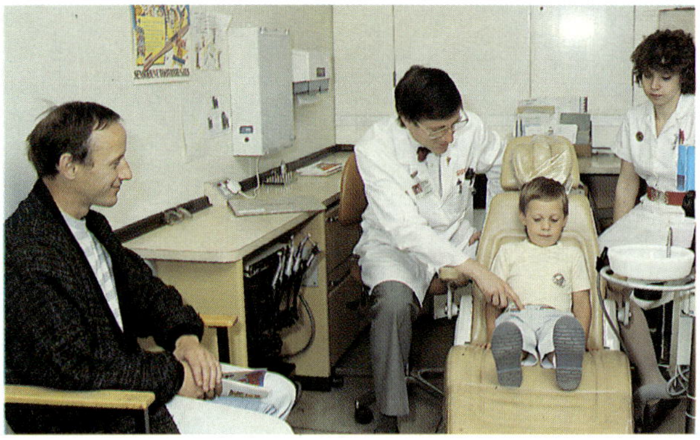

181 Father is strategically placed in full view of his son, who sits in the dental chair. The dental surgeon and dental surgery assistant take up their respective positions each side of the patient, and the dental surgeon then explains to the patient what is to be done, reassuring him as he does so

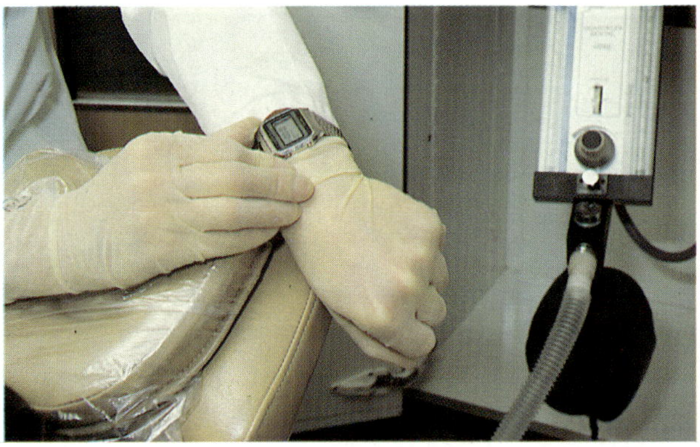

182 As the dental surgeon starts his stop watch, ready to time the 60-second intervals, an increment of ten per cent nitrous oxide is introduced

shoulder, while adjusting the machine with his other hand. The dental surgery assistant, while not appearing to be doing much, is actually keeping a close watch on Mark's respiration, and checking that the reservoir bag is moving in concert with Mark's diaphragmatic movement.

When the dental surgeon gives the instruction, the dental surgery assistant increases the concentration of ten per cent nitrous oxide by rotating the mixture control dial.

The dental surgeon checks the time of induction with his stop watch; Mark, meanwhile, looks very relaxed. The nitrous oxide is set at 35 per cent and four minutes 30 seconds have passed.

Now, the dental surgeon is able to make a thorough examination of Mark's teeth (**184**). This was not possible before because Mark gagged when any instruments were placed in his mouth. The dental surgery assistant passes the local analgesic syringe to the dental surgeon out of Mark's line of vision, using a Sharpsafe technique. The dental surgeon is all the while talking to Mark to reassure him, and Mark for his part continues to look very relaxed: his arms are at his side and his hands are resting gently on his stomach.

The dental surgeon retracts Mark's lip, squeezing it gently to give counter-stimulation. The local analgesic used is an infiltration of the upper right second deciduous molar. The dental surgery assistant, meanwhile, has grasped Mark's hands to reassure him and to prevent him from using them to pull the dental surgeon's hand or the syringe away.

While the local analgesic is taking effect, the dental surgery assistant gently places the aspirator in Mark's mouth so that he can become acclimatized to the 'feel' and the noise of aspiration. Advising Mark that he will feel a shaking sensation, the dental surgeon starts to drill the upper right second deciduous molar. As Mark stretches his mouth wide open there is a tendency for the mask to move slightly, thus causing a leak; however, with Mark now sedated, it is permissible for the dental surgeon to place the thumb of his left hand over the top of the mask to keep it in position and so prevent this happening (**185**).

In due course, Mark lifts his left arm in the air to indicate that he wishes the dental surgeon to stop what he is doing (**186**); Mark clearly feels

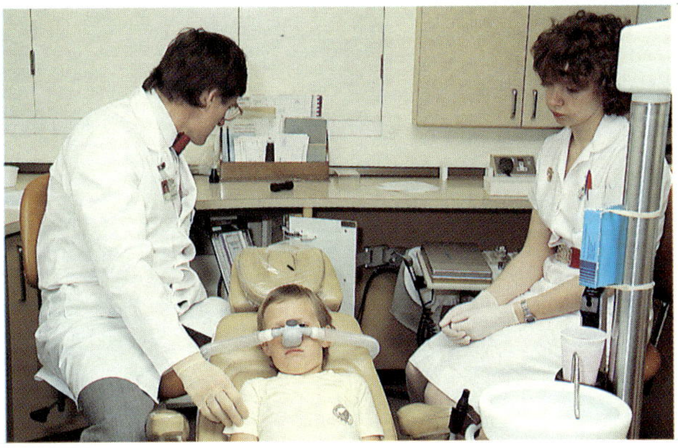

183 The dental surgeon adjusts the machine with his left hand whilst reassuring his patient with his right. The dental surgery assistant watches the patient's respiration and checks that the reservoir bag is moving in concert with his diaphragmatic movements

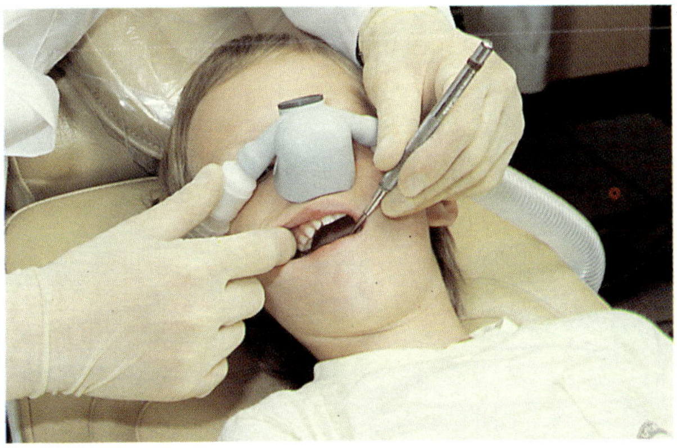

184 With his patient totally relaxed, the dental surgeon makes a thorough and careful examination of his teeth

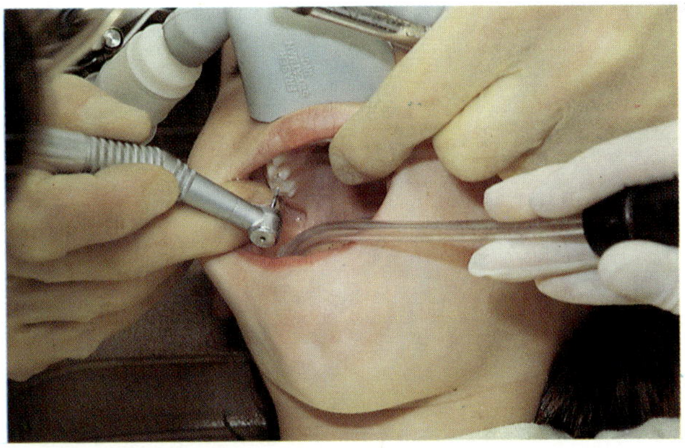

185 While the dental surgery assistant holds the aspirator in position in the patient's mouth, the dental surgeon – holding the nasal hood in place with the thumb of his left hand – proceeds to drill the upper right second deciduous molar

the treatment has gone on too long, or else he is uncomfortable. The dental surgery assistant makes no attempt to restrain Mark, who is merely invoking a pre-arranged stop signal. If the dental surgeon is too engrossed in the operative work to notice the signal, the dental surgery assistant will tell him. Even though Mark is asking the dental surgeon to call a halt, he is not being uncooperative – he has neither closed his mouth nor pulled his head away. After a pause to reassure Mark, the dental surgeon continues drilling the tooth, his patient once more relaxed.

During a preliminary attempt at placing a matrix band, Mark complained of pain 'on the inside', making it apparent that the buccal infiltration is insufficient. A transpapillary injection is therefore given to ensure that the palatal mucosa is made analgesic. The matrix band can now be placed on the tooth and the cavity dried with the air syringe (**187**).

Amalgam is then plugged in place in the cavity with a ball-ended plunger (**188**). Mark is still very relaxed and holding his mouth open sufficiently to enable treatment to progress easily. The dental surgeon checks the fillings to see that they are properly contoured and that the margins are smooth.

Next, the dental surgeon (or dental surgery assistant if instructed) turns the mixture control dial to 100 per cent oxygen to start the period of recovery. He checks his watch to ensure that 100 per cent oxygen is given for two minutes.

While Mark recovers, the dental surgeon writes up the notes. A sideways glance is sufficient to keep an eye on the patient. When he is completely recovered, Mark is helped out of the dental chair by the dental surgeon. Special care is needed at this point because if the patient is not adequately recovered he may stumble and fall.

After another minute, Mark's recovery is evaluated by a modified Romberg's test, to check that he has regained 'street fitness': he is asked to put his feet together and stand up straight with his arms at his side and his eyes closed. Any excessive swaying would mean that he had not adequately recovered.

His recovery complete, Mark is allowed to

186

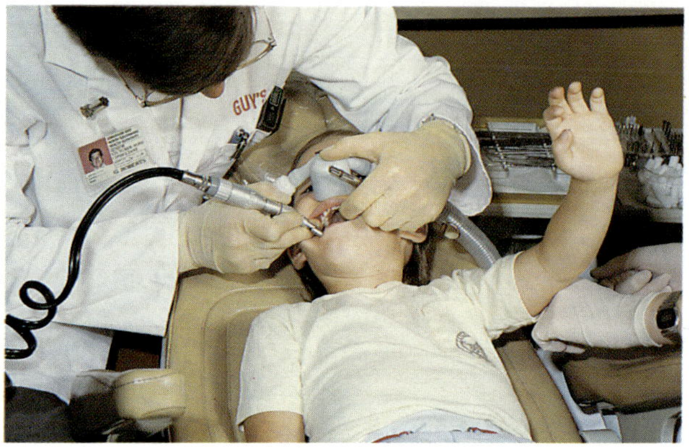

186 Using a pre-arranged signal the patient indicates that he wishes the treatment to cease. If the dental surgeon is too preoccupied to notice the signal, the dental surgery assistant will alert him

187

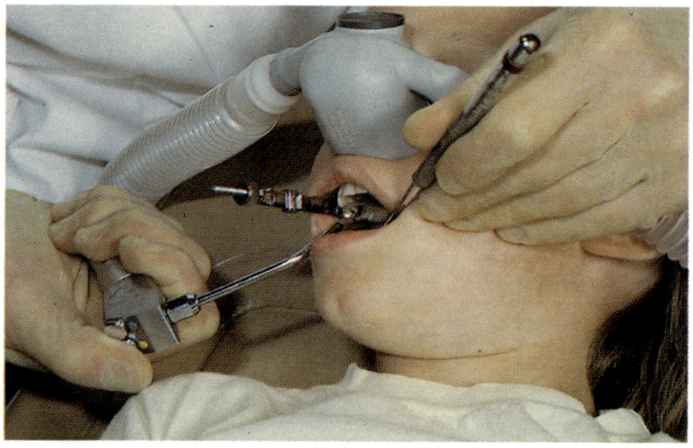

187 Once the palatal mucosa has been made analgesic, the matrix band can be placed on the tooth and the cavity dried with the air syringe

188

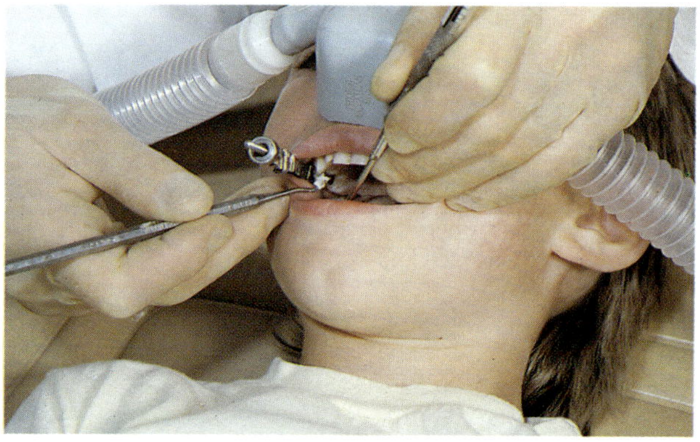

188 A ball-ended plunger is used to plug the amalgam in place in the cavity

choose his favourite badge sticker as reward for having been a good boy; the dental surgeon helps him do this. Finally, with only a few words of persuasion, Mark turns around in his father's arms to say goodbye.

It is important to clean the nasal hood thoroughly and carefully, inside and out, with surgical spirit. It is then set aside for sterilization with a liquid agent.

Technical note: Sedation was achieved using a Quantiflex MDM flow control unit linked to piped oxygen and nitrous oxide. Scavenging was with 2.5cm-wide entrance and exit tubes connected to a 2cm-of-water negative pressure unit in the floor of the surgery. Waste gases were directed via the air-conditioning exhaust outside the building.

The future

It is the belief of both authors that oxygen: nitrous oxide inhalation sedation (relative analgesia) will continue to increase in use wherever modern and sympathetic dental care is practised.

The basic design of the Quantiflex MDM has provided a subtle yet significant shift forward in the technique of administration. The ability to change the flow of gases with a single control without changing the relative proportions represents a distinct advantage in ease of control. Similarly, the single dial to change the proportion of gases without changing the flow is another plus.

The next step seems likely to be the acceptance and widespread use of an electronic MDM. Light and simple to use, this provides audible and visual signals. However, it is too early to say whether it will replace the inertia Quantiflex MDM.

PART 2

INTRAVENOUS SEDATION

Introduction

Intravenous sedation should never be used to mask inadequate local analgesia. Patients who can be reassured and treated normally should be treated not with intravenous sedation but rather by 'verbal' sedation. The dental surgeon's chairside manner and personality can make a considerable difference to the state of anxiety exhibited by a nervous patient. Approaching the patient gently, and explaining the normal dental procedures indicated – and how they can be painlessly carried out under local analgesia – may alone be sufficient to allay the patient's fears. As a result, many patients requesting intravenous sedation can be won over by the dental surgeon and unnecessary intravenous sedation procedures can be avoided.

It is not uncommon for the frightened person to put off a dental appointment until driven to the dental surgery or hospital casualty department by a distorted, swollen face and intense pain. Many of these patients fear that the pain evoked by the dental surgeon will be as bad as – if not worse than – their present distress. But of course, a fair proportion of these apprehensive patients have fears at a more controlled level. As numerous dental surgeons will agree, most patients have no fear of attending regularly at the surgery, which is surely a mark of success for the skill and manner of the dental surgeon and his staff. It is essential that each member of staff at the surgery is well trained and of a friendly and understanding disposition.

As would be expected, a high proportion of children and young adults fall into the acutely anxious and difficult category; but many older people, too, have a deep-rooted fear of going to the dentist. At one time, the only way to complete treatment on severely apprehensive patients, or mentally and/or physically handicapped persons, who can be difficult to control, was by using general anaesthesia, with its attendant dangers. This was most unsuitable, especially for relatively minor dental procedures – although general anaesthesia *is* still indicated for more difficult, totally uncooperative, and prolonged cases.

There is clearly a need for a technique which will relieve anxiety and provide a degree of sedation, so that the patient is conscious but oblivious to what is going on around him. In this state, dental treatment can be carried out under a local analgesic without disturbance. Upon realizing that the dental procedures are not nearly so frightening as he imagined, the patient may then change his attitude towards dentistry and the need for sedation may be reduced or eliminated.

6 THE ORGANIZATION OF INTRAVENOUS SEDATION SESSIONS

Simple sedation is defined in the Report of the Working Party on Training in Dental Anaesthesia (Wylie Report) as follows:

'A simple technique in which the use of a drug or drugs produces a state of depression of the central nervous system enabling treatment to be carried out, but during which verbal contact with the patient is maintained throughout the period of sedation. The drugs and techniques used should carry a margin of safety wide enough to render unintended loss of consciousness unlikely.'

The organization of sedation sessions may be described in three phases: preparation, sedation procedure, and recovery. By giving some thought to a particular procedure and by laying down a set of rules which the dental team must learn and adhere to strictly, a safer and more efficient procedure may be evolved, with minimum stress – not only for the patient, but also for the dental team. The basic structure of these rules remains the same whether in hospital or in a general practice situation. Provided the rules are observed, the likelihood of a medical emergency will be considerably reduced.

Before a sedation appointment can be arranged, preliminary examination of the patient is essential. Written instructions (**189**) are given to the patient prior to the appointment, i.e. no food/drink for an agreed period of time, etc. The patient must arrange for somebody to accompany him to the appointment, and be warned not to drink or drive, or return to work, within a given period of time following sedation.

189

INSTRUCTIONS TO PATIENTS WHO UNDERGO INTRAVENOUS SEDATION

1. No food or drink should be taken for at least four hours before the dental sedation appointment unless told otherwise by your dentist.
2. All patients must be accompanied to the surgery/hospital by a responsible person age 18 or over. In the case of a patient under 16 years, the accompanying person should be a parent or guardian.
3. The accompanying person must be available to sit with the recovering patient if necessary and to escort the patient home.
4. No patient receiving intravenous sedation should drive a vehicle, operate machinery, ride pillion on a motor bike, consume alcohol or undertake any responsible matters for 24 hours following the procedure.
5. It is important to take your routine medicine at the usual times.
6. If you are taking any new medicine or tablets since your last visit, you must inform the dentist.
7. Inform the dentist if you wear contact lenses, hearing aids or have a colostomy bag.

189 Patients must be provided with written instructions *before* the day of their appointment, so that they attend properly prepared

The sedation appointment

It is important to have a pleasant waiting room and good toilet facilities. A friendly welcome by the receptionist and minimal waiting time are also conducive to a calm patient: sedation appointments should be arranged so that the patient is not kept waiting but is seen punctually. Ample time must be allocated for the appointment: dental procedures that are rushed, if not actually promoting a medical emergency, may nevertheless produce stress in the dental team and lead to a lower standard of work. This situation must be avoided at all costs.

When the patient arrives, the receptionist checks on the pre-sedation instructions, i.e. that no food or drink has been consumed for an agreed period of time (usually four hours), and that there is somebody present to accompany the patient when the appointment is over. A visit to the toilet may then be suggested.

When the dental surgeon is ready, the patient is brought into the surgery by the dental surgery assistant (DSA), who again checks that the patient is 'starved'/'toileted'/accompanied. The patient's weight in kilograms may also be recorded, as this information is helpful in the administration of an intravenous drug – the dental surgeon should be aware of the drug company's recommendations recorded on the data sheet. The patient is then settled into the dental chair by the dental surgery assistant.

The dental surgeon carefully identifies the patient with the aid of the case notes and checks that the medical history (**190**) has not changed since the original, pre-sedation visit.

In the case of female patients, handbags or purses should always be placed in front of the patient in her full view. Jackets or other personal belongings of male patients should be treated in the same way. A few words to reassure patients that their belongings will follow them to the recovery area is always comforting. Dentures, contact lenses and glasses may be removed at this stage and put to one side for safe keeping by the dental surgery assistant.

After the dental surgeon has carefully explained the intravenous sedation procedure to him, the patient is asked to sign a consent form (**191**). As well as providing for the patient's consent to the administration of the intravenous sedation, this should also detail the treatment to be carried out.

Once the patient is in the dental chair, the procedure can begin. It is important that only trained and, where possible, experienced dental surgery assistants should be present. Neither general anaesthesia nor sedation should be employed unless proper equipment for its administration and adequate facilities for the resuscitation of the patient are readily available, with both the dental surgeon and his staff trained in their use.

190

BRITISH DENTAL ASSOCIATION

Confidential Medical History

Date ....

Surname .... **First Names** .... **Occupation** ....

Address .... **Sex** .... **Age** ....

Your doctor's name and address ....

Your dentist will be helped in giving you the best possible treatment, if you would kindly answer the following questions. Please state Yes or No.

Are you attending or receiving treatment from a doctor? ....

Are you taking or using any medicines, pills, tablets, ointments, injections or any other drugs, either from a doctor or on your own accord? ....

Are you allergic to or have you ever had any unfavourable reaction to any medicines and in particular, antibiotics, or to food or other substances? ....

Have you had any serious childhood illness? ....

Have you ever been in hospital as a patient or ill at home in bed for a substantial period of time? ....

Do you have or have you had any heart or blood pressure trouble? ....

Have you had rheumatic fever, or chorea (St Vitus' dance)? ....

Have you ever been told that you have a heart murmur? ....

Do you have a heart pacemaker? .... *or have you had any heart surgery?* ....

Do you have chest troubles? ....

Do you suffer from hay fever, eczema, asthma or any other form of allergy? ....

Do you have fainting attacks, giddiness or blackouts? ....

Have you had jaundice, liver or kidney disease or diabetes? ....

Do you bruise easily? ....

Following an extraction, surgery or injury have you or any member of your family bled for such a time as to cause you to be worried? ....

Have you had a general anaesthetic (including dental gas or injection in the arm)? ....

Have you ever had an adverse reaction to a general anaesthetic? .... *or local anaesthetic?* ....

Do you carry a warning card from your doctor or specialist? ....

Are you pregnant? ....

Is there any other aspect concerning your health you think that the dentist should know about such as joint replacements? ....

Has your health changed or have your medicines, injections or tablets been altered? .... Date ....

Date .... Date .... Date .... Date ....

190 The recording of a comprehensive medical history of each patient is extremely important, as it can reveal vital facts affecting suitability for sedation

191

CONSENT TO DENTAL OPERATIVE TREATMENT UNDER INTRAVENOUS SEDATION

Patient's name ....

Address ....

....

....

Telephone no ....

I hereby consent to the treatment stated below. I also consent to such further or alternative measures as may be found necessary during the course of the procedures mentioned below; also to the administration of local anaesthetic procedures for any of these purposes.

Date ....

Treatment ....

....

Extraction of .... teeth.

Conservation of ....

I confirm that the above treatment which I am to undergo, other treatment .... under intravenous sedation, has been explained to me by

Mr/Mrs/Miss/Dr/Ms ....

and that I agree to this treatment. I confirm that I have also received and read my preoperative sedation instructions.

Signed .... patient/parent/guardian

I confirm that I have explained the treatment outlined above.

Signed .... dental practitioner

191 It is important that the consent form should also outline the planned treatment

The intravenous sedation procedure

The syringe is prepared before the patient enters the surgery, the contents of the ampoule or vial having first been checked. All opened vials, empty or full, are retained, as are the needles and syringes, etc. These items must all be kept on a single tray to enable the dental surgeon to check what has actually been used at any stage of the procedure. Drug dosages must always be recorded. It is also helpful to record the batch number of the intravenous drug used, and its date of expiry.

The time the sedation is started is recorded, as is the time it is completed and the patient is escorted to recovery. Finally, the time when the patient is discharged and met by the accompanying person is noted. Any problems occurring during the sedation must also be recorded.

In the event of an incident, the above information can be of prime importance.

Sites of intravenous injection

There are two main sites of injection available to the dental surgeon (see Chapter 8, on Clinical Anatomy, for a detailed comparison):

- The cubital fossa
- The dorsum of the hand.

Choice of drugs

The choice of drugs for intravenous dental sedation is a matter for the dental surgeon to decide on. It is of paramount importance, therefore, that he has up-to-date knowledge of the drugs employed in sedation techniques. Chapter 9 (Pharmacology of Benzodiazepines) includes a detailed consideration of drugs currently in use for intravenous sedation.

7 THE SELECTION OF SUITABLE PATIENTS

Patient assessment

A request from a patient is not in itself an indication for sedation. Unless the patient is in considerable pain, the dental surgeon would be advised to use the initial appointment to decide on the suitability or otherwise of intravenous sedation for the dental procedures under consideration. This will allow the dental surgeon to make alternative arrangements for the patient, should he decide against the use of intravenous sedation; it also means that the patient receives ample notice of whatever the dental surgeon decides – rather than being informed just prior to the operative appointment.

The primary consultation

A careful medical history is obtained from the patient at this appointment. This should give an accurate impression of the patient's fitness for dental treatment and whether or not intravenous sedation is indicated. The medical history-taking commences as soon as the patient enters the surgery. As well as the standard questions and answers indicated by the official form, the perceptive dental surgeon will also notice anything about the patient that might be suggestive of a particular condition; it might be something about the patient's complexion or the way he moves – anything at all. The size of the patient is noted. In the process of taking a medical history, a psychological profile can be built up. The dental surgeon should determine the degree of anxiety and self-control that the patient has. If a patient is very frightened and in an extreme state of agitation, treatment by intravenous sedation may not be advisable.

Patients *not* suitable for intravenous sedation in an out-patient situation include those who:

- Are sensitive to benzodiazepines
- Have an acute pulmonary deficiency
- Have a hepatic dysfunction or insufficiency (**192**)
- Have a renal insufficiency
- Take steroids
- Suffer from a psychiatric disorder even without the medication of psychotropic drugs
- Have hormonal problems which may not be stabilized
- Are pregnant
- Suffer from myasthenia gravis or a similar metabolic disorder
- Have a pathological brain condition (including epilepsy)

Or in whom:

- The venous return is inhibited, i.e. following a total mastectomy or limb injury

Or who belong to one of the following groups:

- The elderly
- The very young
- Alcoholics
- Drug addicts
- Breast-feeding mothers (unless an agreed procedure has been arranged with the patient's obstetrician).

If there is any doubt regarding the medical history or fitness of a patient, the patient's GP must be consulted. Once the patient has been accepted for intravenous sedation, the responsibility will be the dental surgeon's alone should any problem or complication arise due to an unknown or undisclosed aspect of the patient's medical history. This should be borne in mind every time a medical history is taken.

Rather than answering a dental surgeon's sometimes intimate questions out loud, in front of a dental surgery assistant or nurse, some patients – especially those with an infectious problem such as hepatitis B or Aids – will be more forthcoming if left to fill in a medical history form by themselves. However, the dental surgeon must still corroborate this history – it cannot be accepted on its face value alone.

The dental surgeon will ultimately be responsible for the well-being of the patient in his care, so he should always err on the side of safety and refuse to sedate a patient if there is a reasonable possibility of a problem arising.

It should also be noted that highly obese patients, or those who have airway problems due to their skeletal structure, should not be sedated.

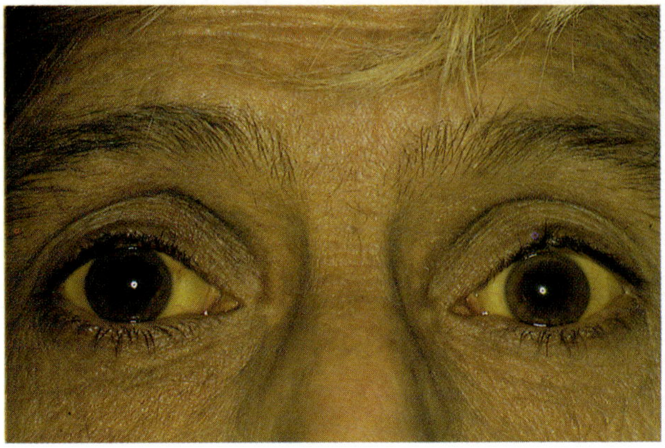

192

192 Patients suffering from hepatic insufficiency are not suitable for intravenous sedation

Unless the dental surgeon feels he can maintain an airway on the patient he is examining, intravenous sedation should be avoided.

Benzodiazepines: dependence and withdrawal symptoms

Dental surgeons who use intravenous sedation techniques with a benzodiazepine as the drug of sedation should note that some patients may be addicted to this group of drugs (BMJ, 1980). Withdrawal symptoms that may be apparent can include anxiety, tremor, confusion, insomnia, perceptual disorders, fits, depression, gastro-intestinal and other somatic symptoms. Whilst it is true that several of these conditions can have other, unrelated, causes, if any of these is suspected – if there is any doubt whatsoever as to the medical fitness of a patient for an intravenous sedation – then the procedure should be postponed at least until the patient has been examined by his own GP.

Dental history

A detailed dental history of the patient should be recorded. In cases where intravenous sedation is to be used for oral surgery, the dental surgeon should examine the patient to see whether there is any swelling present in the floor of the mouth or in the oropharynx, which might interfere with the patient's airway. Any impairment of the airway in a dental patient is an indication for specialist care in hospital.

8 CLINICAL ANATOMY

A knowledge of the anatomy of the cubital fossa and the dorsum of the hand is essential for any dental surgeon carrying out intravenous sedation. With a sound understanding of the anatomical structures relating to the veins to be used in venepuncture, damage to surrounding structures can be minimized. Each site has its own advantages and disadvantages; the decision of which to use must rest with the dental surgeon and may be related to his skill and experience.

CUBITAL FOSSA

Advantages
1. Usually larger veins.
2. If bruising occurs it is easier to be disguised by clothing.

Disadvantages
1. Danger of damage due to moving limb during venepuncture. The arm *must* be supported.
2. Danger of brachial artery injection if aberrant ulnar artery present or medial aspect of arm is used.

DORSUM OF THE HAND

Advantage
1. Easier access.

Disadvantage
1. Any bruising will look unsightly and is difficult to disguise.

Cubital fossa

This is triangular in shape and presents as a slight hollow in front of the elbow joint. It is bounded laterally by the brachioradialis and the extensor muscles of the wrist, and medially by the pronator teres and the flexor muscles of the fingers; the apex is where the two muscle groups meet distally.

Within this area the brachial artery divides into its two terminal branches: the ulnar and radial arteries. The structures covering the cubital fossa are the skin, the superficial fascia and the deep fascia.

Within the superficial fascia are the cutaneous nerves of the forearm, as well as the median basilic vein and also the (lateral) cephalic vein. In about three per cent of limbs the ulnar artery descends superficially to the flexor muscles, a point to remember when considering venepuncture.

The basilic vein runs down the medial aspect of the cubital fossa and may be more clearly defined and more accessible than a less

93

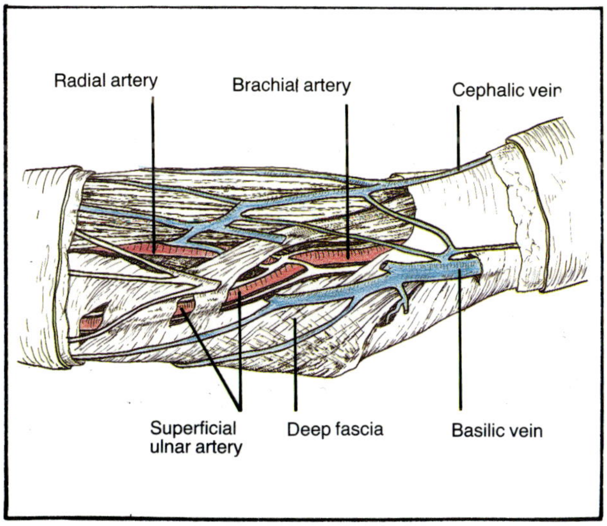

193 Deep anatomical dissection of the cubital fossa showing the relationship of the arteries to the overlying veins

194

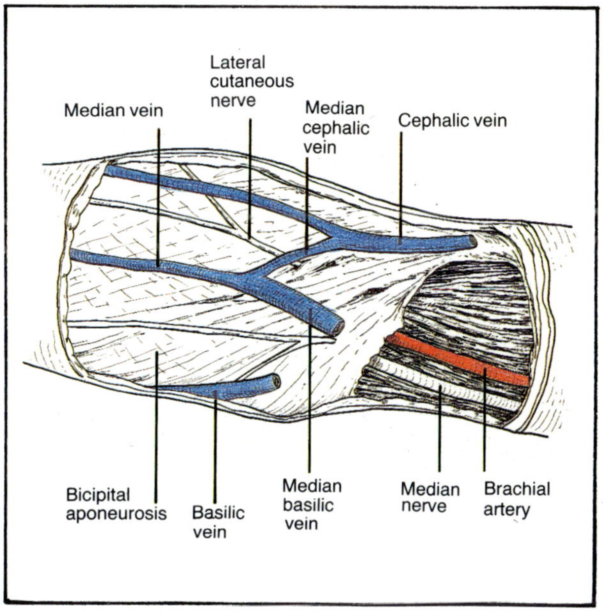

194 Superficial anatomical dissection of the cubital fossa showing the veins. Note the relationship of the basilic veins to the underlying brachial artery

195

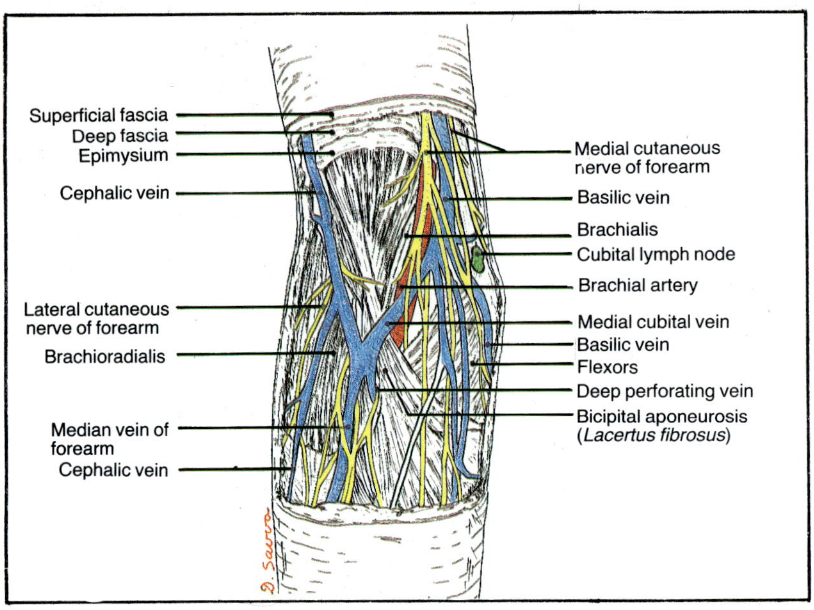

195 A clear anatomical view of the relationship of arteries, veins, nerves and muscles in the cubital fossa

196

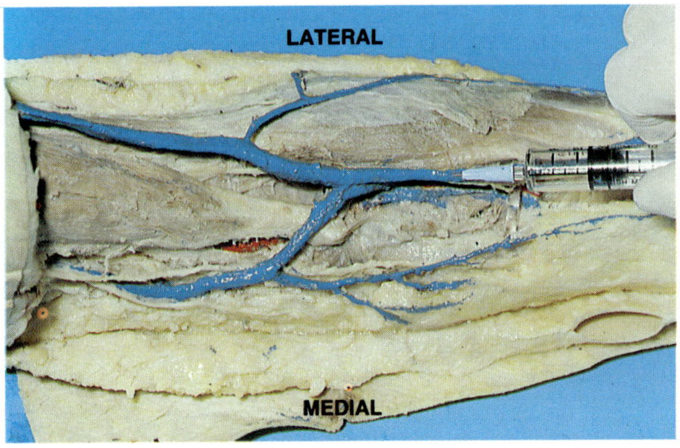

196 Note the straight syringe in the cephalic vein. The bicipital aponeurosis has largely been removed. The brachial artery is seen in red just below the tendon of the biceps and well clear of the injection site

prominent cephalic vein, running down the lateral side of the cubital fossa. Nevertheless, venepuncture into the medial area of the cubital fossa – into the basilic vein or medial cubital vein – is best avoided whenever possible, as there is a danger that the needle may pass through the vein and into the bicipital aponeurosis – causing the patient's arm to flex instantly, thereby increasing the possibility of perforating the brachial artery.

The brachial artery is often quite superficially situated in the medial aspect of the cubital fossa and is closely related to both the medial cubital vein – from which it is separated only by the bicipital aponeurosis – and the basilic vein, which run superficial to the artery. It is easily located by palpating the medial aspect of the cubital fossa. (In fact, it is always advisable to palpate the area chosen for venepuncture even when the vein to be used is not normally found near an artery, for this may locate the arterial pulse of an aberrant artery.)

Invariably, venepuncture is safer when carried out in the lateral cubital fossa, where the cephalic vein and its medial cephalic tributary are located. An aberrant artery is extremely rare in this situation. Furthermore, the branches of the lateral cutaneous nerve of the forearm are fewer and therefore less likely to be pierced by the needle than is the case in the medial part of the cubital fossa, where branches of the medial cutaneous nerve of the forearm abound.

197 A straight needle has been pushed through the medial cubital vein and has entered the fibrous bicipital aponeurosis. (In life, the arm would be bent upwards, and the sudden movement might cause the needle to enter the brachial artery. Anatomy varies from person to person, but in general the insertion of a needle into the middle of the medial aspect of the cubital fossa – that is, into the medial cubital vein or the brachial vein – increases the risk of intra-arterial penetration.)

197

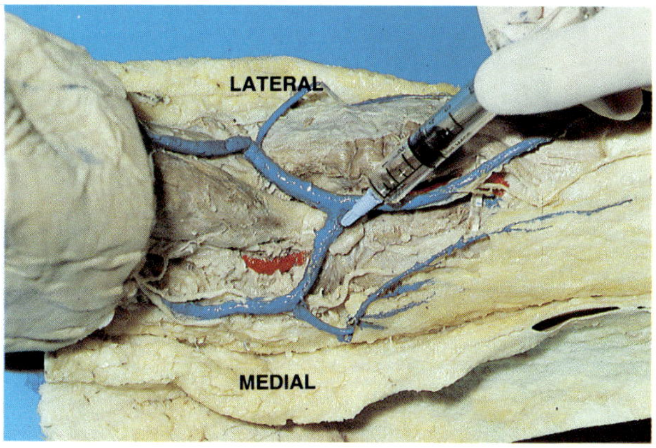

Dorsum of the hand

The dorsal venous network drains proximally into the cephalic and basilic veins and is situated below the surface of the skin.

Arteries present no hazard here. There is a dorsal carpal arterial arch, but it is far removed from the elective region of venepuncture dorsal to the knuckles and metacarpals.

198

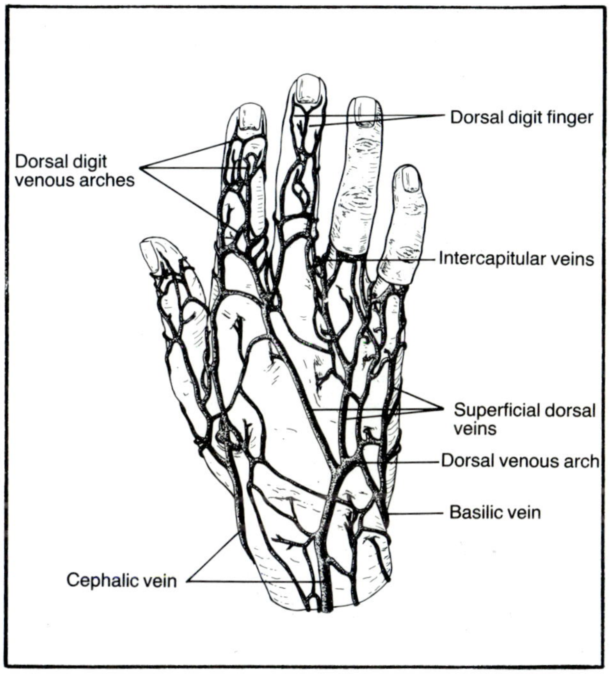

199

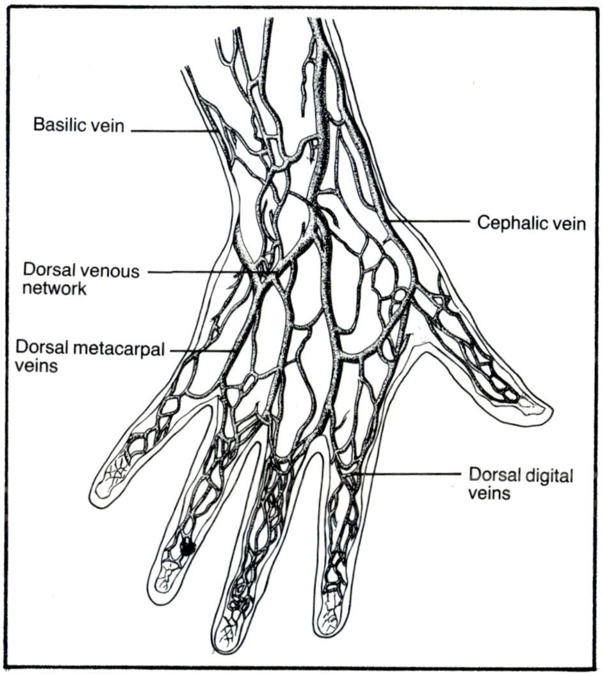

198 and 199 Knowledge of the anatomy of the dorsum of the hand is essential to the dental surgeon, who should also be aware of the variations in the layout of the veins that can occur among individual patients (as illustrated in the two examples here)

200 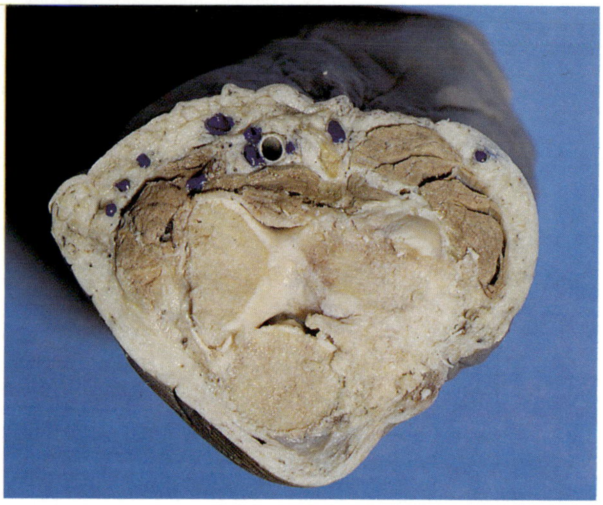

200 Cross-section of the arm at the cubital fossa, showing the relationship of the bicipital aponeurosis and the brachial artery

201 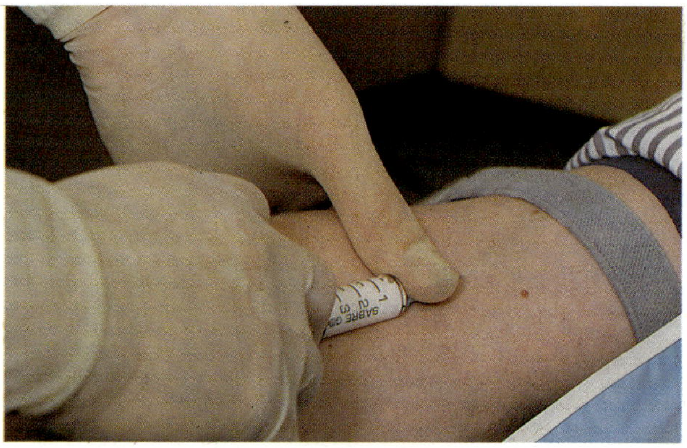

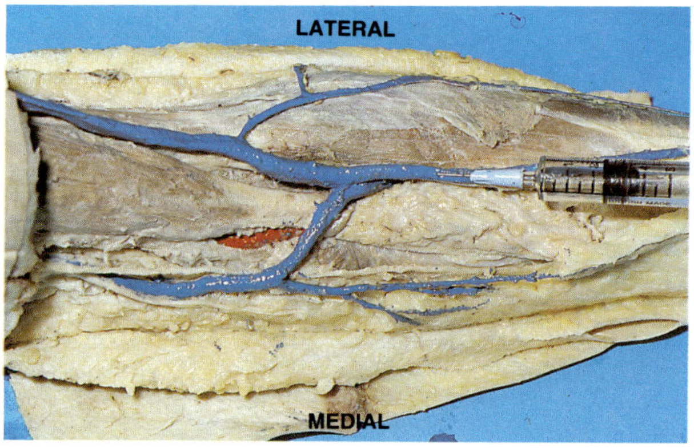 202

201 and 202 The correct site for venepuncture is the lateral aspect of the cubital fossa using a well-defined cephalic vein. Note that the tourniquet would be loosened before the administration of the drug

203 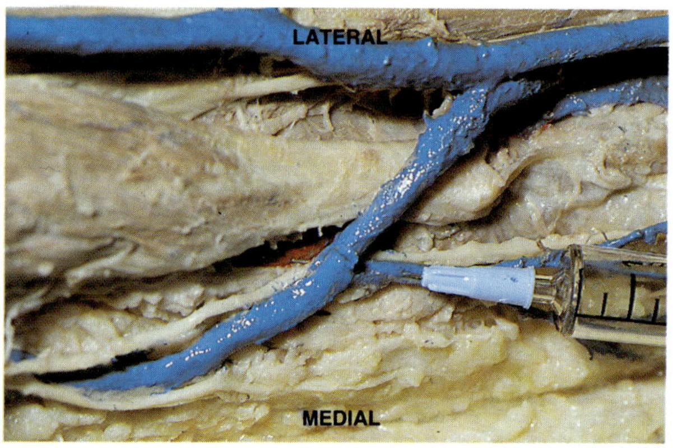

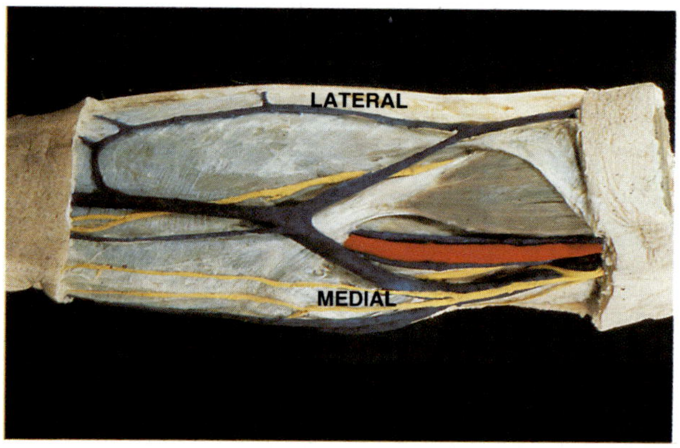 204

203 An accidental intra-arterial injection, the needle having penetrated the brachial vein and entered the underlying brachial artery. The central and medial aspects of the cubital fossa should be avoided when choosing a site for venepuncture

204 In this dissection the fatty tissue has been removed to reveal the relationship of the veins, artery, bicipital aponeurosis and nerves

205

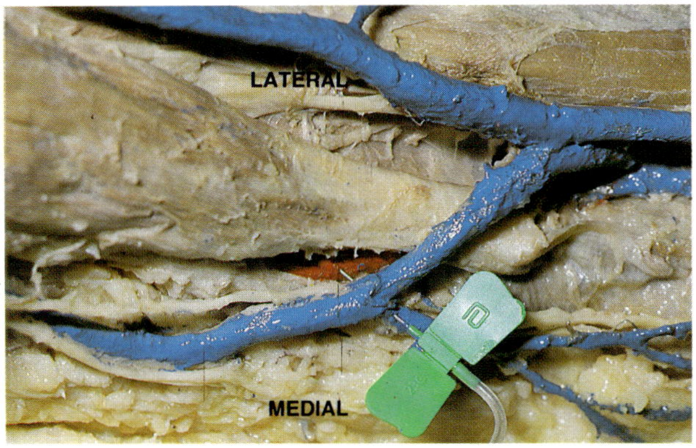

206

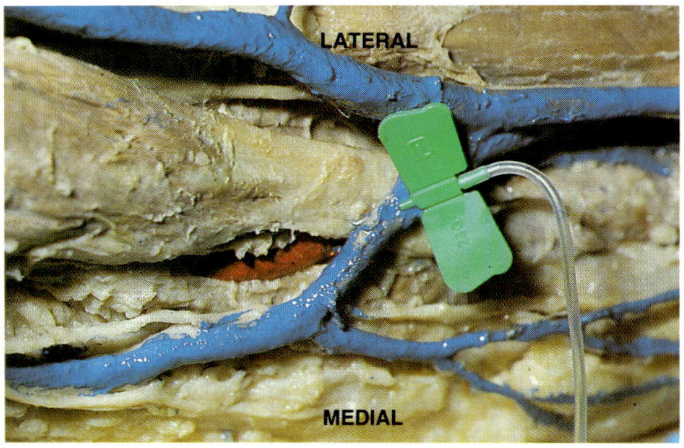

205 and 206 The intra-arterial penetration of badly placed butterfly needles in the medial aspect of the cubital fossa. (The latter is a good site for the insertion of a butterfly or a straight needle, **provided the arm is supported** by a dental surgery assistant or an armboard, and a suitable cephalic vein is used.)

207

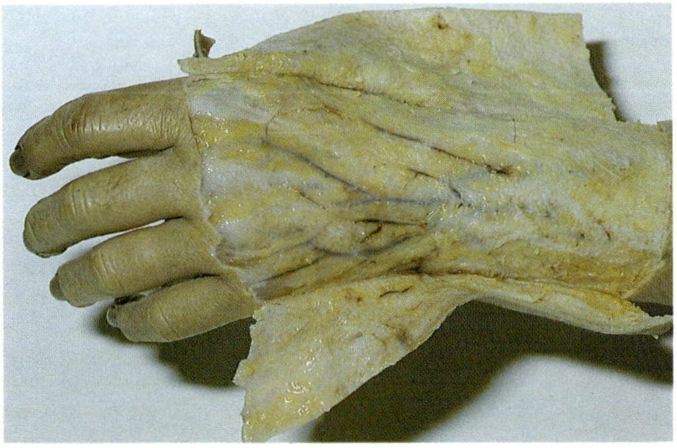

207 Dissection of the dorsum of the hand, showing the sparse fatty tissue which protects the underlying veins and tendons. The superficial dorsal carpal arch is not seen

208

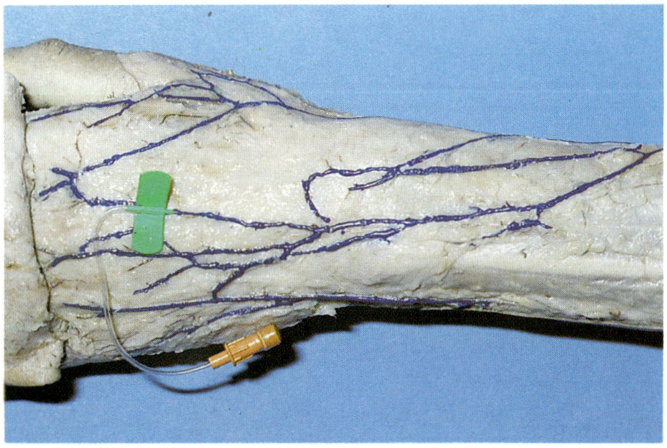

208 The abundance of superficial veins makes the dorsum of the hand suitable as a site for inserting and maintaining a butterfly needle

209

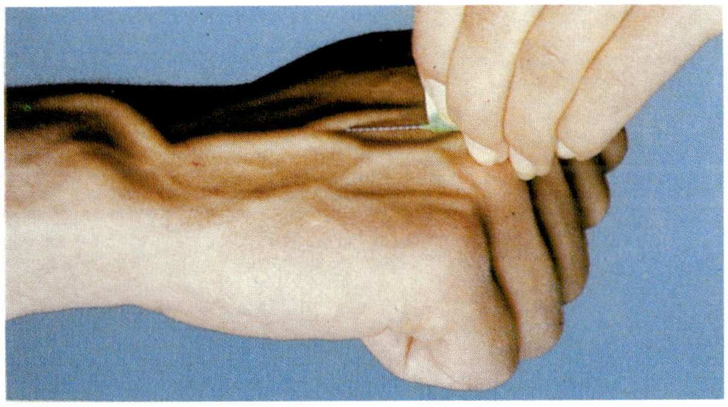

209 Demonstrating the position of the butterfly needle in relation to the veins. Note that the needle is to be inserted where two smaller veins join to form a larger vein

210

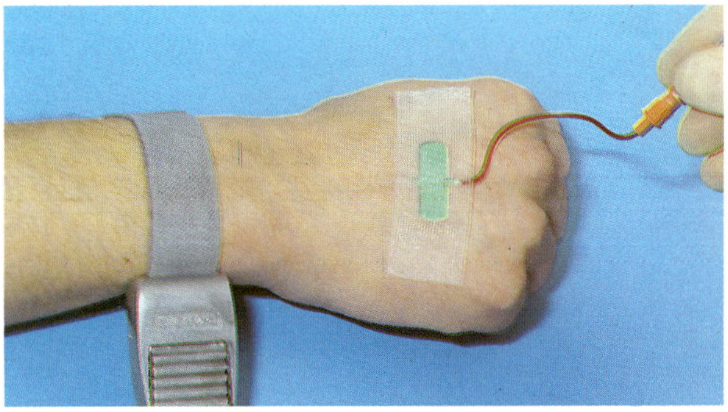

210 Butterfly needle *in situ* on the dorsum of the hand

Summary

The dental surgeon should possess a thorough knowledge both of the anatomy of the region in which venepuncture is to be carried out and of the pharmacology of the drugs that are to be injected. Without this knowledge, complications may arise which could have serious consequences for patient and dental surgeon alike. Local complications that could occur are:

- Mild or massive haematoma
- Sepsis in a haematoma site
- Prolonged and painful fibrosis in the cubital fossa
- Restriction of elbow movement
- Arterial spasm
- Limb ischaemia
- Peripheral gangrene
- Loss of digits
- Painful neuromata.

9 PHARMACOLOGY OF BENZODIAZEPINES

Pharmacokinetics is the study of the rates of absorption, distribution, metabolism and elimination of drugs (ADME). Put simply, it is what the body does to drugs in the course of time, and is but one factor contributing to the understanding of drug action. Of even greater importance are the pharmacodynamics of drug action – what the drug does to the body.

Measuring blood levels of most drugs is now possible, but measuring their concentrations at receptor sites, if these have actually been identified, remains very difficult. The exact modes of action of many compounds, including benzodiazepines, are not yet fully known.

There is no clear correlation between benzodiazepine plasma levels and their clinical effects. It therefore follows that pharmacokinetic parameters calculated from plasma levels are of limited clinical relevance. Half-life is one such parameter.

211

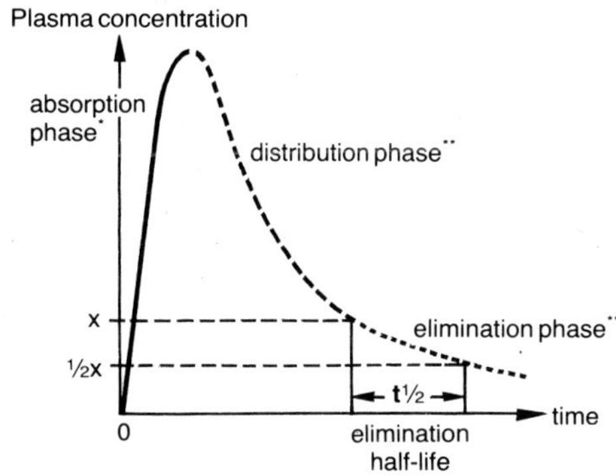

* absorption – blood levels rise as the drug is absorbed into the bloodstream from the site of administration, e.g. GI tract, muscle. The rate is important, as it will play a major role in determining onset of effect.

** distribution – blood levels fall, quite steeply, as the drug is distributed into the body fluid and tissue compartments, e.g. extracellular fluid, organ tissue, fat, etc.

*** elimination – when equilibrium in concentrations has been established between the various body tissues, elimination occurs via the particular routes of metabolism and excretion for that drug. (Some elimination will also be taking place during the distribution phase.)

211 The pharmacokinetics of drugs used in intravenous sedation

Half-life

This is the time taken for the plasma concentration to fall by 50 per cent. (It is *not* the time the drug takes to disappear from the body, nor is it the same as the duration of the effect of the drug!) (*See* **211**.) The terms 'short half-life' and 'long half-life' have become confused with the terms 'short-acting' and 'long-acting' when discussing different benzodiazepines. Such substitution of terms is not only misleading, but also incorrect. For instance, lorazepam is a benzodiazepine with a shorter half-life than diazepam (about half as long), and it has no active metabolites. However, both the onset and the cessation of a relatively easy effect to measure – amnesia after intravenous administration – are considerably longer for the so-called shorter-acting compound (George, Dundee, 1977).

Accumulation

Virtually all drugs accumulate on multiple dosing (Meffin, Wing, 1980). To avoid this, a drug would have to be eliminated before the next dose was taken, and thus – since it takes at least five times the half-life value to do this – only once-a-day compounds with half-lives of less than five hours would qualify.

Most drugs accumulate on repeat dosing to a steady-state level. The blood level reaches a plateau and a 'dynamic' equilibrium is achieved whereby the rate at which the drug enters the blood is the same as that at which it leaves.

Pharmacokinetic anomalies – clinical examples

In overdose cases, where massive amounts of a drug have been consumed, i.e. 400 times the usual dose of diazepam, plasma levels are extremely high, and – because of the long elimination half-life of the drug – will remain so for some days, to the extent that they would cause profound sedation in a previously unexposed individual (Greenblatt *et al.*, 1978). Nevertheless, *clinical* recovery – such that the patient is fully alert and fit to leave hospital – is complete within a few days.

After a single oral dose of, for example, diazepam, subjective and objective effects will be evident, particularly on the upswing of the plasma concentration/time curve (**212**). Yet on later observation, when the curve is on its downswing, the effects will have largely worn off, even though the plasma levels at the time of observation are the same. **It is important to note that the maximum effects of the drug do not always coincide with the peak plasma concentrations.**

Again taking oral diazepam as an example, patients may experience some degree of drowsiness over the first day or two at the start of therapy. This usually abates with continued use, by which time blood levels of both diazepam and its metabolites greatly exceed those measured during the early stages of therapy, when drowsiness was clearly apparent (Greenblatt, Shader, 1978).

These examples highlight two factors of fundamental importance in understanding benzodiazepine pharmacokinetics:

- The effect of any given dose may be related more to the rate of increase of the benzodiazepine in the plasma and/or the generations of its metabolites than to any specific levels.
- A given blood level may have one clinical effect at one time but a different effect at a later time after a period of drug exposure has elapsed.

212

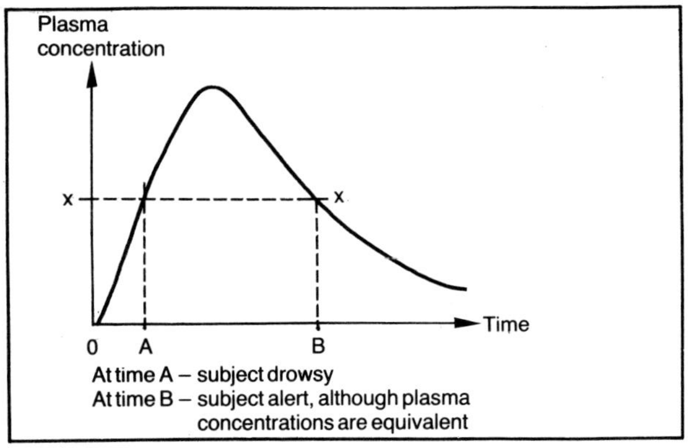

212 Plasma concentration/time curve

Drugs used for intravenous sedation

The drugs most commonly used for intravenous sedation techniques in dentistry are diazepam, midazolam and flumazenil.

Diazepam is available in 10mg in 2ml ampoules. The more recently conceived emulsified preparation (see below) is preferred for intravenous sedation, aqueous diazepam having an irritant effect on veins. Midazolam is available in 10mg in 5ml ampoules, which makes it suitable for intravenous sedation for dental procedures, this concentration giving the dental surgeon reasonable control for drug titration on the patient to be sedated. It is also available in 10mg in 2ml ampoules, but this is too strong a concentration for normal use in dentistry.

Flumazenil is the first benzodiazepine antagonist and is available in 5ml ampoules containing 500mg: that is, 0.5mg in a dilution of 0.1mg per ml. It is essential that the antagonist is always available within arm's reach of the dental surgeon who is using a benzodiazepine for intravenous sedation.

The ampoule of any drug to be used for sedation should not be opened until the patient is on the surgery premises. Pre-loading and storage of the drug ampoule contents can lead to contamination, and septicaemia may result.

Pharmacodynamics

Diazepam, in common with all the other benzodiazepines, has four distinct pharmacological properties: it is sleep inducing (hypnotic) and anxiolytic (sedative), and is a muscle relaxant and anti-convulsant.

It was first synthesized by Roche in 1959. Its mode of action is primarily on the central nervous system and is mainly localized in the subcortical centres and reflexes. The half-life in plasma is 24–48 hours and it can therefore impair a patient's judgment for 48 hours. Because of its long half-life, there is some risk of an accumulative effect with repeated doses.

If a patient already receiving daily therapeutic doses of diazepam is additionally given a high intravenous dose of the same drug, respiratory depression could occur. **It is therefore essential that the dental surgeon, when taking the medical history during the initial consultation, records any drugs the patient is already being prescribed.**

The principal metabolite of diazepam is desmethyldiazepam, which has a half-life of about 100 hours. Oxazepam is rapidly conjugated and excreted. Drug interactions involving diazepines are probably extremely rare in relation to their extensive use. Nevertheless, diazepines can interact with other drugs that have depressant effects on the central nervous system, and will potentiate the effects of other hypnotics and sedatives on the brain. They will also enhance the central effects of alcohol. In addition, they are reputed to enhance anti-depressant drugs.

Uptake, metabolism and elimination of benzodiazepines

In common with other opiates, benzodiazepines have a high specific affinity to certain specific receptors. These receptors are mainly located in the central nervous system. It is believed that the greatest affinity for the benzodiazepines occurs in the cerebral cortex. Although these receptors are highly specific for benzodiazepine agonists or antagonists, they are not receptive to other sedative agents such as barbiturates.

After intravenous administration, diazepam shows a distribution in the body that is typical of markedly lipophilic substances. Central effects appear almost instantaneously but they also disappear relatively quickly in parallel with the metabolism of that substance in that particular organism. Diazepam is transported bound to plasma proteins and is also strongly bound to the tissues.

Following oral administration, diazepam is rapidly absorbed. After a single dose of 10–15mg, a plasma concentration of about 0.2–0.3μg/ml is obtained within two hours. At these plasma levels all patients show signs of drowsiness. Elimination of the drug is rapid at first, but then levels off and becomes increasingly slower. The half-life is 24–48 hours.

The intravenous administration of 10–20mg of diazepam produces a plasma concentration of 1μg/ml within four minutes and an immediate, noticeable sedative effect. The concentration of diazepam then falls to 0.25μg/ml within an hour and the clinical effect decreases at the same rate.

10 INTRAVENOUS SEDATION USING DIAZEPAM AND MIDAZOLAM

Selection of a suitable drug

Previous chapters have been concerned with determining the suitability or otherwise of a particular patient for intravenous sedation. The dental surgeon must now select a suitable drug for use in the sedation.

The ideal dental sedating agent should provide:

- Adequate sedative and anxiolytic properties
- Amnesia for the duration of the procedure
- Ease of administration
- Non-irritant effect on veins, blood and tissues
- Short recovery period
- No effect on cardiovascular or respiratory systems
- Low toxicity
- No side-effects
- Compatibility with other drugs.

Both diazepam in its emulsified form and midazolam fulfil most of the requirements as outlined above, and it is for this reason that they are widely used, both in general dental practice and in hospitals.

Diazepam

Intravenous diazepam has been employed for many years for sedation and premedication, and for the induction of general anaesthesia. The drug is insoluble in water and, initially, the only available injectable formulations contained undesirable solvents such as propylene glycol and ethanol in order to make the drug suitable for intravenous injection. In recent years, however, soya bean oil has been used as a solvent, which is then emulsified to give a preparation which is much safer.

Comparative pharmacokinetic and pharmacodynamic studies show that this new emulsion formulation has a higher margin of safety than an aqueous preparation of diazepam, while plasma concentration and elimination kinetics are very similar. Clinical studies indicate that the emulsified preparation is as effective as aqueous diazepam but has significantly fewer side-effects (pain and/or thrombophlebitis). (Rosenbaum, 1982.)

Dosage of emulsified diazepam

The dosage recommended for intravenous sedation is 0.1–0.2mg per kg of body weight.

The data sheet warns that clinical effects are frequently seen at lower doses in elderly or debilitated patients.

Midazolam

Midazolam is a potent imidiazobenzodiazepine, forming water-soluble salts which are stable and well-tolerated by injection. It possesses the typical pharmacological properties of the benzodiazepines: it is hypnotic, anxiolytic, and acts as a muscle relaxant and anti-convulsant.

In the case of sedative doses given intravenously, the action is rapid on onset and of short duration; anterograde amnesia often accompanies the period of peak sedation.

The ampoule contains midazolam hydrochloride, which is water-soluble. In plasma, midazolam exists as the free base and is lipid-soluble.

The mean elimination half-life of midazolam is about two hours. It is extensively metabolized, undergoing hydroxylation to three metabolites: αhydroxy midazolam, 4-hydroxy midazolam and α4-dihydroxy midazolam. The principal metabolite is αhydroxy midazolam, which has a shorter half-life than the parent drug – about 60–90 minutes on average. All three metabolites are excreted in the urine as glucuronides and none contributes to the activity of midazolam.

Dosage of intravenous midazolam

A dosage of 0.07mg/kg body weight is suggested, and the dose should be titrated against the response of the patient. At the desired sedative end-point, the patient will be drowsy and speech will be slurred, but response to command will be maintained.

As a guide, the manufacturers recommend that 3.75mg of midazolam be administered intravenously over 30 seconds. If after two minutes sedation is not adequate, incremental doses of 0.5–1mg of midazolam should be given. It is recommended that the initial dose should be reduced in patients of low body weight.

The recovery rate is superior to that associated with diazepam, while the incidence of venous sequelae is much lower than with aqueous diazepam and comparable with that reported for the emulsified preparation.

Mode of administration

For the administration of diazepam or midazolam, the patient should be placed in a supine position and remain there throughout the procedure.

A second appropriate person should be present at all times and facilities for resuscitation should always be available. It is recommended that patients remain under the supervision of a suitable member of the staff (or in the presence of the accompanying person, if recovering following the dental procedure) until at least one hour has elapsed from the time of the last injection. They should always be accompanied home by a responsible adult and be warned not to attempt to drive or operate machinery for up to 24 hours after injection.

Contraindications of midazolam and diazepam

- Known sensitivity to benzodiazepines
- Acute pulmonary insufficiency and hepatic dysfunction
- Respiratory depression
- Pregnancy
- Breast-feeding (unless a treatment plan has been agreed with the patient's obstetrician).

Precautions

When midazolam or diazepam is given along with centrally acting drugs such as potent analgesics, the sedative effect may be intensified and the possibility of severe respiratory or cardiovascular depression should be considered. Midazolam should be administered with caution to patients with myasthenia gravis as it may produce airway obstruction, apnoea, hypotension, and/or coma in severe cases.

11 BASIC SURGICAL REQUIREMENTS FOR INTRAVENOUS SEDATION

Equipment

The basic items of equipment for use in intravenous sedation must be in good working order and well-maintained, as their condition is of paramount importance to the safety of the patient.

Dental chair

The dental chair (**213**) must be capable of moving to a flat position very quickly. It is also vital that it can be adjusted so that the patient's head is lower than his feet. Manoeuvrability of the dental chair is critical for all dental procedures, but it is especially important for a sedated patient in the 45–180° position – the purpose of which is to allow for better cerebral circulation, and to place less strain on the patient's heart action in the event of a vasovagal attack or other cardiovascular change brought on by anxiety or drugs.

213

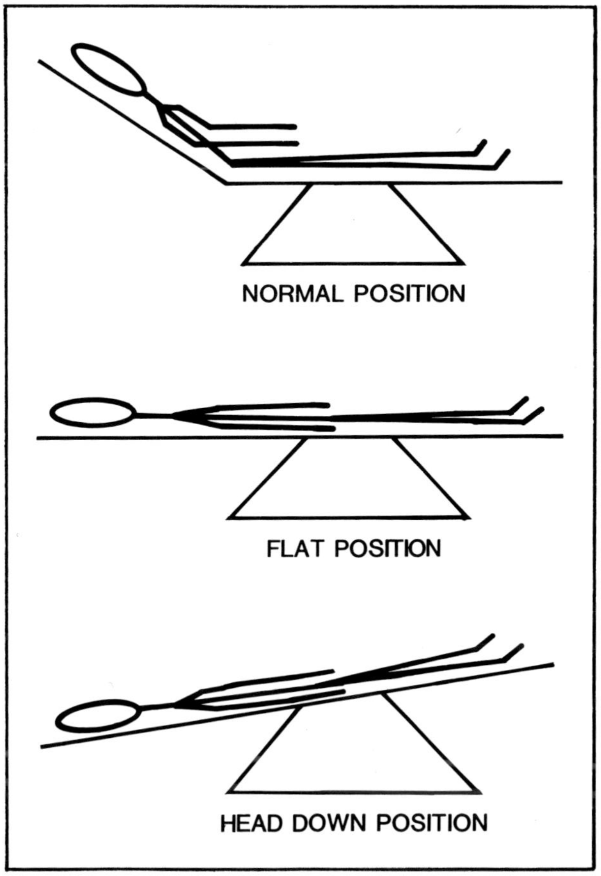

213 The dental chair must be capable of assuming any of the basic positions rapidly

Aspirator

The aspirator (**214**) must be capable of removing fluids and foreign matter rapidly and efficiently. The ideal source of aspiration is central suction or suction that is carried straight into a mains drainage system. These systems are hygienic and easily cleaned. It is absolutely essential that all parts of the aspirating system in the surgery can be dismantled without difficulty for frequent cleaning and disinfection.

It is important to have a spare aspirator available as back-up. This should be of a mechanical type (**215**) which can be used if a power failure or mechanical fault occurs. Disposable aspirator tips, suckers and a range of saliva ejectors (**216** to **218**) should also be kept in the surgery for use.

214

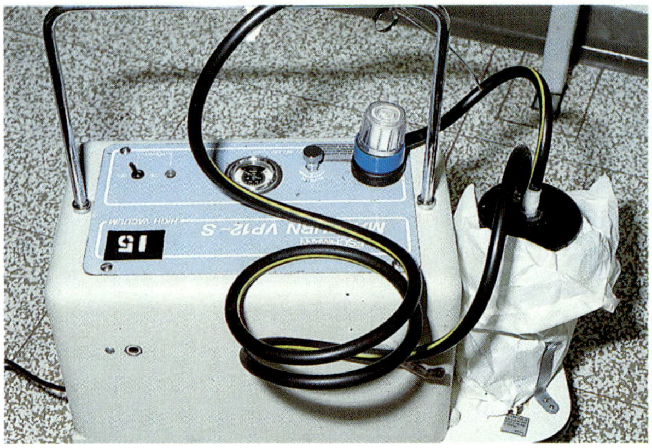

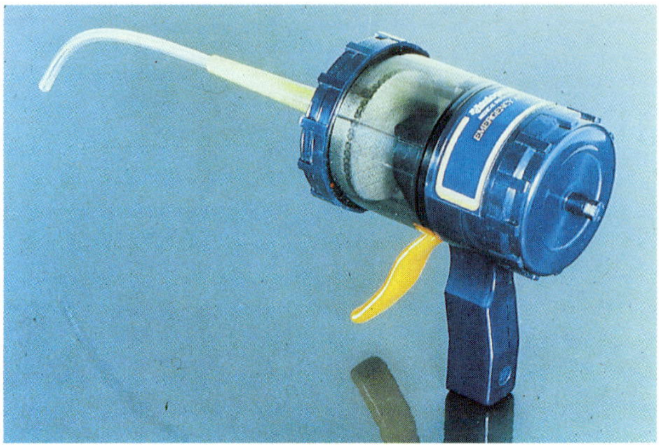

214 A typical aspirator

215 Always have a mechanical aspirator on hand, as a spare in case of emergencies

216

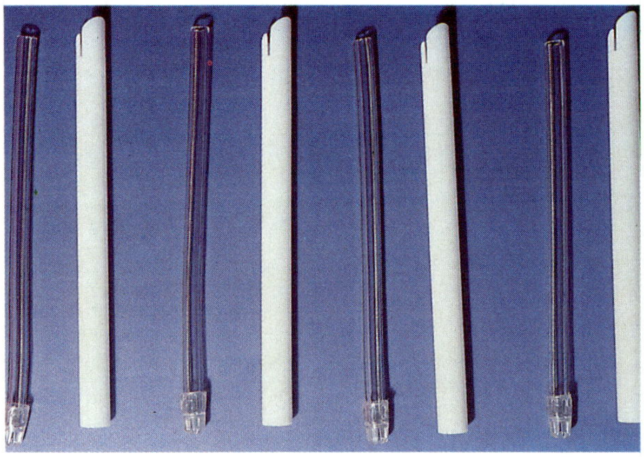

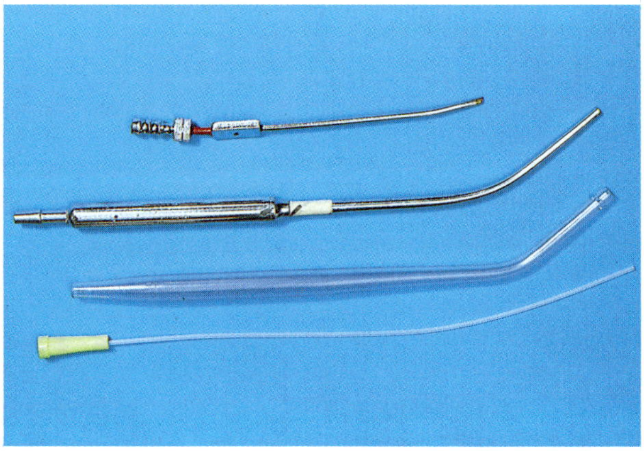

216 and 217 Disposable aspirator tips, suckers and a selection of saliva ejectors

218

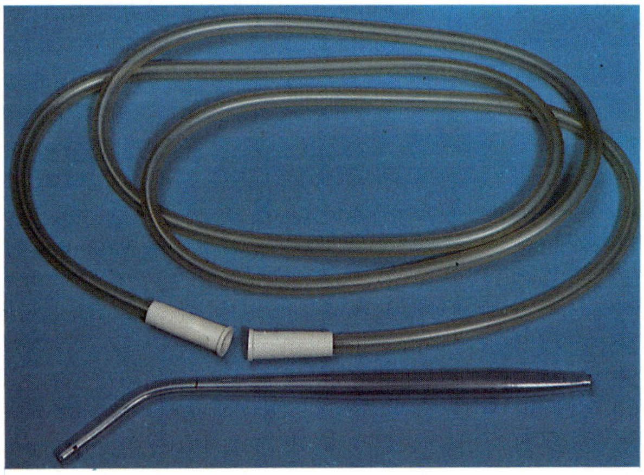

218 An aspirator tube and Yankee sucker. This type of aspiration disposable kit (here removed from its pre-sterilized packaging) is particularly suitable for oral surgery

Syringe

For use in intravenous sedation, the syringe (**219**) should always be of the disposable type – the same goes for all needles and accompanying materials. It would obviously be very dangerous to re-use any of these items on another patient, due to the high risk of infection and/or cross-infection. Syringes should be clearly marked in millilitres, the ideal size being 5ml. It is the responsibility of the dental surgeon to know the dosage in milligrams per millilitre of the drug that is being administered.

219

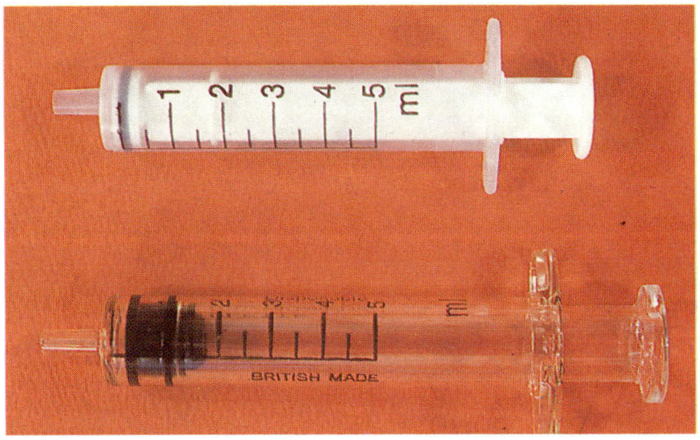

219 Disposable 5ml syringes suitable for the administration of drugs for intravenous sedation

Needle

The disposable needles used in intravenous sedation for dental purposes are of two varieties: straight, and butterfly type (**221** and **222**), each varying in size and length. For easy identification the needle hubs are colour-coded.

Needles destined for clinical use must not be bent (**220**), as this inevitably weakens them. If a needle should accidentally become bent, it should be disposed of straightaway. Otherwise, if it happened to be used on a patient and broke, the dental surgeon would be clearly at fault and might have to assume liability for any harm caused to the patient as a result.

220

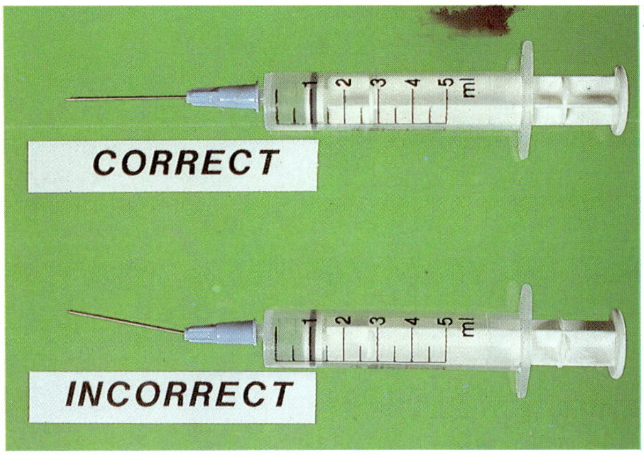

220 A bent needle is not just 'incorrect', it is potentially dangerous, and must be thrown away immediately

221

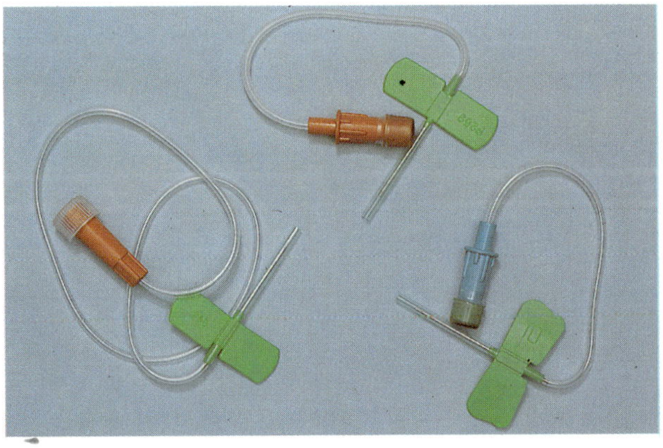

222

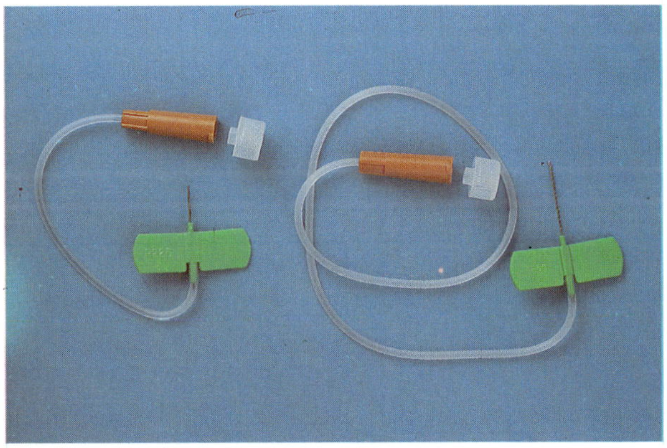

221 and **222** Butterfly needles have either a rubber diaphragm (**221**) or a removable plastic bung (**222**) at their end. The dental surgeon will decide which type of needle he prefers according to his intravenous sedation technique

Surgical tape

It should be remembered that some patients have sensitive skin, and in these cases permeable non-woven surgical synthetic adhesive tape ('surgical tape' for short!) should be used. (See **223** and **224**.)

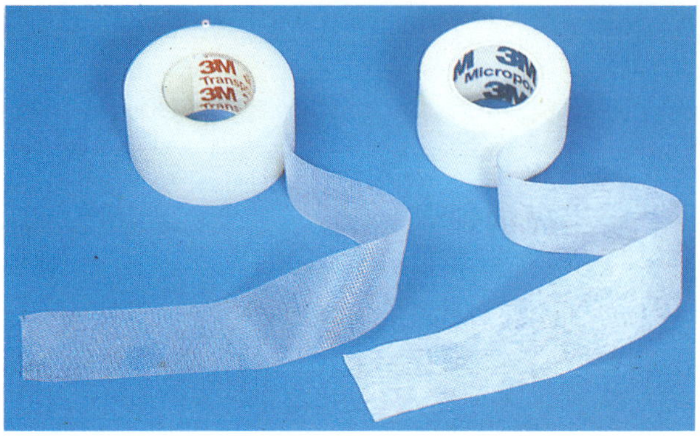

223 Surgical tape should be used where patients have a sensitive skin

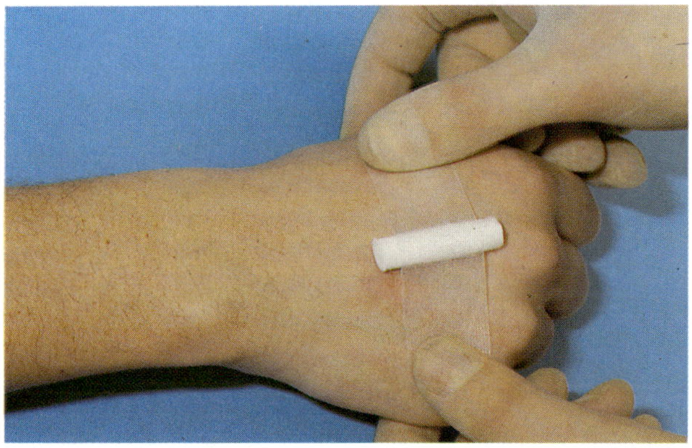

224 Surgical tape is used to hold a cotton wool roll in place over the venepuncture site

Armboard

A simple armboard (**225**) may be helpful in the case of dental surgeons who prefer to use the cubital fossa for venepuncture. The armboard's use prevents any sudden movement of the patient's arm, which might otherwise push the inserting needle into deeper anatomical structures, with resultant damage.

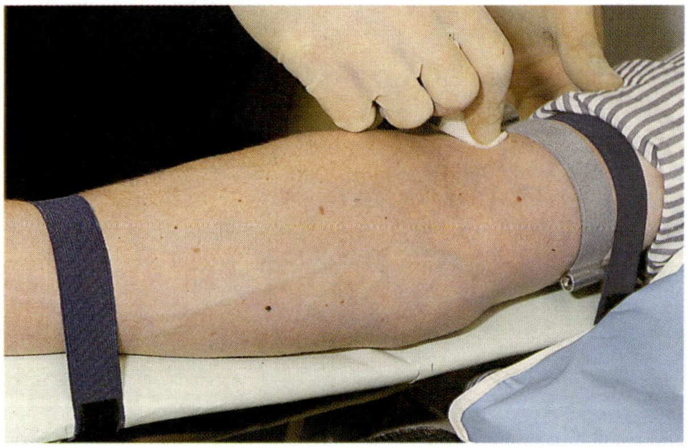

225 Armboard, made from 5mm-thick plywood with a cloth covering and a short length of Velcro tape

Safety glasses

Safety glasses (**226**) must be available for use by both patient and staff, for damage can occur even during short, simple procedures. The slower reflexes of the sedated patient mean he is more at risk than the non-sedated patient. Some patients also prefer to remove contact lenses for intravenous sedation procedures.

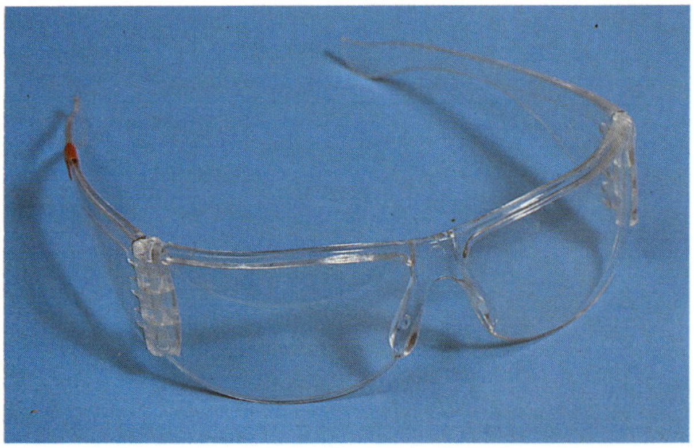

226 Safety glasses must be available for both patient and dental surgery staff

Weighing scales

Although the administration of drugs is titrated against the individual patient's requirement, it is helpful from the point of view of the dental surgeon's own records (and also for the manufacturer's data sheet recommendations) to weigh patients before intravenous sedation.

Lighting

The surgery lighting should allow both the dental surgeon and the dental surgery assistant to see clearly. The 'daylight' variety reveals the colour of the patient's face accurately and places less strain on the eyes of the surgery staff.

Means of administering oxygen

It is essential that there should exist in the surgery the means to administer oxygen under pressure through a suitable face mask. The laryngeal mask (227) is an easy-to-insert airway consisting of an inflatable silicone ring attached diagonally to a flexible tube. The ring forms an oval mask which fills the space around and behind the larynx, achieving a low-pressure seal between the tube and the trachea without penetration of the larynx, resulting in a perfectly clear airway. The laryngeal mask can be autoclaved and reused. The oxygen delivery system must be regularly maintained and checked by the dental surgeon, so that it will be in good order in the event of its use.

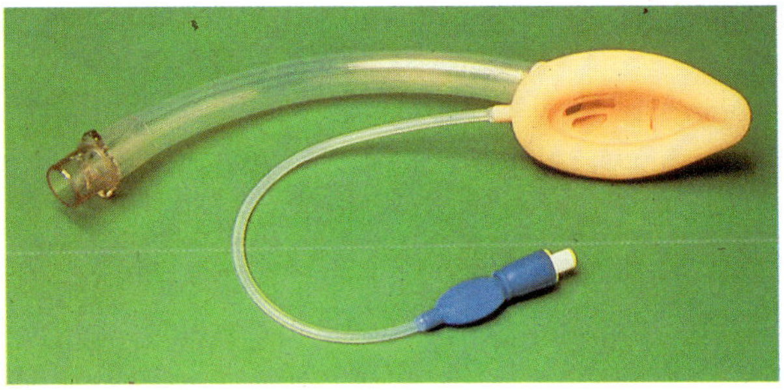
227

227 Laryngeal mask, an effective alternative to the endotracheal tube as a means of administering oxygen

An oxygen cylinder (230), too, must be available in the surgery, where the intravenous sedation is carried out; the oxygen content of the cylinder must be checked before each sedation session.

Oropharyngeal airway

All sizes and types of oropharyngeal airway should be on hand and the dental surgeon should be trained in their use and insertion. The Laerdal pocket mask (228) is an alternative to mouth-to-mouth resuscitation, providing for effective ventilation through the mouth and nose simultaneously. This type of mask has a valved oxygen inlet to permit oxygen enrichment during ventilation.

228
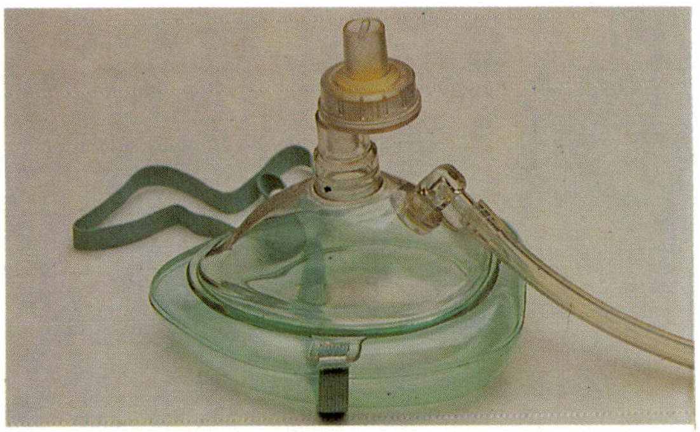

228 Laerdal pocket mask, designed to provide the non-breathing patient with effective mouth-to-mask ventilation. It is held in place by the dental surgeon with both hands, making an airtight seal easier to achieve

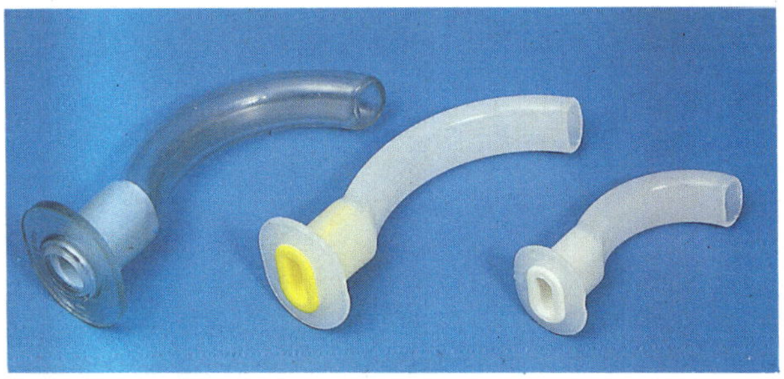
229

229 Disposable Guedel airways

Resuscitator bag

The resuscitator bag (**230**) is able to administer atmospheric air which contains 20 per cent oxygen. In a dental surgery, where oxygen must always be available, the oxygen can be connected to the resuscitator's inlet valve.

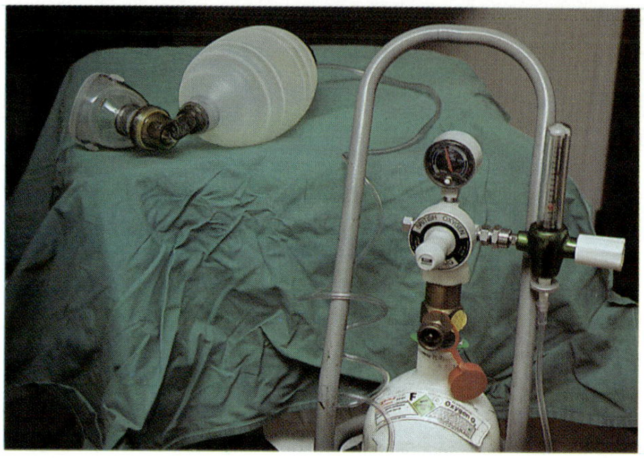

230 Resuscitator bag, connected to an oxygen cylinder

Disposable tray

There are different sizes of disposable tray available to suit the needs of the individual dental surgeon, but basically it should hold all drug ampoules, needles and syringes for use during the intravenous sedation procedure (**231**). Keeping the tray and its contents on hand until completion of the procedure means that – in the event of an emergency – the dental surgeon will have evidence at his fingertips of exactly how much of each drug has been administered to the patient up to that point. Only when the patient is recovered should the dental surgery assistant dispose of the contents of the tray via a Sharps container.

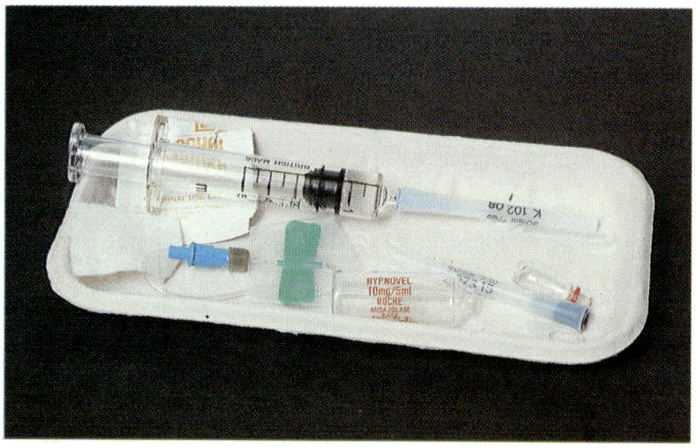

231 Disposable tray containing items that have been used in the dental procedure. Only when the patient is well on the way to recovery are the items disposed of via a Sharps bin

Tourniquet

This is used to obstruct venous return and thereby help identify a suitable vein and assist in venepuncture. The tourniquet must be loosened before any drug is injected (**232**) or else vein damage can occur: always check that this has been done before proceeding.

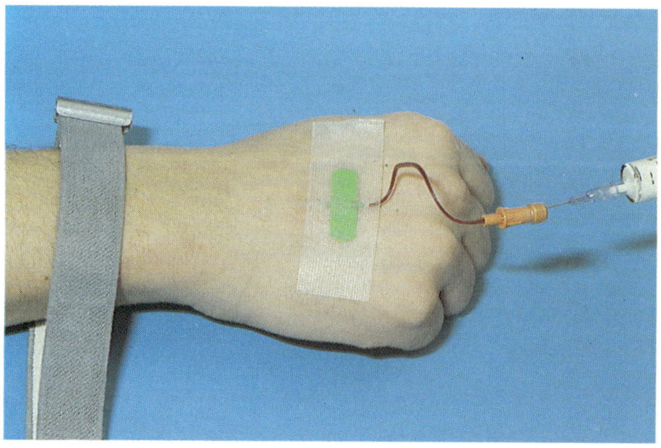

232 Tourniquet is loosened before injection commences

Mouth prop

Maintaining the patient's opening with a suitably sized mouth prop (**233**) facilitates some dental procedures.

233

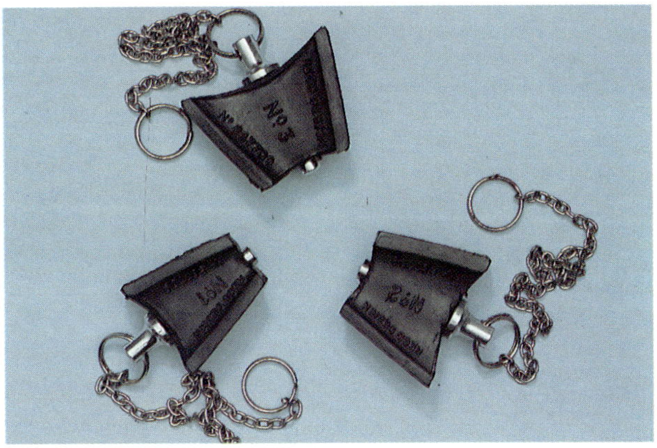

233 Mouth props

Mouth pack

When excessive debris in the form of water, blood or tooth material is anticipated, it is advisable to use a mouth pack. If a post-surgical pack is used, at least 7.5cm of the pack must extend outside the mouth. The use of a mouth pack merely facilitates aspiration; it does not mean that less aspiration is required.

234

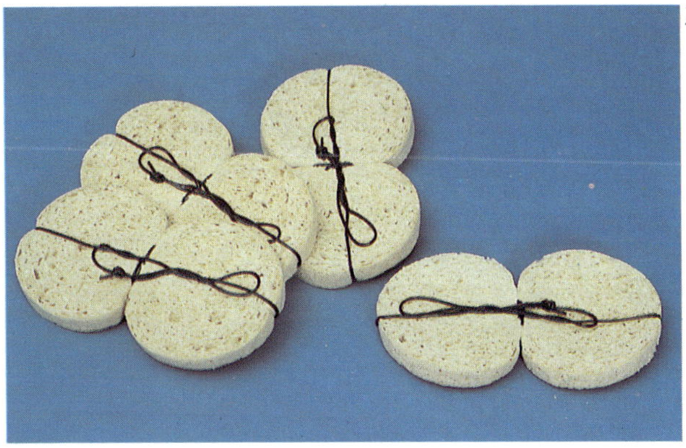

234 Absorbent mouth packs

Surgical gloves

Where contact with blood or body fluids may occur, surgical gloves must be worn. They are always worn for intravenous procedures in dental practice and hospital situations.

Swab

Swabs come impregnated with isopropyl alcohol and are available in sealed containers.

Drugs for use in emergencies

Many different combinations of drugs are available to make up an emergency drug kit. It must be the responsibility of the dental surgeon to consult with his senior medical and dental colleagues on what drugs to keep in such a kit, but among those which might be included are:

- Chlorpheniramine maleate: 5x1ml ampoules each containing 10mg
- Hydrocortisone sodium succinate injection B.P.: 5x100mg vials with water for injection
- Adrenaline injection B.P.: 5x0.5ml ampoules of 1000 solution
- Diazepam: 5x2ml ampoules (5mg in 1ml)
- Atropine sulphate: 5x1ml ampoules (0.6mg in 1ml)
- Phentolamine mesylate: 5x1ml ampoules each containing 10mg
- Dextrose injection, strong B.P.C. 50 per cent in 50ml
- Water for injection, 5 ampoules each containing 10ml.

Resuscitation drugs

Cardiovascular	*Amount*	*Purpose*
Smelling salts (sealed)	2 bottles	Fainting
Atropine 1mg in 2ml	2x2ml	Bradycardia
Sodium bicarbonate 8.4 per cent = 1 m. eq. per ml	4x50ml	Acidosis following cardiac arrest
50ml 'Min-i-jet'	4x50ml	
Methoxamine 20mg in 1ml	2x1ml	Hypertension
Amyl nitrite	2 brisettes	Angina
Isosorbide dinitrate 5mg sublingual (chewable sorbitrate Stuart)	4 tablets	Angina
Practolol 10mg in 5ml	2x5ml	Tachycardia
Ouabain 0.25mg in 1ml	2x1ml	Cardiac failure
Heparin 5000 IV in 1ml	1x4ml (refrigerator)	Intra-arterial injection
Lignocaine 1 per cent 100mg in 10ml		Extravenous injection Intra-arterial injection Ventricular arrhythmia
Calcium chloride 1 per cent 50mg in 5ml	1x5ml	Cardiac massage
Respiratory		
Aminophylline 250mg in 10ml	2x10ml	Bronchospasm
Isoprenaline 0.1mg in 2ml	1x2ml	Bronchospasm
Nikethamide 25 per cent	2x2ml	Respiratory stimulant
Doxapram 100mg in 5ml 1gm in 5000ml	2x5ml 1x500 ml IV pack	Respiratory stimulant
Naloxone hydrochloride 0.4mg in 1ml	2x1ml	Opiate antagonist
Allergy		
Chlorpheniramine 10mg in 1ml	2x1ml	Antihistamine
Adrenaline 1:10,000 1mg in 10ml	2x10ml	Anaphylactic shock
Endocrine		
Hydrocortisone 100mg and 2ml water	2x2 ampoules	Persistent bronchospasm allergy steroid treatment
Dextrose 5 per cent 500ml IV pack	2x500ml	Hypotension
Dextrose 50 per cent 50 ml	2x50ml	Hypoglycaemia
Nerves		
Dexamethasone 5mg in 1ml	2x1ml	Cerebral oedema following cardiac arrest
Diazepam 10mg in 2ml	1x2	Sedative Anti-convulsant
Thiopentone 500mg in 20ml water	1x2 ampoules	Anaesthetic
Succinylcholine 100mg in 2ml	2x2 (refrigerator)	Muscle relaxant

The author keeps the following within easy reach of patients undergoing intravenous sedation in his surgery:

- Atropine 0.6mg in 1ml
- Adrenaline 1 in 1000 in 0.5ml ampoule
- Hydrocortisone succinate 100mg
- Promethazine hydrochloride 10–40mg
- Naloxone hydrochloride 0.4mg in 1ml
- Flumazenil 0.5mg
- Dextrose
- Glyceryl trinitrate
- Oxygen.

It cannot be stressed too strongly that all emergency drugs must be on hand *in* the dental surgery, and within arm's reach of the dental surgeon when a sedation is to be undertaken – not outside or merely near the surgery to be used. It is essential that the expiry dates of drugs are checked and that equipment maintenance is carried out on a daily basis before a sedation is started.

Monitoring the sedated patient

The safety and well-being of the sedated patient are of paramount importance and are the responsibility of the dental surgeon and his qualified assistants. All patients undergoing intravenous sedation must, therefore, be adequately monitored. There is no excuse for not having one's staff trained in the use of basic monitoring equipment or for suggesting such equipment is too expensive. The dental staff must be trained also in the interpretation and comprehension of recorded data produced by the monitors, and must know how to act when a problem is indicated.

The most efficient monitors of all are the eyes and ears of the dental surgeon and his dental surgery assistant: by observing the patient closely at all times, many problems may be avoided. Electronic monitoring, although essential, cannot replace the human senses.

Pulse and blood pressure

A variety of pulse and blood pressure monitors are available (235). These can provide early warning of severe cardiovascular activity by monitoring any changes that may occur in a distressed patient's vital signs. Early warning of respiratory depression or of other causes of cardiovascular problems enables the dental surgeon to take immediate, potentially life-saving action to remove or treat the cause of the problem.

235

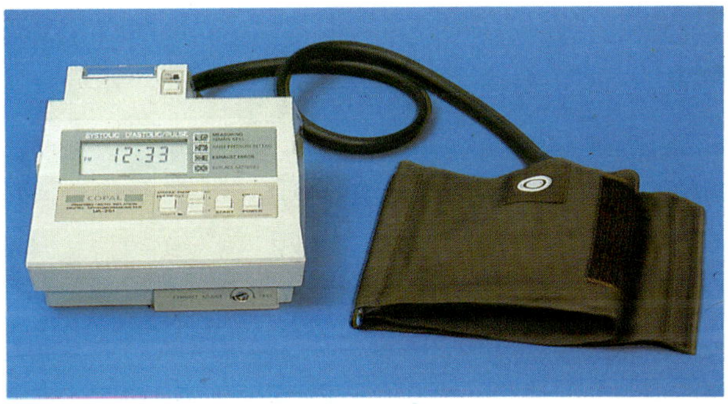

235 Pulse and blood pressure monitor with print-out facility

Pulse oximetry

This is the most accurate form of non-invasive monitoring of a patient's saturation status. Its operation is based on the difference in the light absorption characteristics of haemoglobin when it is oxygenated and in its reduced form. The pulse oximeter calculates the percentage of oxygen saturation, i.e. the ratio of oxygenated haemoglobin to total haemoglobin, by measuring the absorption of selected wavelengths of light passing through a sample of living tissue (for example, a finger or an ear lobe).

Oxygenated haemoglobin and reduced haemoglobin absorb light in known functions of wavelengths and it is thereby possible to calculate the relative percentage of these two constituents. The sensor converts the light

236

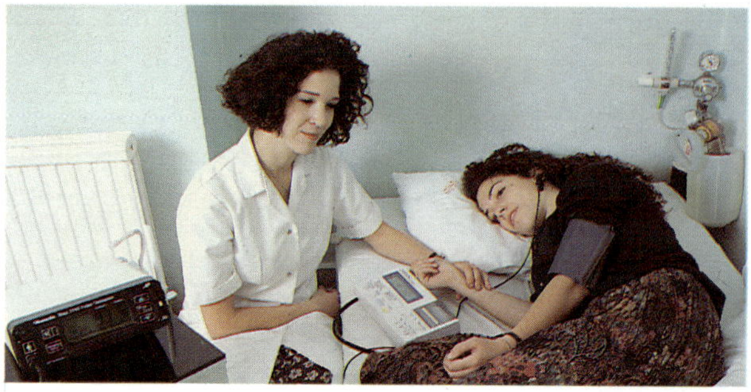

236 A patient in recovery following intravenous sedation. Note that she is in a supine position under the watchful care of an experienced dental surgery assistant, who is taking a radial pulse. Within easy reach are an oximeter and print out, a sphygmomanometer/pulse monitor, a supply of oxygen and an aspirator. This patient, although well on the way to recovery, must still be monitored. As the sedation wears off the patient's escort may sit with the patient. A bell push to summon assistance is placed next to the recovering patient

passing through the tissue sample into an electrical signal, which is transmitted through the sensor cable to the monitor, where a microcomputer calculates the oxygen saturation level and the pulse rate. The oxygen saturation level is the ratio of oxygen-saturated haemoglobin to total (that is, saturated and reduced) haemoglobin multiplied by 100.

In order to eliminate light-absorbing effects of other blood and tissue components, one pulse oximeter uses a method based on the pulsation of capillary blood. The blood pulsation itself modulates the light detected by the sensor. Light passing through the sample is affected both by the pulsation and by other tissue components. However, by electronically filtering the resulting signal to register only the pulses, it is possible to cancel out signals that arise from other components of the sample.

Pulse oximetry is of particular value in the management of patients with any possibility of compromised respiration and oxygenation. Hypoxaemic situations can be spotted earlier than by conventional arterial blood gas analysis, and the effect of any therapeutic measures which have an influence on the patient's oxygenation can be detected rapidly.

Safety parameters of oxygen saturation can be set as well as parameters of pulse rate (pulse volume is also measured and visually displayed). Should the oxygen saturation fall below or rise above the parameters set by the dental surgeon, an alarm will sound. This also applies to the pulse monitoring of the patient. The use of this simple but accurate type of monitoring makes intravenous sedation in the dental surgery situation considerably safer, providing the dental surgeon and his surgery assistant with advance or instant warning of any problem affecting the patient, thus enabling immediate remedial action to be taken.

Oximeters are available which produce a pulsatile waveform (**237**). The waveform display acts as a representative of the detected signal, so that it is possible to determine when interference is present and take corrective action. The waveform's indication of interference assists in the better identification of potentially invalid readings. This type of oximeter can also store recorded information of up to eight hours' monitoring, and possesses a facility to enable it to operate off an inbuilt battery in the event of a power cut. It can be used with an ear lobe attachment (with or without an ear support) or with a finger probe (**238** and **239**).

237

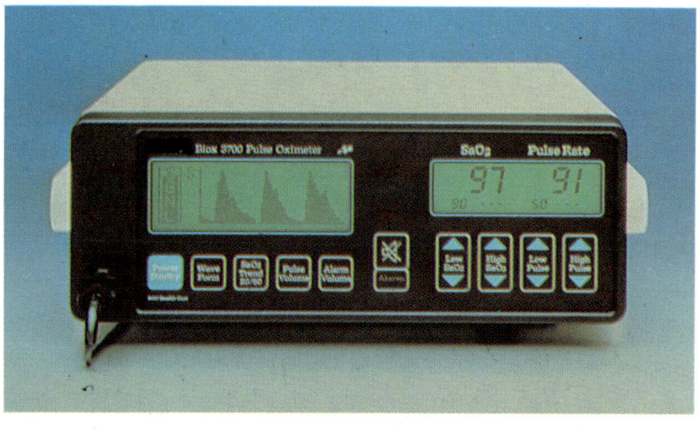

237 Pulse oximeter with waveform display

38 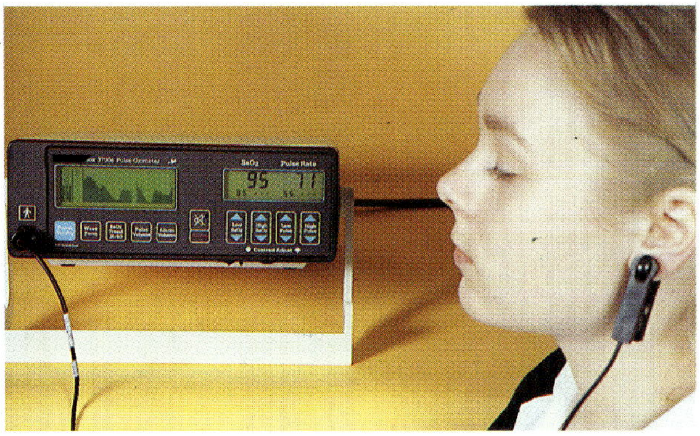 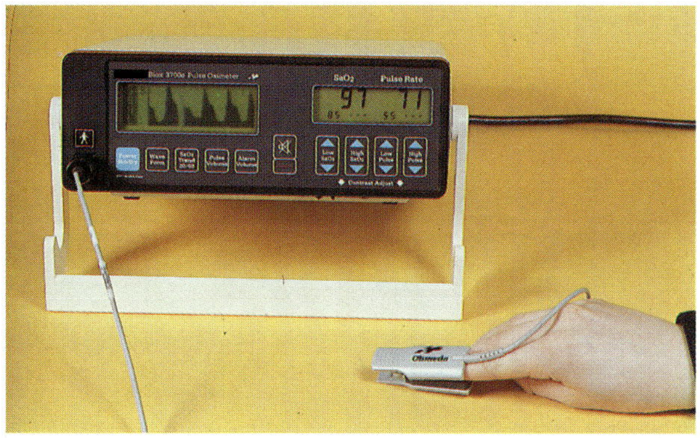 239

238 and **239** Oximeter can be connected to either an ear lobe or a finger

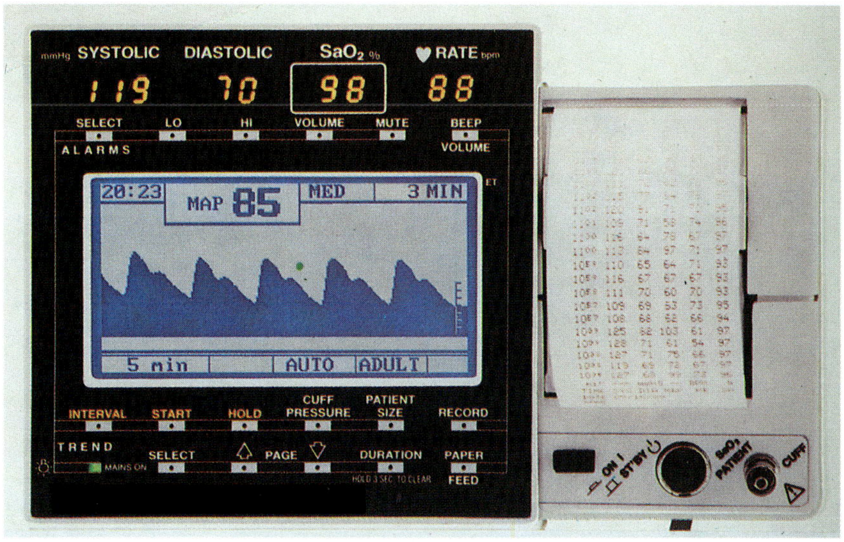

240

240 Combined blood pressure monitor and oximeter with recorder facility; in the event of a power failure it will run off a built-in battery

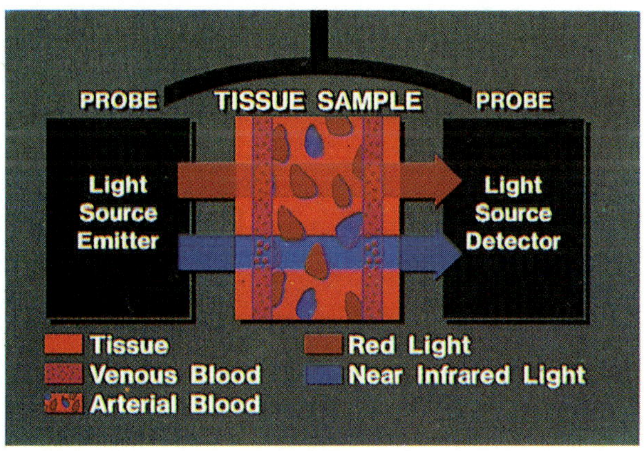

241

241 The oximeter shown in **240** works on the principle illustrated here. Light is emitted by the probe at two discrete wavelengths (red and near infra red). It is partially absorbed and modulated by the pulsing arterial blood, and passes through the tissue sample, after which it is converted into an electronic signal by the probe's detector. Because oxyhaemoglobin and reduced haemoglobin allow different amounts of light to reach the detector at the selected wavelengths, the electronic signal will vary in proportion to the SaO_2 (arterial haemoglobin saturation). This type of oximeter possesses a printing facility which can record measurements taken by the oximeter at any time during its use – very useful should a problem occur

Arterial oxygen saturation and pulse oximetry

THREE WAYS TO MEASURE BLOOD OXYGEN

PaO_2 – Tension exerted by dissolved oxygen in plasma
(O_2) – **Oxygen saturation** of haemoglobin
O_2 content = Xml oxygen per 100ml blood

As depicted in the familiar oxygen dissociation curve (**242**), blood oxygenation information can be represented by the partial pressure of oxygen molecules (PO_2) dissolved in the plasma, and by oxygen loosely bound to the haemoglobin molecule as compared to total haemoglobin (per cent oxygen saturation SO_2). An accurate measurement of arterial PO_2 (PaO_2) is usually accomplished through laboratory analysis of arterial blood. Pulse oximetry technique enables the assessment of arterial haemoglobin saturation (SaO_2) non-invasively and continuously, allowing analysis of patient oxygenation during intravenous sedation procedures or in any other situation in which patient oxygenation monitoring is useful.

The dental surgeon could imagine a car parked with its brakes on at the point of 90 per cent oxygen saturation on the illustrated graph (**242**), this being the lowest acceptable patient oxygenation. If the oxygen saturation decreased below this point (90 per cent), the car would clearly fall over the steep cliff of oxygen dissociation – possibly to disaster. It is therefore imperative that the patient's oxygenation is maintained well over 90 per cent. If the alarm on the oximeter sounds, instant corrective action must be taken; the alarm must never be turned off or ignored.

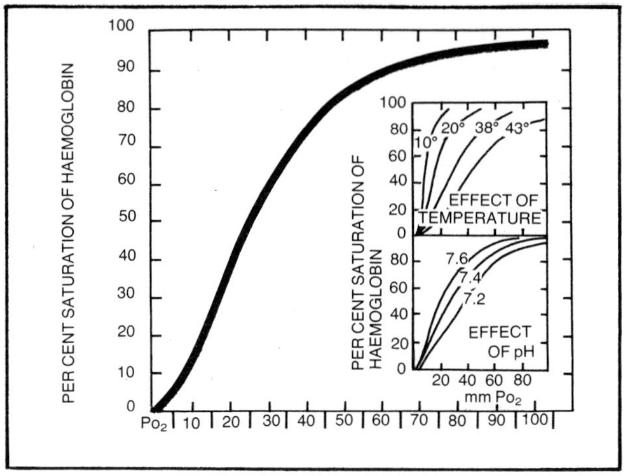

242

242 Graph showing oxyhaemoglobin dissociation curve (assuming adult haemoglobin, 38°C and pH of 7.40)

Remember:

- The routine use of pulse oximetry on all patients undergoing sedation or analgesia represents a **major** improvement in safety
- Lack of oxygen not only stops the machine, it also wrecks the machinery!
- Unrecognized hypoxia inevitably leads to irreversible brain damage within just a few minutes
- Higher mental functions are most sensitive
- Accidental hypoxic brain damage has led to many of the largest medico-legal settlements in both the UK and the USA.

As already stated, it is up to the individual dental surgeon to decide on how he will equip and maintain his surgery for intravenous sedation use – but even to attempt sedation without the basic items mentioned in this chapter would be dangerous. It is also essential that both the dental surgeon and the dental surgery assistant are adequately trained, not only in the administration of intravenous sedation but also in emergency procedures.

Fire precautions

It is vital that the dental surgeon should be aware of his responsibilities to a patient who, while in a sedated state, will be unable to care for himself in an extrinsic emergency. Whilst it is reasonable to expect surgery or hospital staff to take adequate fire precautions and to have fire-fighting equipment on the premises, it is nevertheless important to check that the sedated patient is well safeguarded in the event of such an emergency. An emergency fire drill should be carried out by surgery personnel at regular intervals and this should include the evacuation of sedated patients.

12 THE TECHNIQUES OF INTRAVENOUS SEDATION

Before starting an intravenous sedation session, the dental surgeon must first check that all resuscitation equipment is at hand and that the oxygen cylinder is turned on and is adequately filled. The oxygen delivery system is checked to see that it is in working order. The expiry dates of drugs for sedation are checked, as are emergency drugs.

Intravenous sedation technique using the cubital fossa

A consent form (**191**) is signed by the patient, the procedures having been carefully explained by the dental surgeon; the form is then witnessed by the dental surgery assistant.

A less experienced practitioner, using the drug data sheet as a guide on how much of a drug to use, may choose to weigh the patient as the information provided can be useful. Drug administration should always be titrated against a patient's response rather than according to a fixed dosage of mg/kg weight.

Before the patient enters the surgery a disposable tray is prepared containing:

- A 5ml syringe
- A butterfly needle, in this case orange-coded gauge 25
- A green needle gauge 21
- An isopropyl alcohol swab
- An ampoule of the intravenous sedation drug
- A tourniquet.

After being weighed, the patient is settled in the dental chair with his possessions clearly in sight. He is placed in the supine position and a tourniquet is applied by the dental surgery assistant. The assistant places a finger under the tourniquet to help achieve the required pressure on the patient's arm; it should not be so tight as to obstruct the arterial flow but tight enough to inhibit venous return. That is somewhere between the systolic and diastolic blood pressure. A sphygmomanometer makes a good tourniquet for a less experienced dental surgeon; it can be left in position and used as a blood-pressure monitor during the procedure. The pulse oximeter is attached to the patient's finger or ear lobe.

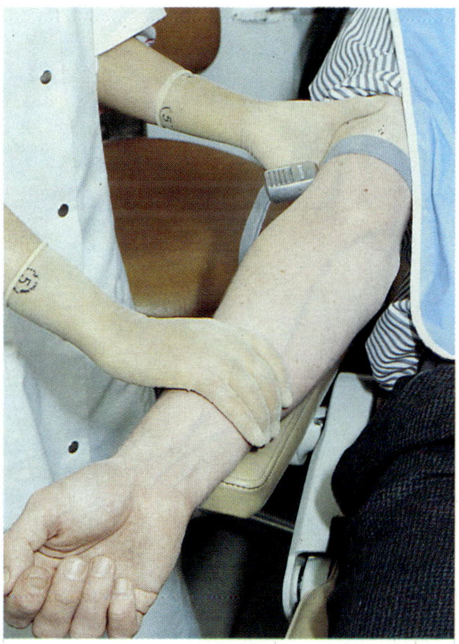

243

243 The patient's arm is supported by the dental surgery assistant: one hand is placed over the wrist and the other under the arm, above the elbow. This prevents the patient making any sudden movement which could displace the needle. An armboard is normally used to provide support (see **245**)

244

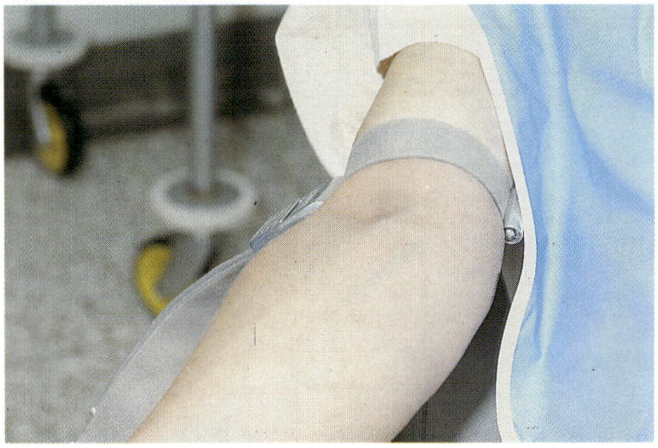

244 The tourniquet *in situ*. The brachial vein, though prominent, should generally be avoided if venepuncture is to be employed in the cubital fossa, as it is closely related to the brachial artery. Rather, the lateral or cephalic vein should be used

245

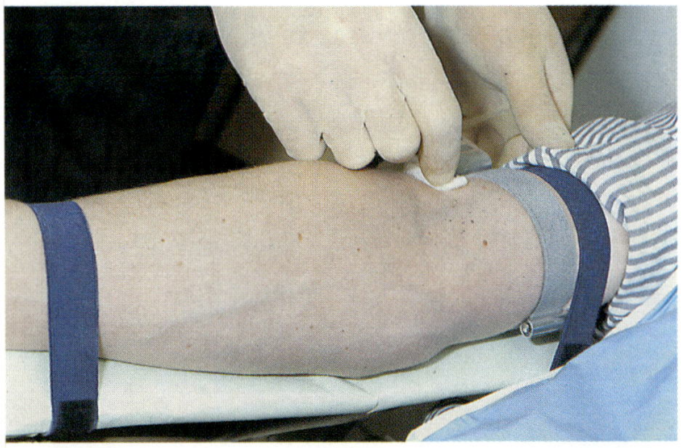

245 The lateral (cephalic) vein of the arm is cleaned using the isopropyl swab prior to venepuncture. The assistant's support is not necessary if an armboard is used

246

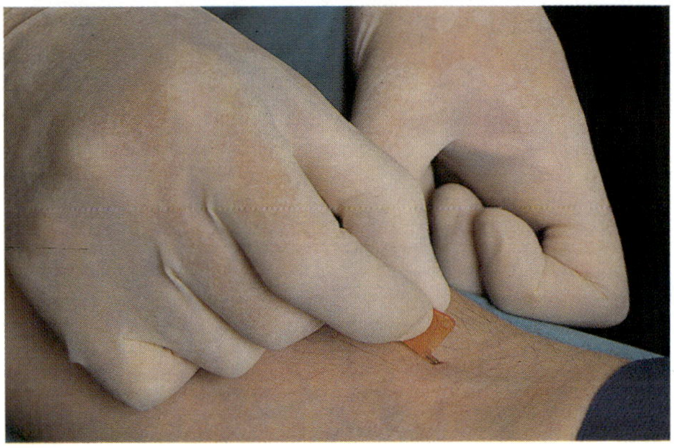

246 The skin overlying the vein is gently stretched to help immobilize the vein and prevent its movement away from the needle on penetration. The patient is always warned just prior to venepuncture that he will feel a small scratch, and should always be given a moment of preparation so that he knows what to expect. This helps build an atmosphere of trust between patient and dental surgeon

EVE signs

Before any drug of sedation is administered, the patient is asked to touch the tip of his nose with his forefinger. This constitutes an 'objective control movement', and is known as an 'EVE Sign Negative' (**247**). After slow titration of the sedation drug, a stage is reached when the patient, when asked to repeat the movement, responds slowly and/or performs the movement inaccurately. This is known as an 'EVE Sign Positive', and is the point of minimal adequate sedation for that patient (**249**). Combined with the patient's slurring of speech, it is a very useful sign for the dental surgeon.

Although the straight needle is still widely used, it is now generally accepted that it is safer to use an indwelling butterfly needle for administering drugs of sedation. Should a problem arise, an open vein is available for using an antagonist or other required drugs.

Depending on the dental procedure to be carried out, the sedation may be deepened. But for normal dental treatment, the dosage

247

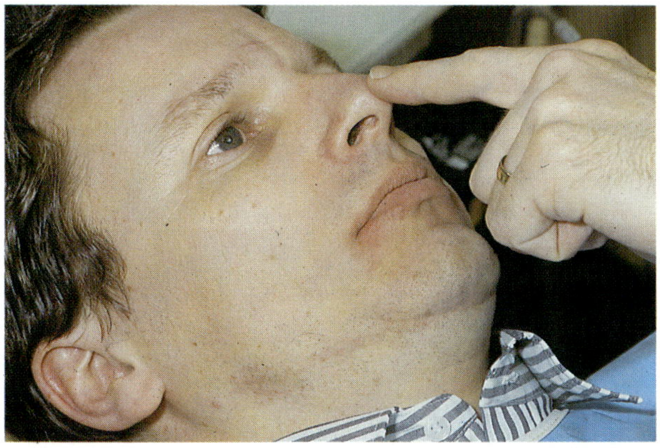

247 Prior to the administration of the drug of sedation, the patient is asked to touch the tip of his nose with his forefinger. Successfully undertaken, this action is described as an EVE Sign Negative

248

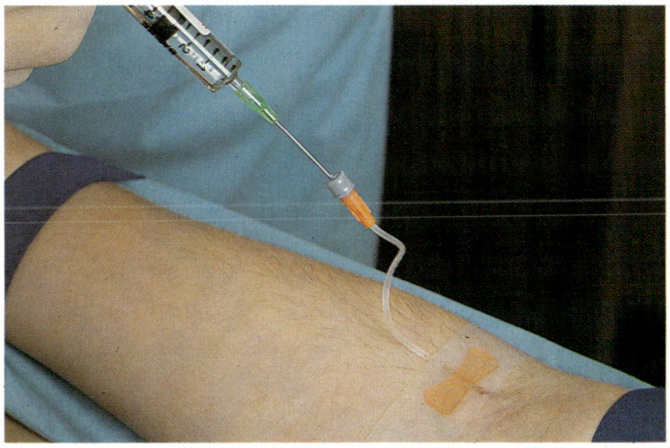

248 The drug of sedation is slowly titrated against the individual requirements of the patient. Note that, when a butterfly needle is employed for venepuncture in the cubital fossa, an armboard can provide beneficial support

249

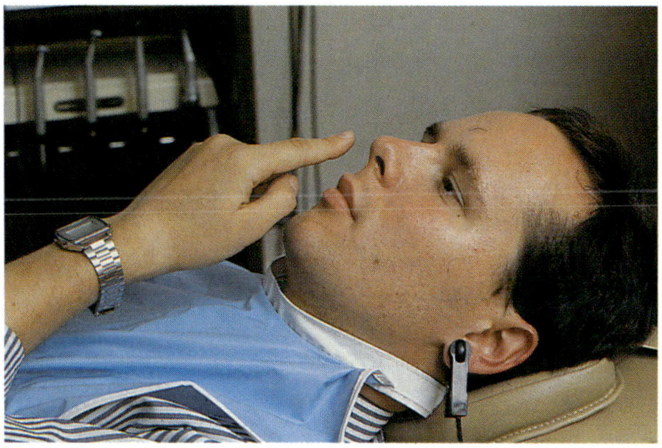

249 Asked again to touch the tip of his nose, the patient this time is unable to comply and thus performs an EVE Sign Positive – indicating that the point of minimal adequate sedation has been reached

required to give an EVE Sign Positive tends to be lower rather than higher. The EVE Sign is, therefore, helpful in avoiding over-sedation.

The drug is gently and slowly titrated against the patient's individual response (**248**). The local analgesic injection may be given after the first few milligrammes of the sedation drug have been injected. This allows time for the local analgesic to take effect before the EVE Sign Positive is reached. Patients do not usually remember the local analgesic injection being given.

The patient wears protective glasses, the dental surgeon and the dental surgery assistant wear surgical gloves. A mouth pack is in place, as well as a saliva ejector. The dental surgery assistant is also aspirating.

As explained in Chapter 11, all drugs are kept in a disposable tray until the patient is well on the way to recovery, enabling a double check to be made against the patient's recorded data in the case notes.

After recovering, it is usual in general dental practice to give the patient a cup of tea or coffee before he is placed in the care of his escort.

Before leaving the surgery, the patient's escort is given a night telephone number in case there are any problems. The latter, where they do occur, are usually related to the patient's treatment rather than the sedation. Post-sedation instructions should always be written down and handed to the escort, who should pass them on to the patient only when the latter has recovered from the effects of the sedation. The fact that the patient will then know where the dental surgeon can be contacted has a reassuring effect.

250

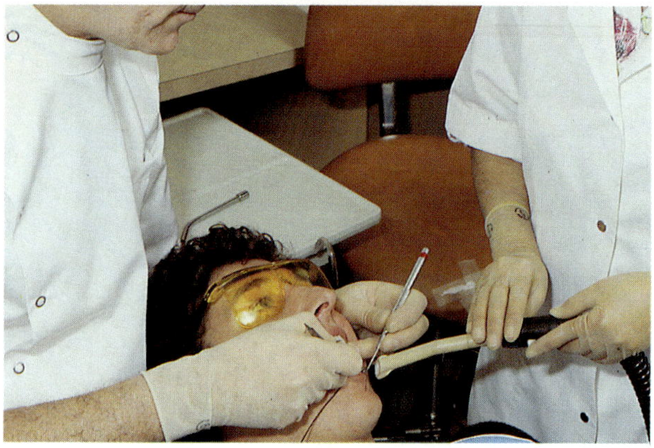

250 Conservation treatment can be carried out once an EVE Sign Positive has been obtained. Note that the patient, although sedated, has his eyes open and is looking at the dental surgery assistant on his left

251

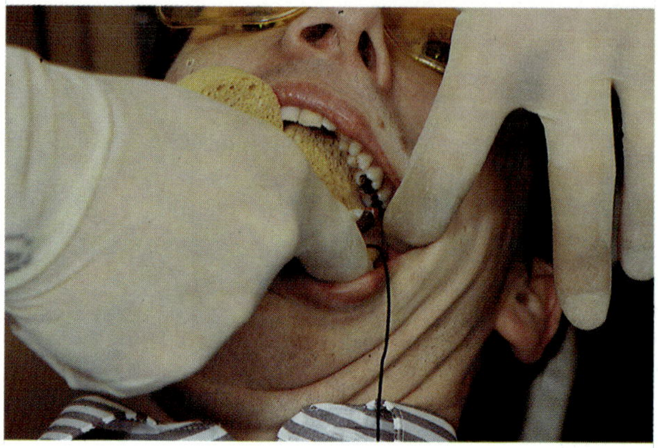

251 The patient here underwent tooth extraction as well as conservation treatment. Note that his eyes are open even though the EVE Sign is still positive

252

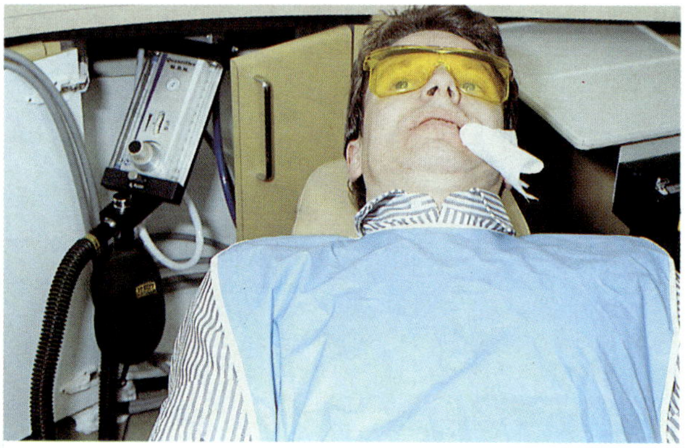

252 The patient is given a few minutes to recover before being taken to the recovery room. Note that oxygen is available just behind the patient

253

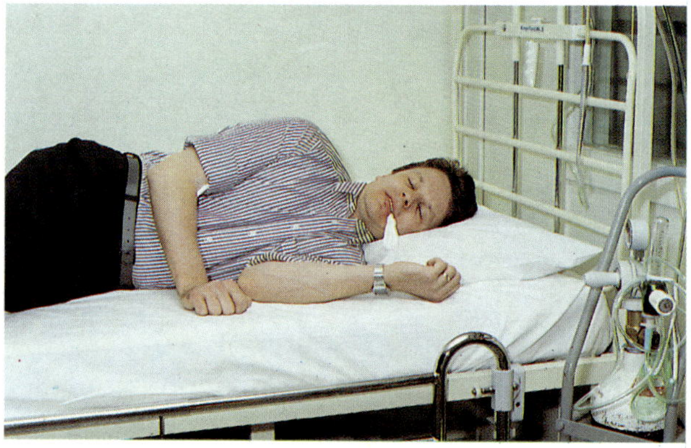

253 The patient is allowed to rest in the recovery room having been placed on his side in the lateral position. If a mouth pack is used in recovery following an oral surgical procedure, at least 7.5cm of it must be outside the mouth. The patient will invariably fall asleep during the recovery period, which should normally be not less than one hour. He should not be left unattended while recovering – the escort can join him in the later stages

Intravenous sedation technique using the dorsum of the hand

The procedure is initially the same as for the cubital fossa technique: the patient signs a consent form, is weighed and then made comfortable in the dental chair in a supine or semi-supine position (*not* upright).

254

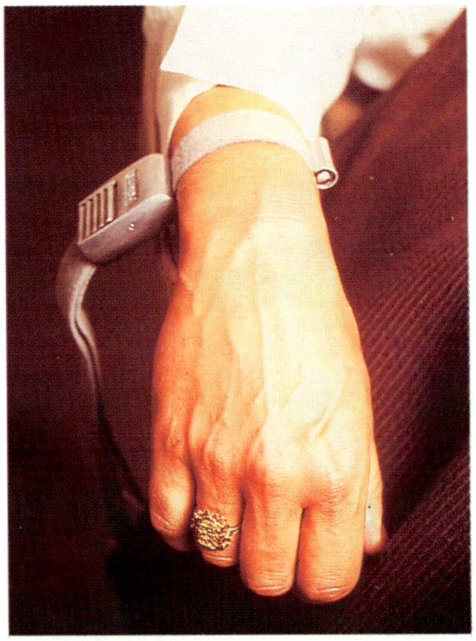

254 The tourniquet is applied and the hand to be used is lowered below arm level, allowing gravity to make the veins more pronounced and to stretch the overlying skin. The dental surgeon should feel for an aberrant artery on the dorsum, although it is unlikely that one will be found

255

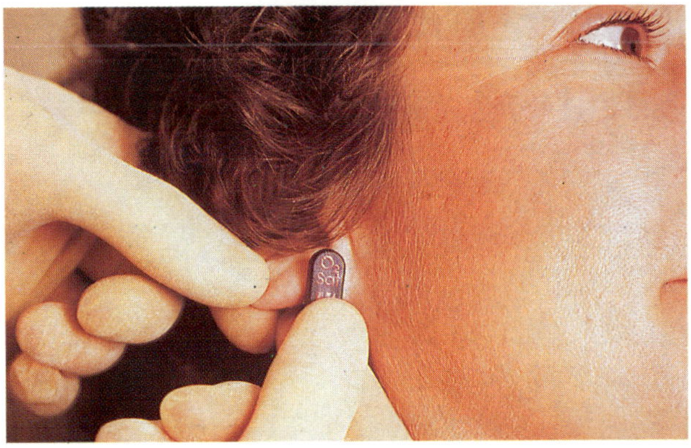

255 An ear-lobe contact is used for monitoring the patient

256

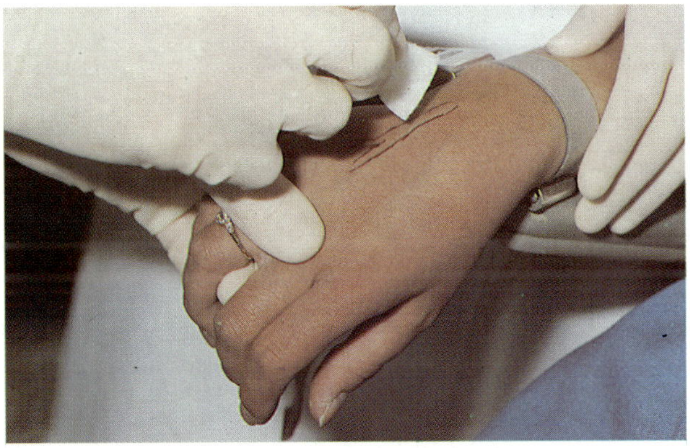

256 The area for venepuncture is first cleaned with an isopropyl alcohol swab. (The vein to be used on the dorsum of the hand has been outlined with a marking pen for clarity during photography. This is not normal procedure.)

257

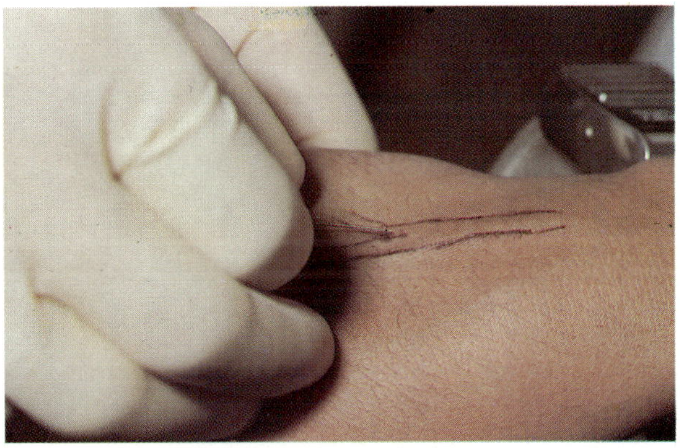

257 Keeping the overlying skin taut, venepuncture is then carried out. Note that the venepuncture is made where two veins have joined to make a larger, clearer and more accessible vein. The hand is angled downwards slightly, the effects of gravity thus making the vein a little more prominent

258

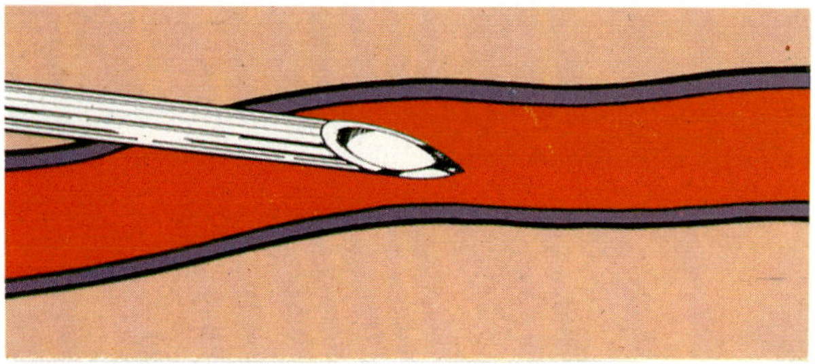

258 The correct positioning of the needle within the lumen of the vein

259

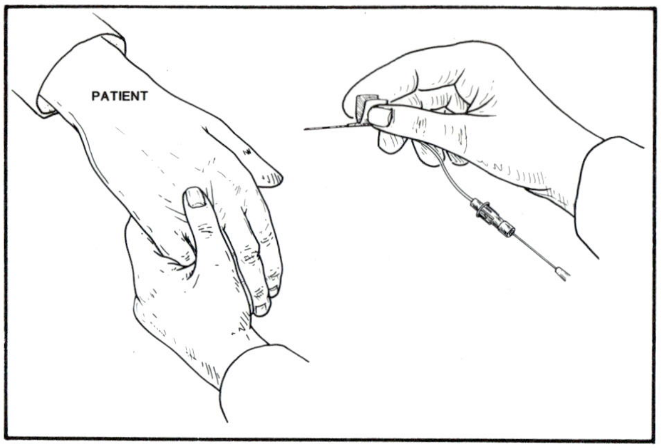

259 How to hold the butterfly wings and – with the other hand – immobilize the underlying vein to be used for venepuncture by stretching the tissue overlying the vein with the thumb

After inserting the needle along the vein the butterfly is spread out and taped to the dorsum of the hand (**260** and **261**). Before venepuncture, the patient is warned to expect a small scratch: alerting him will aid cooperation, and help prevent a rapid withdrawal of the hand. By inserting a needle into the rubber cup of the butterfly, the patient's blood will run down the plastic tubing – showing the dental surgeon that the needle of the butterfly is within the vein's lumen. The blood flow can be stopped either by removing the open-ended needle or by connecting the syringe containing the sedative drug.

Before the sedation drug is administered, the patient is asked to touch the tip of her nose with a forefinger of the hand that is not being used in the venepuncture (EVE Sign Negative). This is the control movement of an unsedated patient. When successful venepuncture has been achieved the tourniquet is loosened.

After the patient has become relaxed and before adequate sedation has been achieved, some dental surgeons may wish to inject a local analgesic. This not only encourages slower administration of the drug of sedation, but also makes that administration safer. Very few patients remember the injection of local analgesic when benzodiazepines are used.

If an incremental dose is required, the syringe needle is simply injected into the rubber bung of the butterfly (which is one definite advantage of the butterfly compared with the previously described direct syringe needle administration into a vein). The syringe needle is then withdrawn, leaving the butterfly needle within the vein. Further doses may be administered as required.

The availability of venous access at all times during the procedure is obviously an advantage, especially if an emergency situation arises and other drugs have to be administered. In the case of a cardiovascular collapse, the superficial

260

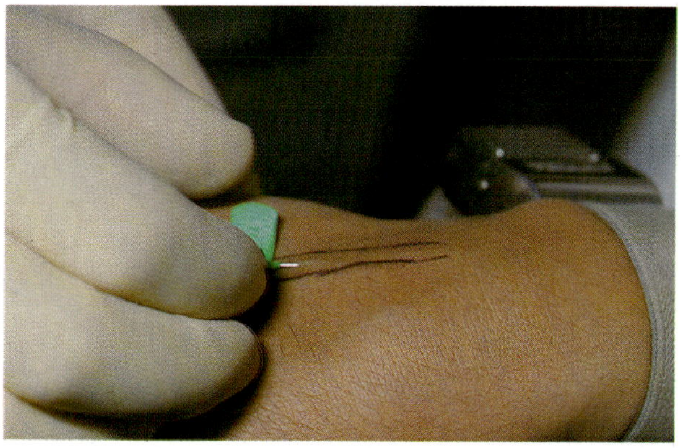

261

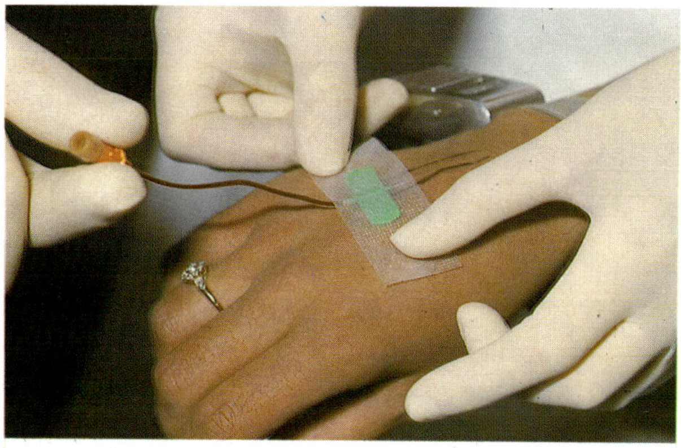

260 and 261 The butterfly needle is inserted and the wings of the butterfly opened and secured by the dental surgery assistant with a strip of permeable non-woven surgical synthetic adhesive tape

262

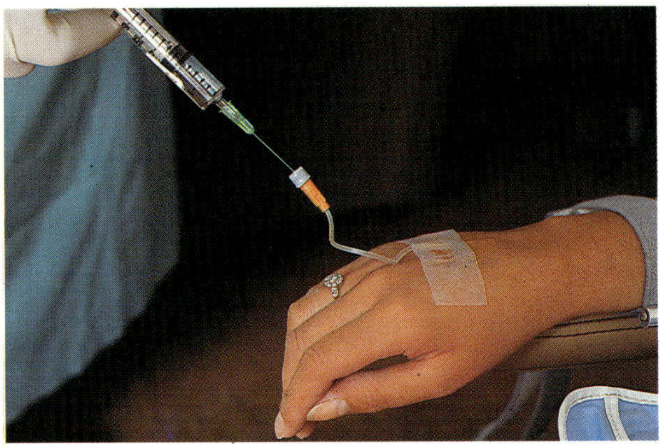

263

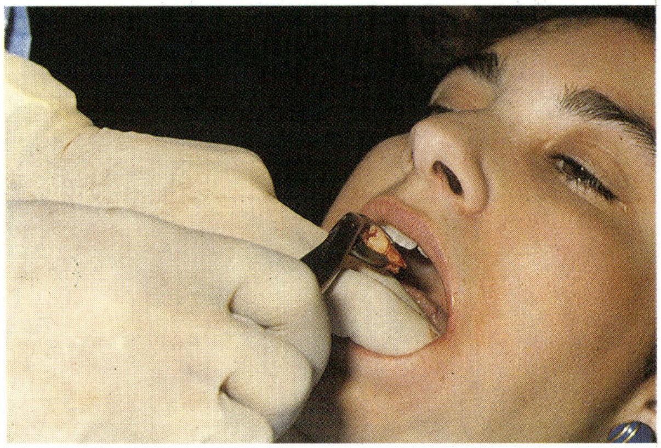

262 The sedation drug is administered slowly, bearing in mind the recommendations of the drug data sheets, to allow the dental surgeon time to assess the patient and – through an individual titration of the drug – to consider the patient's requirements for that particular course of treatment. The point of minimal adequate sedation may be obtained by using the EVE Sign

263 The patient, though sedated, has her eyes open and appears relaxed as the dental procedure is carried out. Should the patient become unsettled, an incremental dose of the sedation drug may be administered through the butterfly

veins invariably become difficult to find; but when a butterfly is in position, easier access is available through the patent vein.

It is not uncommon for patients to cross their legs during sedation. Over a lengthy period the pressure of the overlying leg may produce numbness, which can be unpleasant and cause the patient to fall on leaving the dental chair. The dental surgery assistant should therefore uncross the patient's legs.

To avoid a 'needle stick' injury to the dental surgeon, the withdrawn needle should be inserted into the butterfly's own rubber diaphragm and secured with the attached adhesive tape.

As explained earlier, the syringe and all the opened drug vials are kept in a disposable tray until the patient is well on the way to recovery. Only then can the remains be disposed of into a Sharps container. The final dosage of the drugs administered should always be entered in the patient's records, together with the time that the intravenous sedation was commenced and that the operative procedure was completed – and the time it took the patient to recover.

The patient's escort is given verbal and written instructions on how to care for the patient. The patient should be discharged only by the dental surgeon, never by the dental surgery assistant.

264

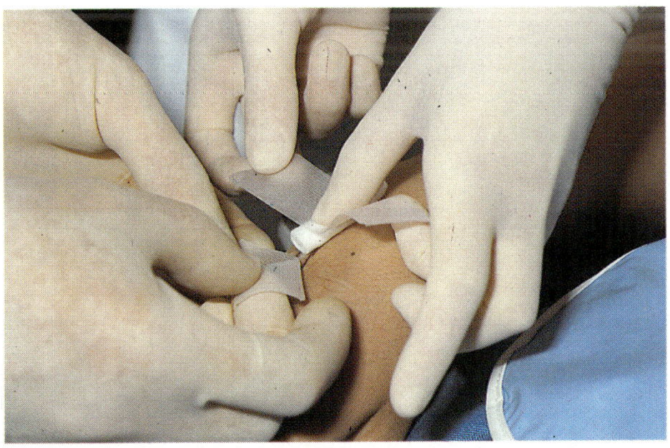

265

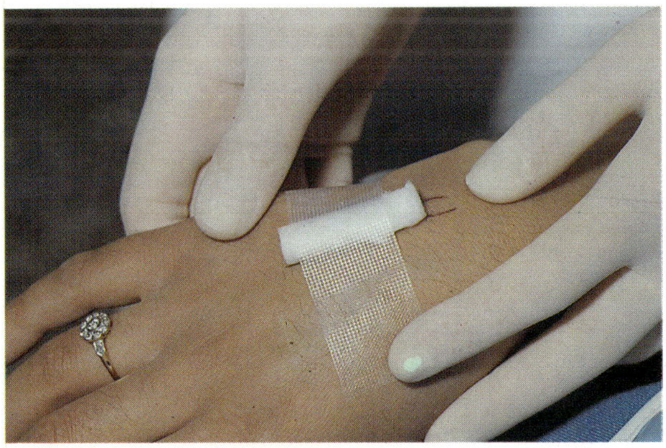

264 and **265** At the end of the procedure a cotton wool roll is placed over the venepuncture site and held in position by surgical tape. The dental surgery assistant places the dressing *in situ* as the dental surgeon withdraws the needle. The patient is taken to a supervised recovery area and discharged 45 minutes to one hour later

266 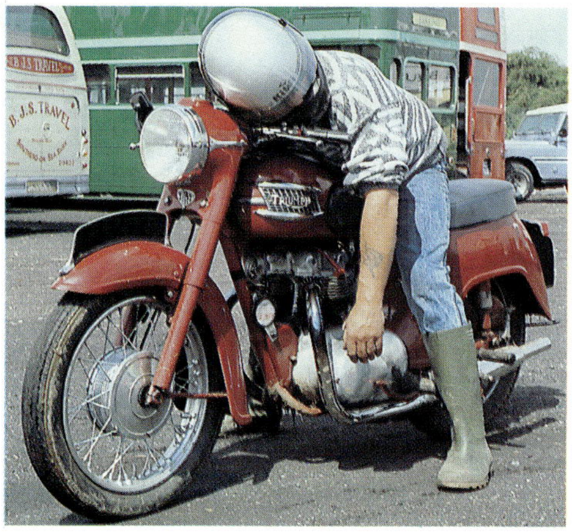

266 The dental surgeon should check that the sedated patient will be escorted home and not left alone in a car park; the patient will be unfit to drive or to travel home alone. The mode of transport home should also be verified – a patient recovering from intravenous sedation could easily fall off the back seat of a motor bike!

Minimal adequate intravenous sedation

The point of minimal adequate sedation for a patient is not necessarily dose-related in the mg/kg weight; it should be determined by slow and careful administration and titration of the drug of sedation against the individual patient's response (**262**). The variable factors that may affect response to a drug of sedation are:

1. The age of the patient.
2. His sensitivity to the drug of sedation being administered.
3. His psychological profile.
4. His state of anxiety.
5. His weight.
6. The dosage of the drug of sedation that has been administered to the patient.
7. The speed at which the drug of sedation is administered to the patient.
8. The discomfort that may be caused to the patient by the dental procedure involved and the length of time that it takes.

Painless venepuncture

A small but significant number of patients are reluctant to undergo intravenous sedation due to their fear of needles and the pain or discomfort produced by venepuncture. However, this fear can be conquered by the use of a new topical local analgesic, which has been found to be effective in eliminating the offending pain or discomfort. The analgesic is a mixture of 2.5 per cent lignocaine plus 2.5 per cent prilocaine and can be applied to the skin prior to venepuncture. Each gramme of the white cream contains lignocaine base 25mg and prilocaine base 25mg in a eutectic mixture as an oil–water emulsion.

Contraindications for topical application

These include patients who are hypersensitive to analgesics of the amide type or who suffer from atopic dermatitis. Mucous membranes and open wounds should also be avoided.

Transient paleness, redness and occasional oedema have all been reported, while – when given parentally – prilocaine has been known to cause methaemoglobinaemia.

Although the systemic availability of prilocaine by percutaneous absorption is low, caution should be exercised in patients with anaemia, congenital or acquired methaemoglobinaemia, or with those receiving concomitant therapy known to produce such conditions.

The only drawback to the cream is that it has to be applied to the patient's intended venepuncture site (such as the dorsum of the hand or the cubital fossa) for one hour before the injection is to be undertaken (see below). The occlusive dressing containing the cream at the injection site sometimes produces a slight redness on the patient's skin and the cream itself on occasion produces some transient blanching of the skin. Generally these minor drawbacks are outweighed by the efficiency of the topical skin analgesia produced.

After 60 minutes the dressing is removed, the cream is wiped off and the area is cleaned with alcohol. The venepuncture may then be carried out without any discomfort to the patient.

Of all the techniques available for reducing the pain of venepuncture – such as spraying the skin with ethyl chloride prior to venepuncture – that described here is the most effective and painless.

Technique for painless venepuncture

267

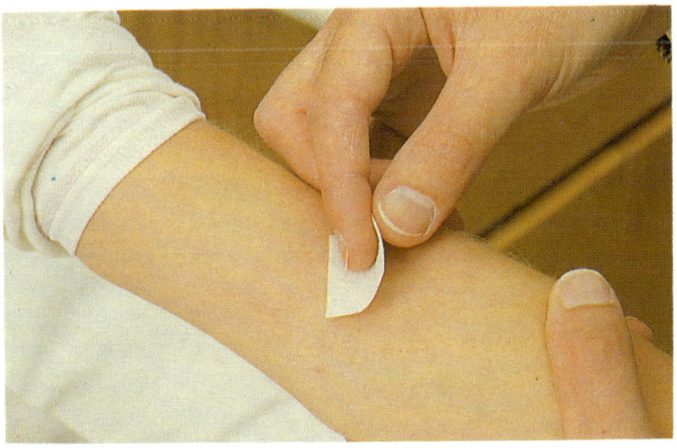

268

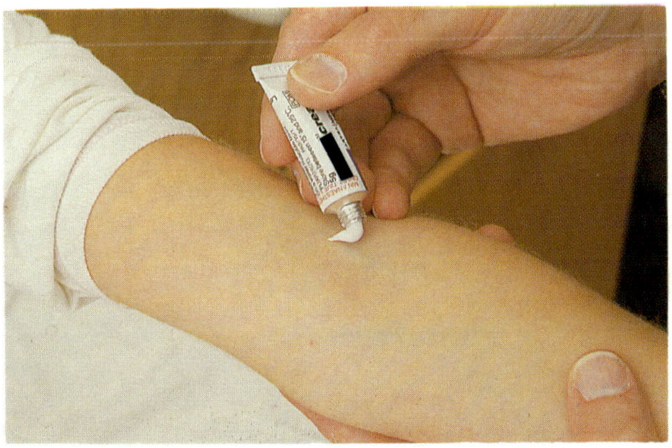

267 The site of the application of the cream is cleaned by wiping the intended venepuncture site with an isopropyl alcohol swab. Here, the cubital area above the cephalic vein is being cleaned on the lateral area of the patient's cubital fossa

268 About 1cm of cream is squeezed out in a mound on the area to be made analgesic

269

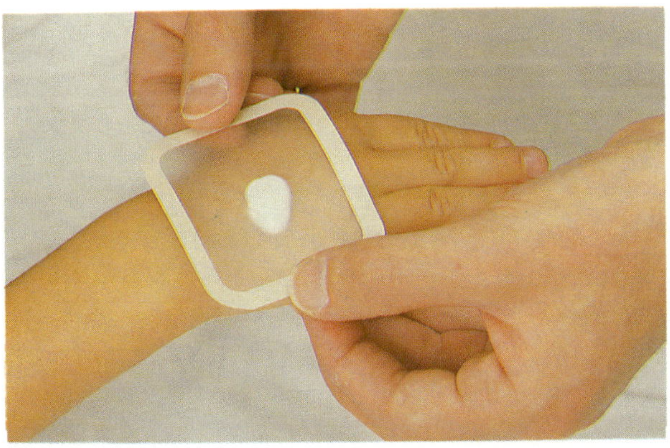

270

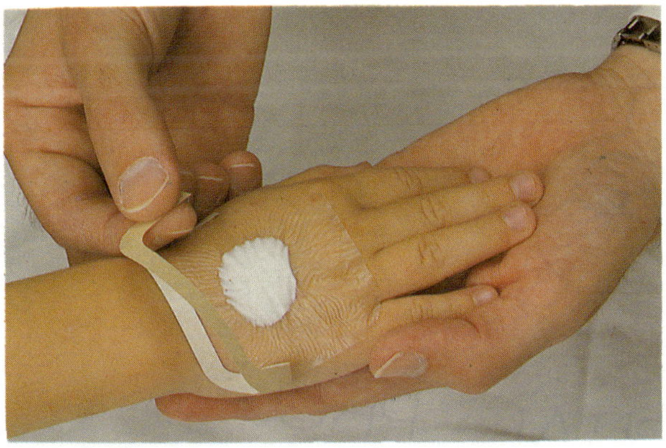

269 A peeled dressing is applied, covering the cream, which should not be spread

270 The paper frame is removed from the dressing, the edges of which are carefully smoothed down. The dressing is then left for 60 minutes. The time of application of the cream and dressing can be written on the occlusive dressing

Intravenous cannulation

This may be used as an alternative to the insertion of butterfly or straight metal needles for the administration of drugs of intravenous sedation. When a cannula is used in the cubital fossa it is still wise to use an arm support.

Insertion procedure

The selected site for cannulation is cleaned with an isopropyl alcohol swab and the cannula's container is checked to see that the contents are intact and that the expiry date has not been exceeded.

Dental surgeons should use this type of cannula only after being trained by an experienced colleague.

271

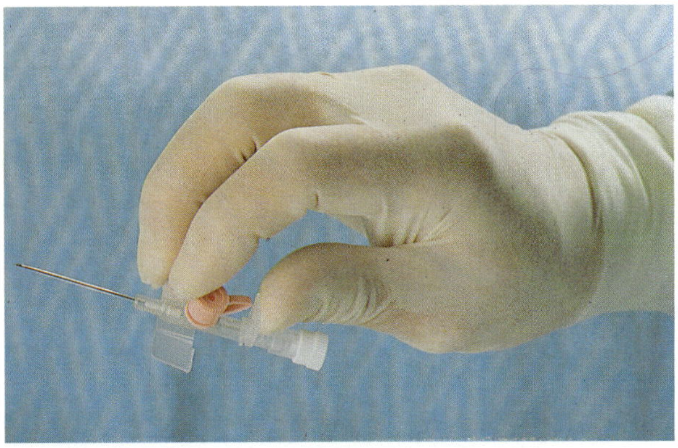

271 The design of the intravenous cannula enables a firm three-point grip to be used, minimizing the risk of touch contamination and allowing for accurate positioning between the needle point and the cannula

272

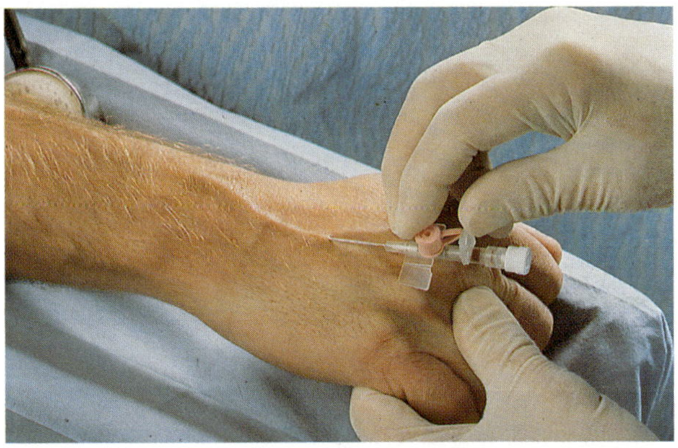

272 The cannula is inserted into the vein. Entry of the tip of the needle into the vein is indicated by the entry of blood into the flash-back chamber. The flow of blood is stopped by a control plug

273

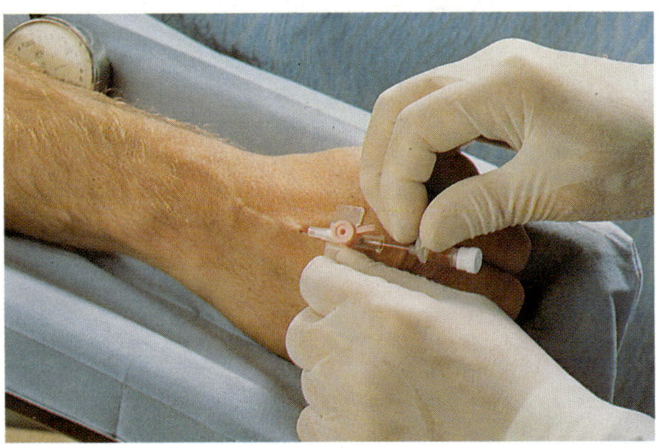

273 Before the cannula is advanced a few millimetres into the vein, the needle is partially withdrawn – by about 5mm – to avoid it emerging through the other side of the vein. After partial removal, the needle must never be reinserted while the cannula is in the vein, as this could result in the cannula being severed completely

274 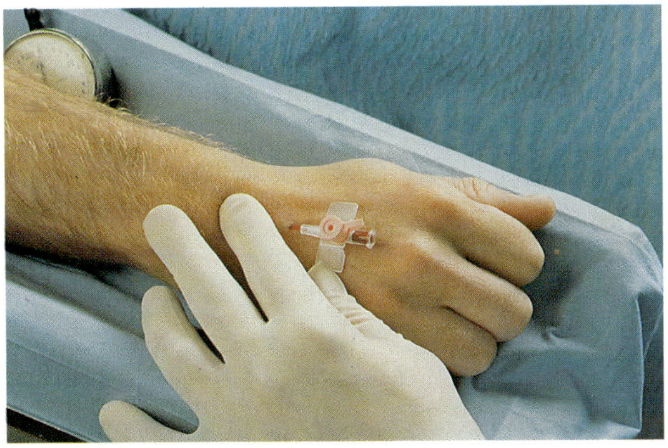

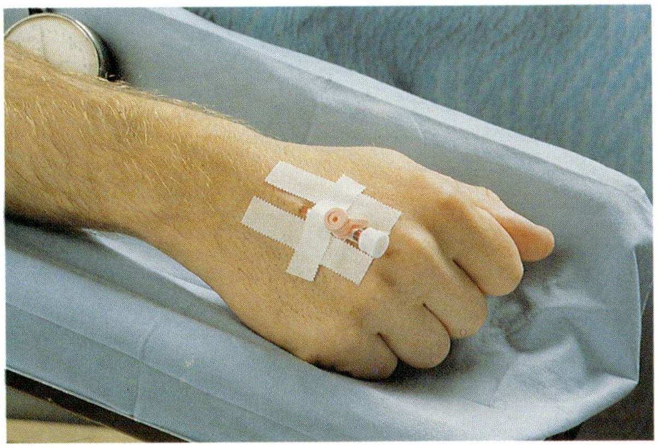 275

274 The needle is withdrawn completely. A finger pressed on the vein or below the cannula tip will prevent blood spillage

275 The cannula is sealed off with the luer lock plug. The flexible wings of the cannula are then secured to the patient's skin

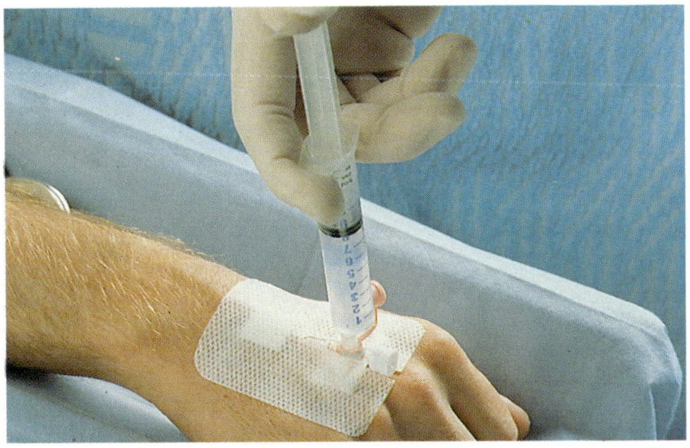 276

276 The puncture site can be covered with a sterile dressing. A safe and convenient way of administering drugs and/or flushing the cannula is via the injection valve

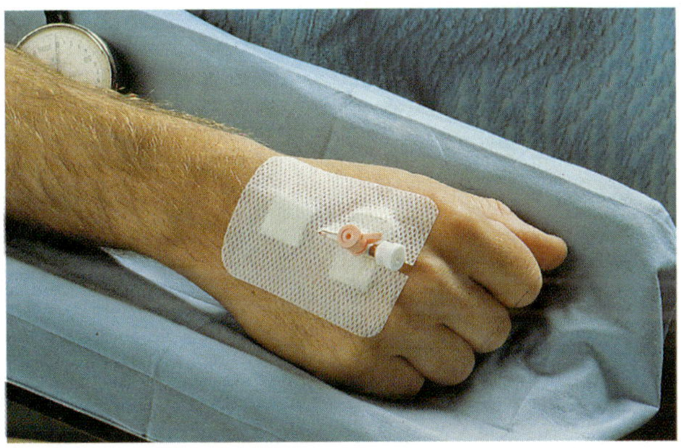 277

277 The injection valve must remain covered by protection caps when not in use

13 THE REVERSAL OF SEDATION

The availability of the benzodiazepine antagonist flumazenil within arm's reach of the dental surgeon and patient is a prerequisite to intravenous sedation when a benzodiazepine is used. Two practical examples of the use of the benzodiazepine antagonist are illustrated below.

278

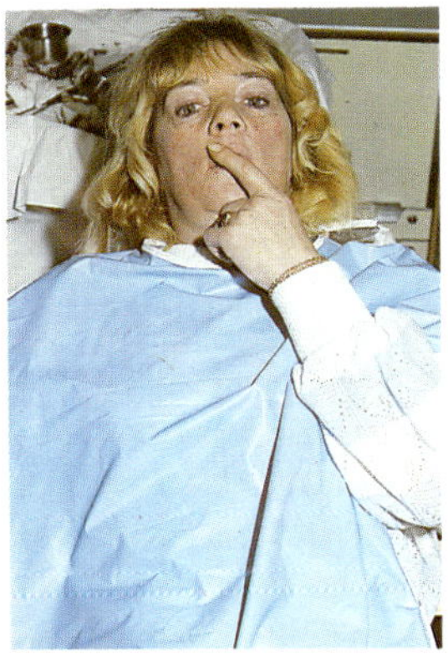

278 This patient has been sedated with 7mg of midazolam, and has reached the point of minimal adequate sedation. The objective observation was made when the EVE Sign was positive and slurred speech occurred. Note that the patient's eyes are wide open and that there is no drooping of the eyelids

279

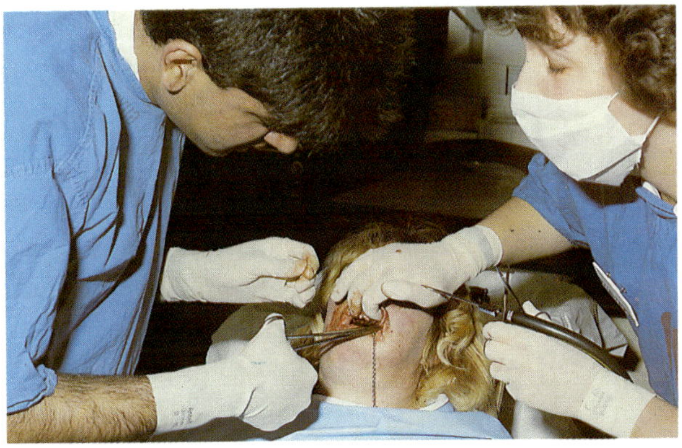

279 After completing the removal of buried roots under local analgesia, the dental surgeon sutures the wound

The patient is then taken to a recovery area to rest under observation. She is unsteady on her feet and needs to be supported by the dental surgery assistant. Within 20 minutes of the initial administration of the sedation it was decided (with the patient's prior consent) to use the benzodiazepine antagonist.

The administration of flumazenil (Anexate)

An initial dose of 0.2mg of flumazenil was administered through the butterfly, which was *in situ* on the dorsum of the patient's hand. The butterfly should always be retained in the vein throughout the procedure and not removed until the patient is well-recovered. There is no local reaction between midazolam and flumazenil and it is therefore quite safe to use the same indwelling butterfly needle.

Within seconds of receiving 0.4mg of flumazenil, the patient blinked her eyes and sat up. The EVE Sign was negative and normal speech had returned. The patient was allowed to stand and was completely stable on her feet. She could not recall the surgical procedure and in fact remembered nothing since the initial venepuncture had been carried out.

Fully recovered, the patient was allowed to sit down with her escort for a few minutes and the latter was given written and verbal post-operative instructions.

280

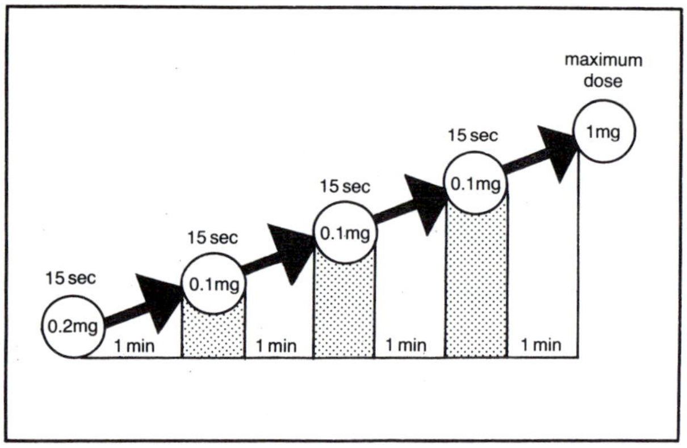

280 After the initial dose of 0.2mg flumazenil, which is given over 15 seconds, a minute is allowed to elapse. A further 0.1mg flumazenil may then be given, once again over a 15-second period. Using this form of titration, an optimum dosage of the antagonist of 0.4mg was found

The patient who was to be treated under intravenous sedation with midazolam first had the procedure explained to her and then signed an informed written consent.

She was requested to sign her name on a large art paper pad before the procedure commenced (**285**), and then to perform a control finger-to-nose movement to establish an EVE Negative Sign. The drug of sedation was then slowly titrated until the patient's finger-to-nose action became uncoordinated and/or inaccurate. Together with slurred speach, this display of EVE Sign Positive is a useful guide to when the point of minimal adequate sedation has been reached, occurring well before ptosis. In this case, 7mg of midazolam was titrated against the patient's response to obtain an EVE Sign Positive. The patient's eyes were open normally and there was no sign of ptosis.

Following sedation, the patient was again asked to sign her name (**285**). Her scrawled signature indicated a lack of coordination.

Flumazenil was administered using an initial dose of 0.2mg, which is given through the same retained butterfly needle through which the original midazolam was injected. This initial dose is administered slowly over 15 seconds; one minute is allowed to elapse before a further 0.1mg is titrated over 15 seconds. Using this form of titration, the optimum dosage of flumazenil was found to be 0.4–0.5mg. At this dosage, the patient was able to perform an EVE Negative Sign and no slurred speech was in evidence.

Next the patient was again requested to stand up, and this time was able to do so without any help.

It should be clearly understood that there is

281

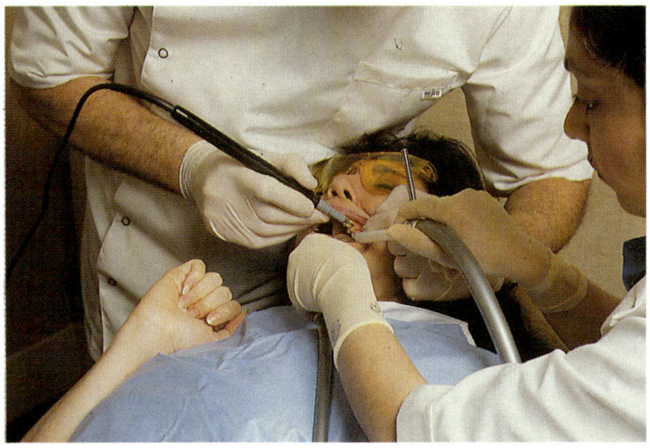

282

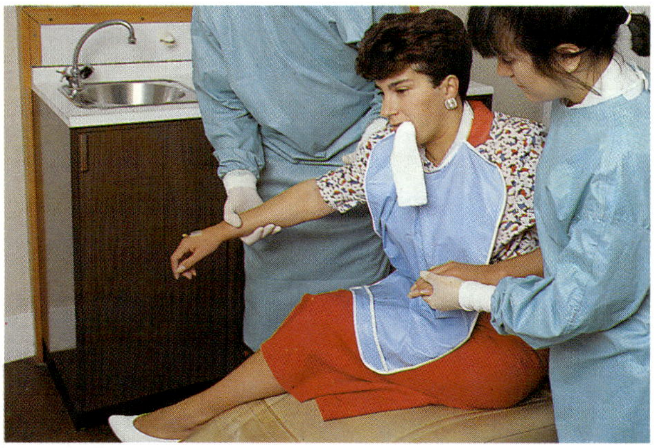

281 The dental procedure. The treatment in this case was periodontal. The patient raised her hand at one point and the dental surgeon asked her to repeat the EVE Sign. The result was positive; the patient's speech, too, was slurred, so no more midazolam was administered

282 On completion of the dental procedure, the patient – whose prior consent had been obtained – was asked to stand up carefully. She, being quite uncoordinated, was unable to carry out the instruction successfully, and had to be helped back into the dental chair

283

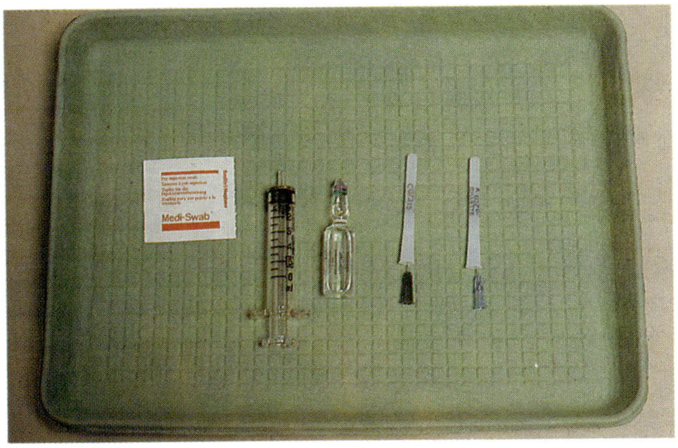

284

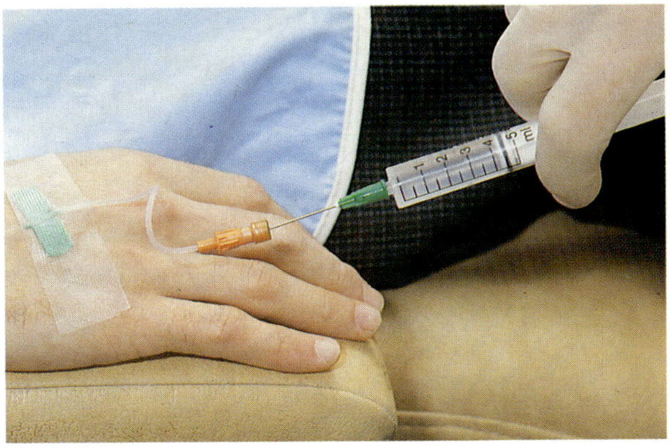

283 The flumazenil has been laid out on a separate disposable tray

284 Twenty minutes after the initial administration of midazolam, and following the successful completion of the dental procedure, the benzodiazepine antagonist was administered through the indwelling butterfly needle

no set dosage for sedation or for recovering a patient. All drugs used in intravenous sedation must be titrated slowly and carefully against the individual patient's response, and oversedation must be avoided.

Finally, the patient signed her name again, and the result this time closely matched her pre-sedated signature (**285**). This clearly demonstrates the excellent amnesic properties of midazolam and shows how the antagonist does not affect the amnesia in any way.

Although it is possible to discharge the patient into the care of a suitable accompanying person, the post-operative instructions remain unchanged; in particular: no alcohol, no driving, and no attempting to carry out complex procedures. These restrictions should be observed for the rest of the day.

The advantages of the benzodiazepine antagonist in the dental surgery are:

1. Its use as an emergency drug for oversedated patients
2. Full patient cooperation
3. A safer recovery phase.

Use as an emergency drug. Flumazenil's use as an antagonist to the overdosage of benzodiazepines such as midazolam makes it a drug of prime importance to the dental surgeon carrying out intravenous sedation techniques. It should be kept close to any patient undergoing sedation with midazolam; occasionally, a patient is found to be hypersensitive even to low doses of benzodiazepine, in which case the antagonist may actually save the patient's life.

It is well known that elderly patients are more sensitive to midazolam's potent effects. However, where its use is unavoidable – as when oral surgery is required and general anaesthesia is contraindicated due to respiratory insufficiency

285

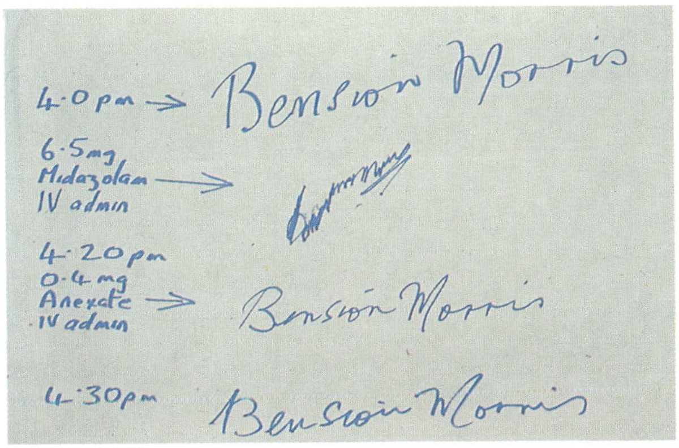

285 The patient's signature: before sedation (4 PM); after sedation, following administration of 6.5mg of midazolam; on completion of the dental procedure and following the reversal of the benzodiazepine (4.20 PM); and when fully recovered and resting in the recovery room with the accompanying person

or other medical reasons – then the presence of flumazenil must make the sedation safer. But whatever the circumstances, as a general rule elderly patients should not be submitted to sedation procedures as out-patients.

Full patient cooperation. When a patient is under sedation, he is in a state of disorientation and would be unable to cooperate effectively with the dental surgeon, as may be required in certain dental procedures, were it not for the antagonist. This enables the patient to be recovered fully, so that he can provide the dental surgeon with his invaluable assistance (**286** and **287**).

The preparation of extensive crown and bridge work is another procedure which benefits from the reversal of sedation. The anxious patient may be sedated with a benzodiazepine (midazolam) and, following the administration of a local analgesic, the crown preparations may be carried out. The traumatic part of the treatment over, the less unpleasant bite registration and accurate impression-taking can be proceeded with. A patient requiring surgery prior to the fitting of an immediate denture may first be sedated. Then, once the teeth have been removed, the sedation can be reversed to enable bite correction and the fitting of the denture to be carried out. These tasks are carried out more accurately with the patient's cooperation – which the use of an antagonist will make possible.

286

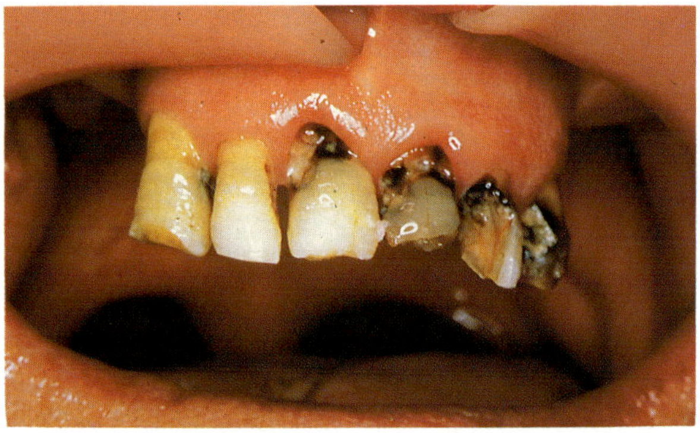

286 The mouth of an extremely nervous patient who requires the removal of teeth prior to the fitting of an immediate denture. The method of removal is to be under the administration of local analgesia which will be injected while the patient is sedated with midazolam

287

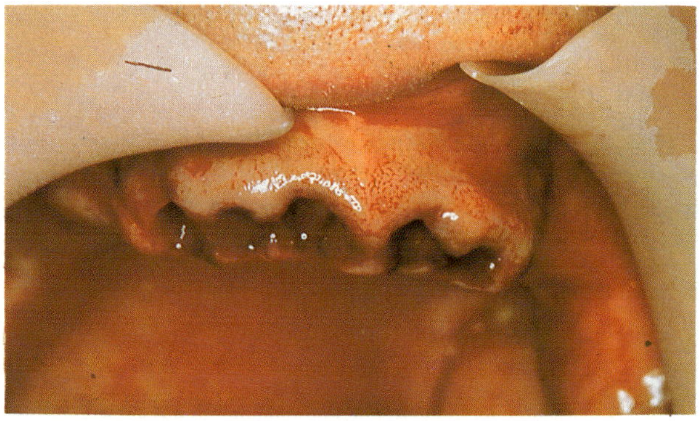

287 The teeth have been removed and the dental surgeon proceeds to fit the dentures. It is at this stage that the patient's cooperation is an advantage: having recovered fully by use of the antagonist, he can now indicate to the dental surgeon any areas of discomfort produced by the newly fitted dentures. Their occlusal relationship can also be improved if necessary, as the patient – being fully cooperative – can bite in a normal manner

Safer recovery phase. The patient who has undergone intravenous sedation with a benzodiazepine and – following completion of his dental treatment – has had his sedation reversed by flumazenil, may then be recovered in a sitting position. By virtue of the fact that the recently sedated patient is now fully aware and oriented, the final recovery phase is much safer.

The presence of the accompanying person sitting next to the treated patient is of psychological benefit: the patient has someone he knows to whom he can express relief or pleasure on completion of the supposedly traumatic dental procedure!

288

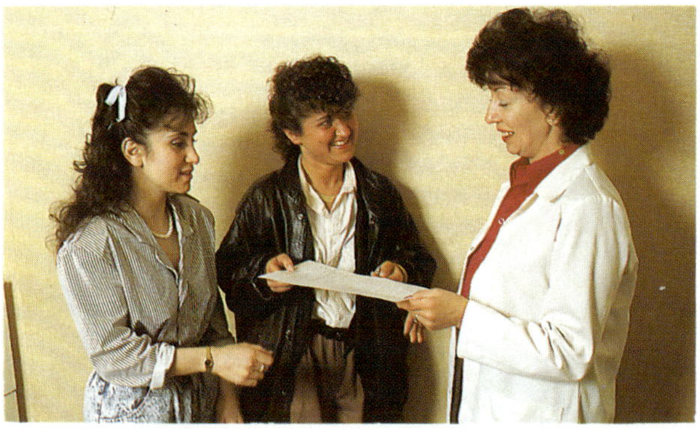

288 Following the patient's discharge by the dental surgeon, the dental surgery assistant hands the post-operative instructions to the accompanying person (rather than the patient herself – this despite the reversal of her sedation)

Basic principles to remember when using the antagonist

Only patients who have been carefully screened for their medical history and who fulfil the requirements for undergoing an intravenous procedure should be sedated. If any doubt exists about the safety of administering a benzodiazepine drug of sedation to a patient, the fact that an antagonist is available must not in any way influence the decision of the dental surgeon.

Precautions to be observed – the reversal of intravenous sedation

Following the introduction of any new drug, problems may arise with its usage. During the initial clinical trials of flumazenil, the author formed the impression that some patients preferred to recover lying down and that, during the recovery period, they should be allowed to fall into a natural sleep: some patients are simply not happy to be returned to normality immediately after their dental treatment.

This reasoning may also apply to patients who have undergone more extensive or painful procedures such as the removal of difficult teeth. To recover such patients suddenly, even though they have had local analgesia administered to them, may be very traumatic. Suddenly to become aware and to find a blood-soaked pack in the mouth may not be pleasant.

In normal circumstances, therefore, it would be better for patients who have had traumatic dental treatment to be allowed to recover naturally and in a supine position.

Some patients who recover following the use of an antagonist have said that their mind has recovered before their body. This is possibly due to the rapid reversal effect of the drug. Nevertheless, the patient must be allowed to sit for a few minutes with the accompanying person so that the dental surgeon can see and hear from the patient that he is fully normal before being discharged.

It would be most unwise for a dental surgeon to use the antagonist routinely to increase the patient work-load beyond the normal capabilities of the dental surgeon and his team. It would also be inadvisable to risk administering intravenous sedation to patients who would not normally be sedated due to their age, psychological make-up or medical history, merely because the antagonist is available.

Monitoring of the patient is highly desirable – but electronic monitoring must never replace that undertaken by a trained and observant dental surgery assistant.

Oxygen and all emergency equipment must be within an arm's length of the dental surgeon and second appropriate person.

Separate disposable trays are recommended to hold different drugs, so that there can be no possibility of any confusion in an emergency.

The post-operative instructions are explained verbally and given in writing to the patient's escort. The pre-arranged mode of transport home is rechecked (to exclude the possibility of the patient travelling on something unsuitable, such as the pillion of a motocycle – or even riding a bicycle!).

The recovered patient is then allowed to leave the dental surgery, in the company of the responsible adult escort. Both patient and escort are provided with a night and day telephone number where the dental surgeon may be contacted should any problems arise relating to the patient's dental treatment or the sedation procedure.

To recap: The availability of a benzodiazepine antagonist such as flumazenil (Anexate) should greatly increase the safety of intravenous sedation in the dental surgery, and its presence is therefore of paramount importance, providing for the reversal of oversedation in sensitive patients, and – where desirable – for a more controlled recovery.

14 FLUMAZENIL: THE FIRST BENZODIAZEPINE ANTAGONIST

Flumazenil (which is the generic name) is a specific benzodiazepine antagonist, and is one of the imidazobenzodiazepines. When one of this group of drugs is used, it brings about the rapid controlled reversal of sedation.

One of the most commonly used drugs for intravenous sedation in dentistry is midazolam, which is very potent and can easily produce oversedation if not handled carefully. As a result, the availability of flumazenil as an emergency drug is of great value to all dental surgeons using midazolam for intravenous sedation.

Flumazenil was discovered in 1978, through the investigation of a number of compounds which had a high *in vitro* affinity for the benzodiazepine receptor, but very weak intrinsic activity. A concerted effort was made to find an explanation for this apparent discrepancy using one of these compounds, Ro 14 – 5974.

Receptor binding experiments, as well as electrophysiological and behavioural drug-interaction studies, revealed a benzodiazepine antagonizing property. New tests for detecting such properties were set up, novel derivatives synthesized, and within a short time Ro 15 – 1788 (flumazenil) was selected as a reasonably pure benzodiazepine antagonist.

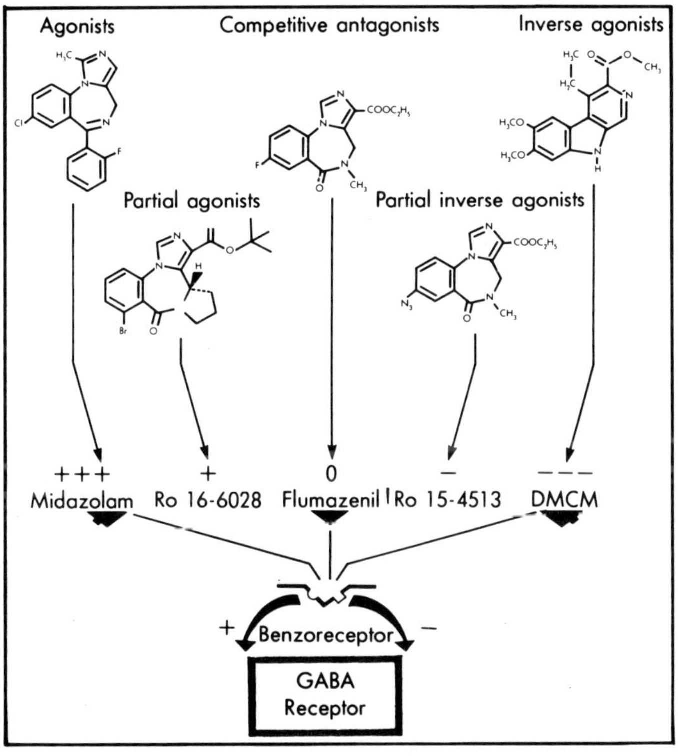

289

289 Schematic presentation of the various classes of ligands of the benzodiazepine receptor, amongst which flumazenil was isolated

The structure of flumazenil (Anexate)

The molecular structure of flumazenil has been determined by single crystal X-ray analysis. It was first synthesized by Dr. W. Hunkeler in 1979 in Basle. *See* **290** and **291**:

290

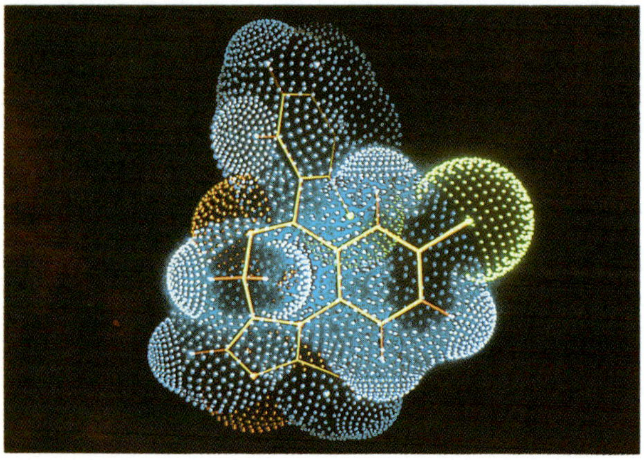

291

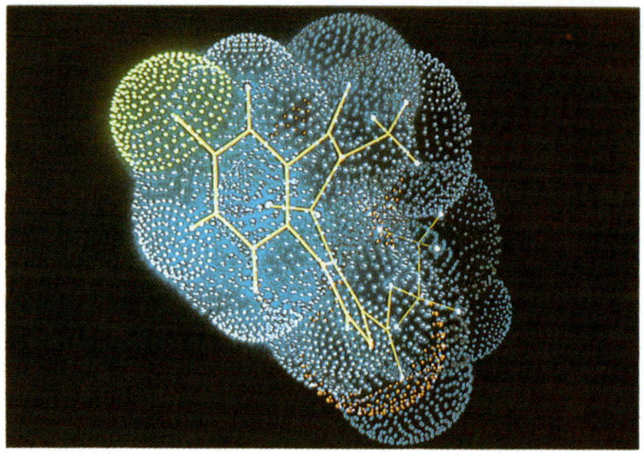

290 and 291 Midazolam and flumazenil, respectively. Atoms of each have been specifically colour-coded, and the dotted surface representation superimposed on the X-ray structure. KEY: white for hydrogen, yellow for fluorine, red for nitrogen and blue for oxygen

292

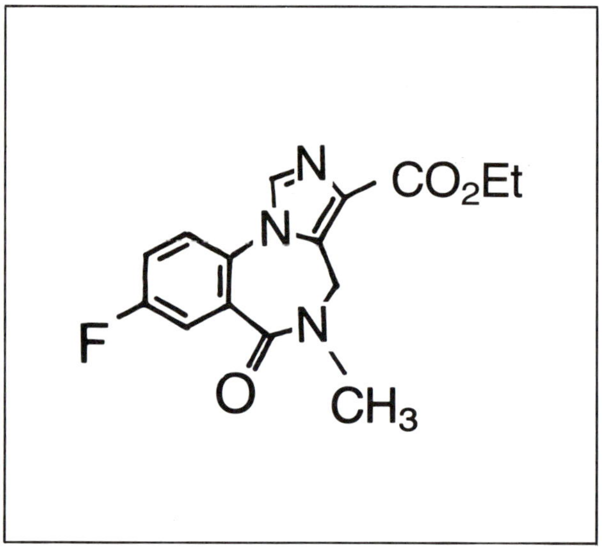

29

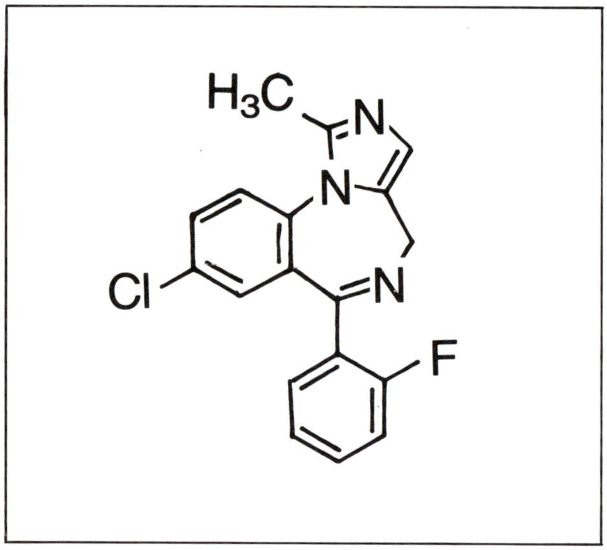

292 and 293 The benzodiazepine antagonist flumazenil is itself a benzodiazepine. It differs from classical benzodiazepines in the absence of the phenyl group, this being replaced in flumazenil by a carbolyn group

The principal properties of flumazenil

Biotransformation

Flumazenil is completely metabolized in the body to the free carboxylic acid Ro 15 – 3890 and the corresponding glucuronide. Carboxylic acid has no affinity with the benzodiazepine receptor.

Physicochemical data

Flumazenil is a crystalline, colourless powder with a melting point of 200°C. The pk of 1.7 indicates that it is a very weak base. The solubility in water is 0.4g per litre, which is sufficient to prepare aqueous solution for ampoules. The partition coefficient (n-octanol/aqueous phosphate buffer, pH 7.4) is 14.

Mode of action of flumazenil

Flumazenil competitively displaces the agonist from the benzodiazepine receptor. It has the effect of partly or completely reversing the action of agonists on the central nervous system.
Specificity of action. Flumazenil blocks only those pharmacological effects that are mediated by the benzodiazepine receptor.
Short elimination half-life (53 minutes). Flumazenil is easily controlled. The effect lasts 60–180 minutes, depending on the case. As midazolam has a half-life of 90–150 minutes, biliary circulation is unlikely. It therefore follows that on smaller dosages of midazolam, up to a maximum of 10mg, the return of sedation is most unlikely. But it is of the utmost importance that the dental surgeon should titrate the midazolam slowly and carefully against the individual patient's response. The total dosage of midazolam used is usually well below 10mg.
No intrinsic action. The action of flumazenil is limited purely to inhibiting or abolishing the effects of benzodiazepine agonists.
Tolerability. There appears to be good local and systemic tolerability. No impairment of liver or kidney function is known. Its use in anaesthesiology may in rare cases produce nausea and/or vomiting.
Controlled recovery. This can be achieved with appropriate dose titration. It can be useful in some cases where the dental surgeon wishes to lighten the sedation, such as in overdosage, but still have the patient in a sedated state.
No effect on pharmacokinetics. The pharmacokinetics of the benzodiazepine agonists remain unchanged, as do those of flumazenil.
Good local tolerability. Venous irritation is unlikely to occur – indeed, flumazenil may be considered to be as non-irritant as midazolam.

294

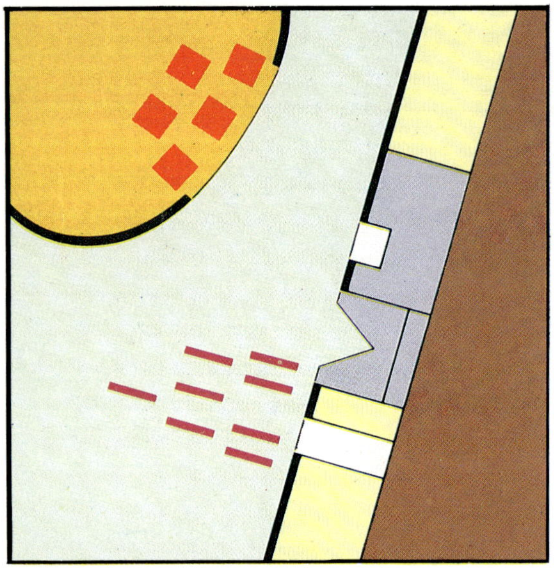

295

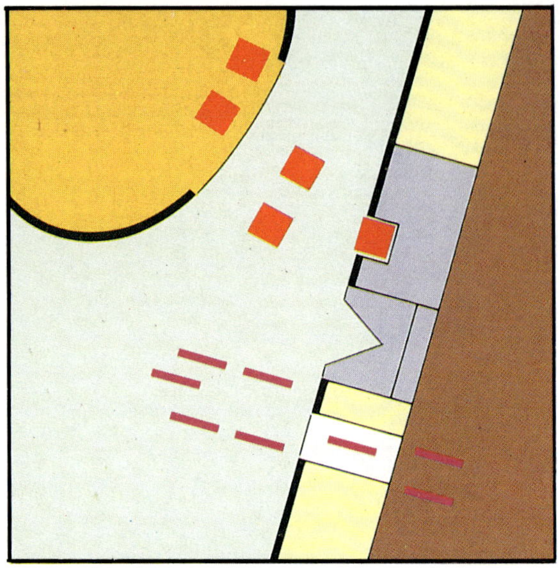

294 GABA (gamma-aminobutyric acid) is a major inhibitory neurotransmitter in the central nervous system. It is released from the presynaptic end of the neurone into the synaptic cleft and from there to the GABA receptor of the adjacent excitatory neurone

295 This has the effect of increasing the permeability of the neurone to chloride ions, thereby reducing its excitability

296

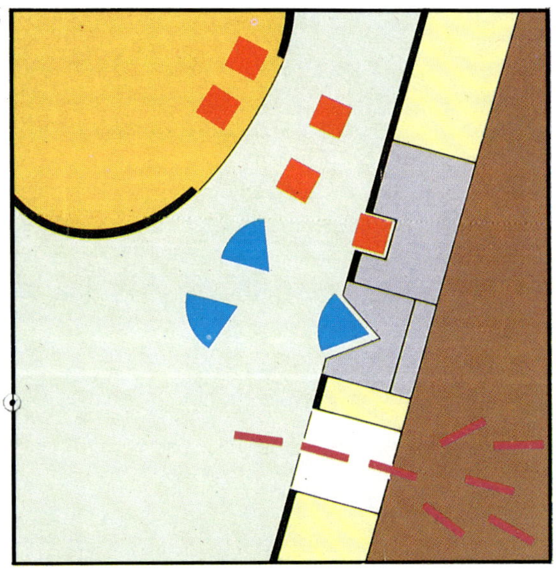

297

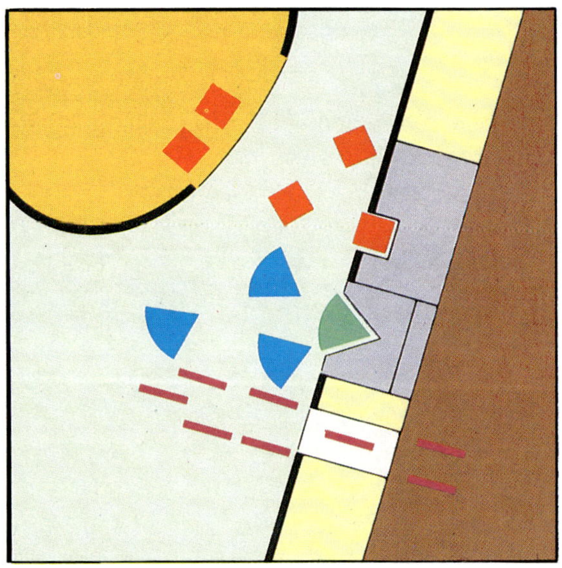

296 Benzodiazepines produce their therapeutic effect by potentiating the inhibitory action of GABA. This occurs at the benzodiazepine receptor, which is closely associated with the GABA receptor. When benzodiazepine agonists bind to the benzodiazepine receptor, the effect of GABA is increased and more chloride ions pass into the neurone, further reducing the excitability

297 Flumazenil has a high affinity for the benzodiazepine receptors and therefore displaces the benzodiazepine agonists from their sites. It has no significant intrinsic activity at the recommended dosage

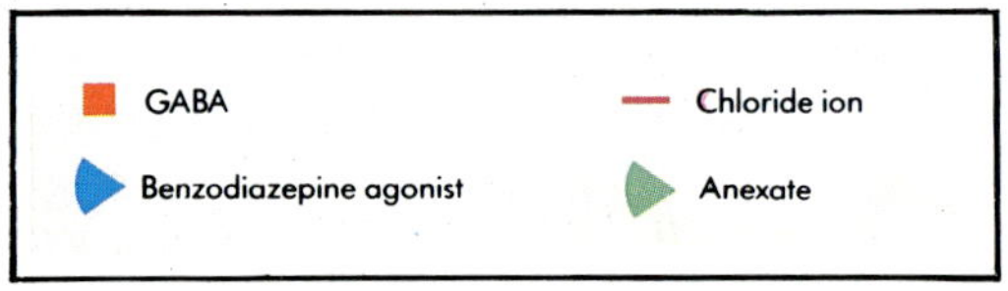

Simple dosing

The use of flumazenil to reverse the sedative effects of midazolam formed the subject of a dental study (Rosenbaum, Hooper, 1988) whose purpose was:

A To assess the efficacy of flumazenil in terms of:

1. The reversal of sedation
2. Increased cooperation
3. Increased coordination

B

1. To assess the effect of flumazenil on the patient's memory of the procedure
2. To assess the safety of flumazenil.

The efficacy of flumazenil was tested in a double blind placebo controlled study of 40 patients undergoing dental procedures. At five minutes and 30 minutes, respectively, flumazenil patients were: less sedated post-operatively, better orientated, and more cooperative.

None of the patients in either the placebo or the flumazenil group could remember operative events. It was felt that the flumazenil made recovery in the supine position unnecessary and post-operative monitoring easier.

No adverse reactions occurred in the trial. The authors concluded that reversal of sedation produced:

1. More cooperation on the part of the patient
2. A more coordinated patient.

This could lead to:

1. Recovery of the patient in the sitting position
2. Less monitoring during the recovery stage.

The amnesic properties of midazolam are well known and the study showed that flumazenil does not effect amnesia. It is therefore recommended that flumazenil be included in the armamentarium of any emergency drug kit when benzodiazepines are used intravenously.

15 THE DENTAL SURGERY TEAM

* It is recommended that any members of the dental team who are or who may be actively engaged in hands-on treatment of patients should consider being vaccinated against hepatitis B (Department of Health, 1990).

The receptionist

The receptionist is an important member of the dental team, being the patient's first contact at the surgery. In the event of an emergency occurring, the receptionist should be informed by a pre-arranged buzzer or light signal, or by internal telephone: **the second appropriate person must never leave the dental surgeon alone with a patient** under any circumstances whatsoever. The receptionist will keep the name and telephone number of the local consultant physician close at hand; also the number of a pre-arranged local hospital casualty department and ambulance facilities.

The receptionist should also participate in the routine practice of cardiopulmonary resuscitation, together with the rest of the dental team: in an emergency, every member of staff should be equipped and ready to act as resuscitator.

The dental surgery assistant

The dental surgery assistant's responsibility begins when she receives the patient in the waiting room. She should be of a pleasant disposition so as to place a nervous patient at his ease. She should ask the patient if he would like to visit the toilet and should check when food and drink were last consumed. The dental surgery assistant should confirm that a second accompanying person is present and that a suitable mode of transport has been laid on to take the patient home.

It is advisable also to check whether the patient is taking any new medication or has suffered any illness since the initial visit when the intravenous sedation procedure was arranged. The dental surgery assistant should report any adverse findings to the dental surgeon prior to the sedation being administered.

As Second Appropriate Person: training necessary

An adequately trained dental surgery assistant may act as the Second Appropriate Person when intravenous sedation is to be carried out. The definition of a second appropriate person was provided by the General Dental Council in its Notice for the Guidance of Dentists (Professional Conduct and Fitness to Practise, November 1989):

'Where intravenous or inhalation sedation techniques are to be employed a suitably experienced practitioner may assume the responsibility of sedating the patient, as well as operating, provided that as a minimum requirement a second appropriate person is present throughout. Such an appropriate person might be a suitably trained dental surgery assistant or ancillary dental worker, whose experience and training enable that person to be an efficient member of the dental team and [who] is capable of monitoring the clinical condition of the patient. Should the occasion arise, he or she must also be capable of assisting the dentist in case of emergency.'

The training of the dental surgery assistant is the direct responsibility of the dental surgeon.

She can reasonably expect to receive regular tuition in how to monitor and look after patients, and also in what to do and how in emergency situations – this must include regular practice in cardiopulmonary resuscitation. A basic training manual, in which practice procedures are laid down, should be kept in all dental practices. After reading the procedures, staff should sign a staff training book designed for the purpose. The same book should be signed and dated by members of staff following cardiopulmonary resuscitation training sessions.

Monitoring

Although it is desirable to use monitoring apparatus on a sedated patient, its use should always be in conjunction with direct monitoring by the dental surgery assistant. She must monitor the patient visually as well as physically from the time he arrives in the waiting room until when he is discharged by the dental surgeon into the care of a suitable accompanying person. This direct monitoring means that the dental surgery assistant will be observing the patient's colour and vital signs constantly and will be capable of accurate pulse recording (**298**).

She may prevent a patient suffering a fear-induced vasovagal attack or, possibly, from experiencing a hypoglycemic episode from lack of food. The latter can be remedied by a small glucose drink – subject to the dental surgeon's agreement. An experienced dental surgery assistant may notice an allergic reaction or a change in vital signs long before the preoccupied dental surgeon realizes a complication is arising: it is important that the dental surgeon takes immediate notice of any information provided by the dental surgery assistant.

In the event of the patient collapsing, the dental surgery assistant's training should equip her to carry out cardiopulmonary resuscitation, should the dental surgeon be otherwise engaged. She must also be capable of monitoring pulse oximetry and recording blood pressure, and be able to understand the recorded information provided by the monitors and know how to act should a problem be observed (**299**).

298

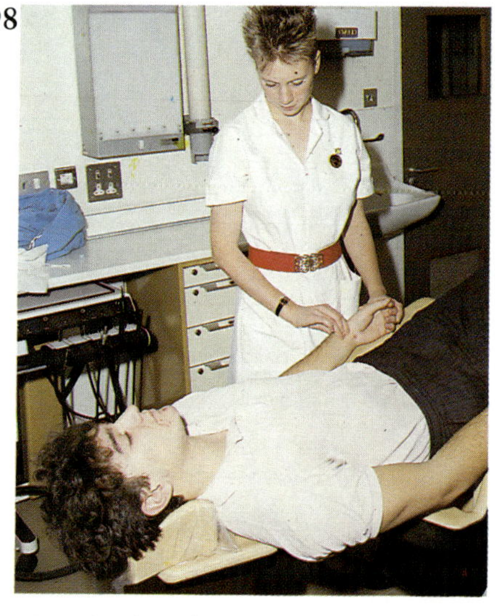

298 The dental surgery assistant must be capable of taking a radial pulse by the direct method

299

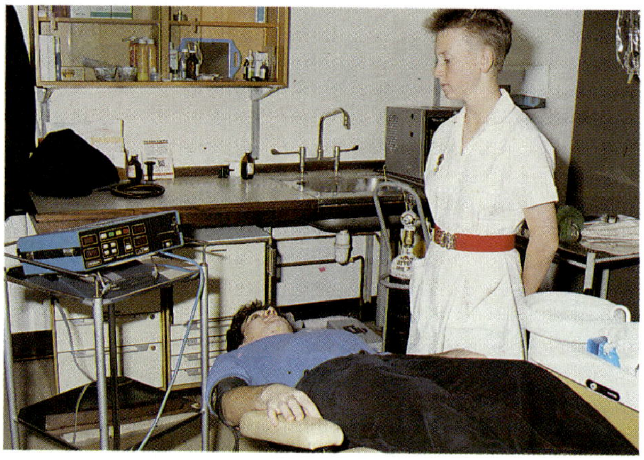

299 The dental surgery assistant must also be able to operate and understand the monitoring apparatus. Here, she observes a machine which records blood pressure and pulse rate at pre-set regular intervals

300

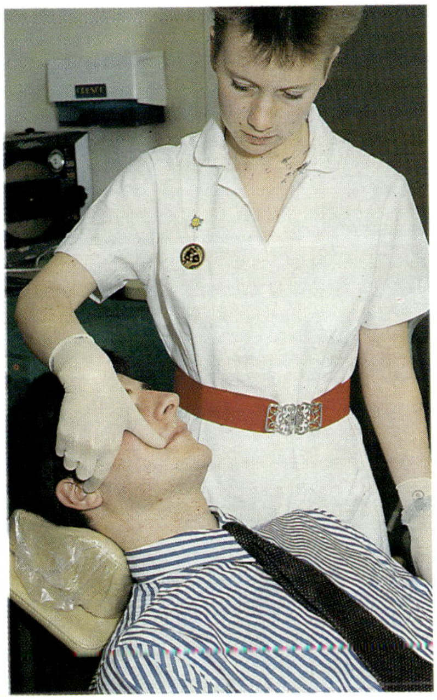

301

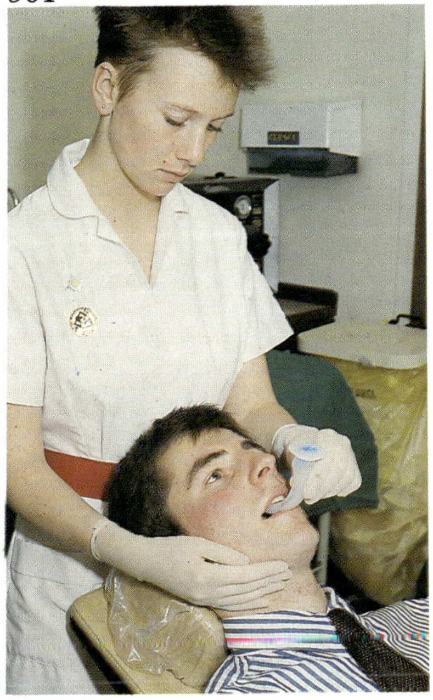

302

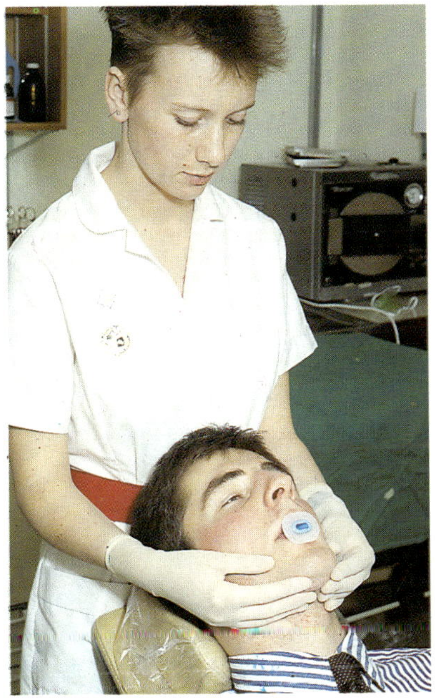

300 The dental surgery assistant measures from the tragus of the ear to the angle of the mouth to find the size of a suitable disposable oropharyngeal (Guedel) airway

301 The Guedel airway is inserted over the tongue, and then rotated 180° over the dorsum of the tongue into the oropharynx

302 The airway in place, the dental surgery assistant supports the patient's jaw upwards and forwards

303

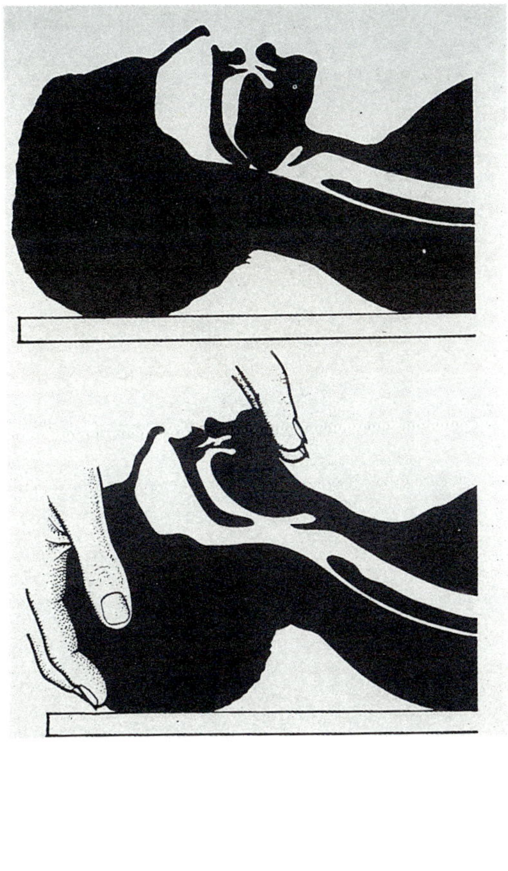

303 **Right:** the correct maintenance of the airway. The chin is directed forwards and upwards, and the front of the head is pushed gently back, so that the oropharynx is clear. The oropharyngeal airway can then be inserted. **Above right:** the collapse of an unsupported airway. The tongue and soft palate fall back to block the oropharynx, and thereby obstruct the airway. **Death from anoxia will occur within three minutes if the airway is not cleared**

304

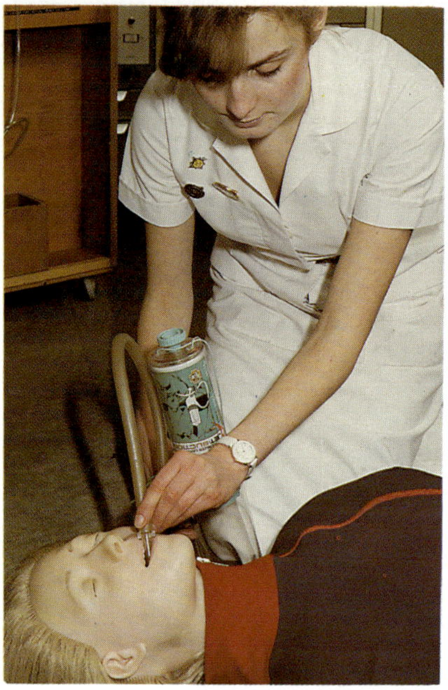

305

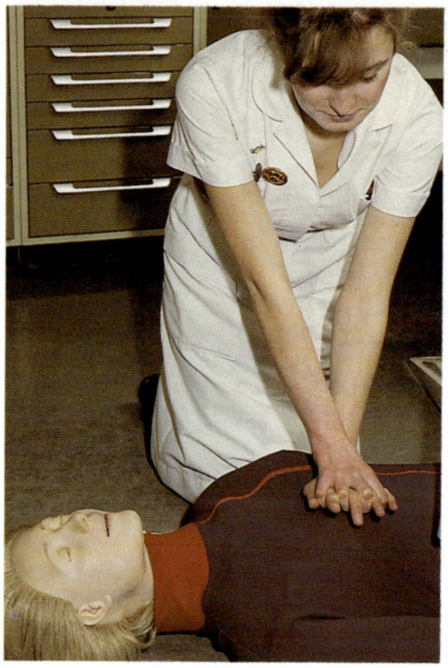

304 The dental surgery assistant practising on a manikin. She has laid the collapsed 'patient' flat and is aspirating the oropharynx using an emergency aspirator which works off a vacuum can and which can therefore be used in the absence of electricity

305 The dental surgery assistant practising external cardiac massage. When cardiopulmonary resuscitation is carried out correctly, a bulb connected to the manikin lights up. Note the dental assistant's straight arms and linked fingers

306

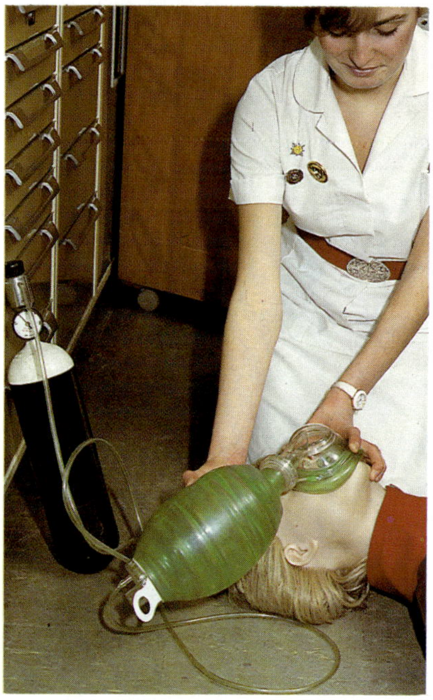

306 The dental surgery assistant is taught how to administer oxygen whilst maintaining the patient's airway

307

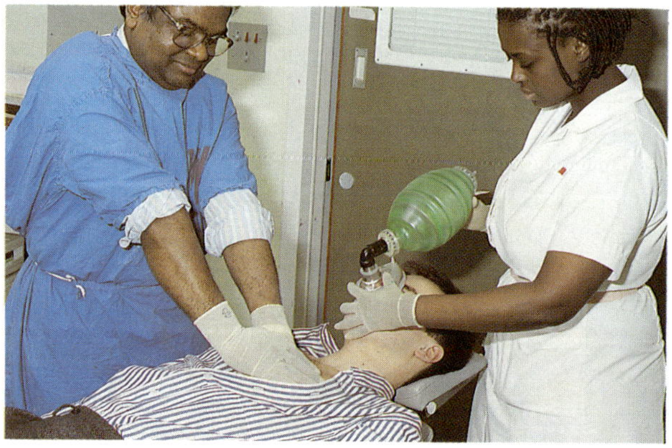

307 A practice session involving cardiopulmonary resuscitation. The dental surgery assistant administers oxygen via an ambu bag, which delivers oxygen under pressure

308

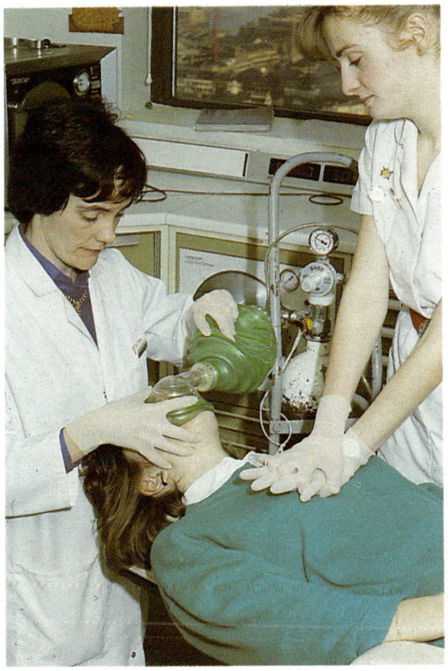

308 The dental surgeon administers oxygen while the dental surgery assistant carries out external cardiac massage

309

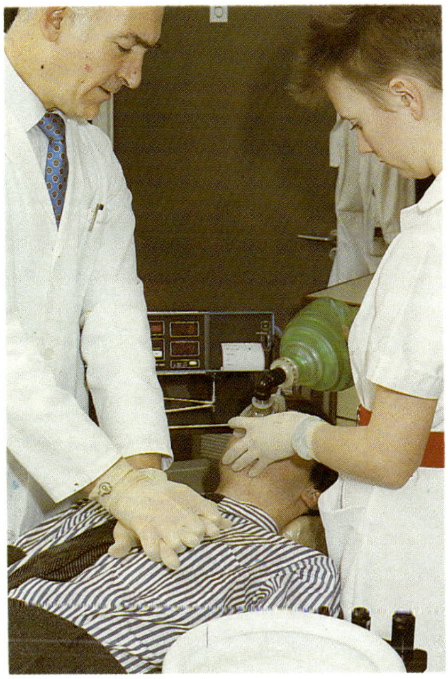

309 All cardiopulmonary resuscitation practice sessions should be made as realistic as possible. A dental chair in the supine position makes an adequate enough firm base upon which to carry out external cardiac massage – it is not always necessary to place the patient on the floor. (In fact, the height and support of the dental chair make cardiopulmonary resuscitation less difficult than carrying out the procedure at floor level.)

310

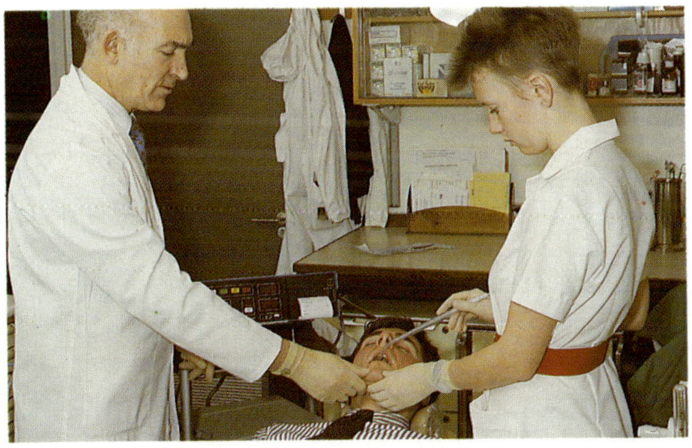

310 The dental surgeon demonstrates the maintenance of the airway while the dental surgery assistant clears the oropharynx with an aspirator. The technique required to perform two procedures simultaneously, such as maintaining the airway while operating or delivering oxygen via an ambu bag, is one that requires practice

311

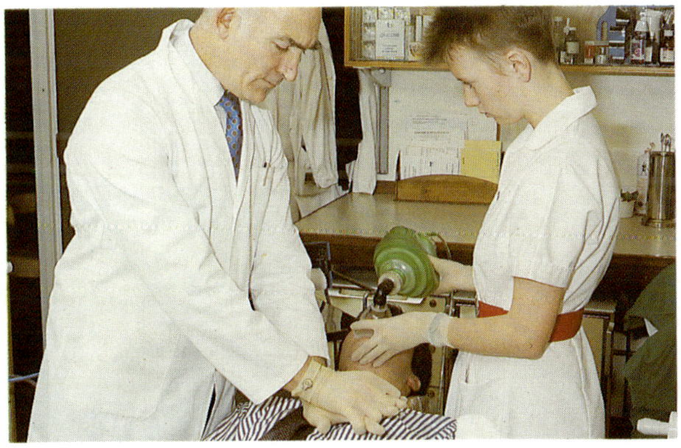

311 The dental surgeon's confidence in his dental surgery assistant to carry out two procedures in a competent manner leaves him free to perform external cardiac massage

Summary

As has been demonstrated, a trained dental surgery assistant, acting as a second appropriate person, should be able to carry out *any* of the preceding procedures. Where necessary, she should be competent enough to take over such tasks from the dental surgeon – be it external cardiac massage or maintaining the airway and administering oxygen under the direction of the dental surgeon. The dental surgery assistant should also be familiar with drugs that may be required during an emergency situation.

With the emergency practice drill being carried out at regular intervals, the dental surgery assistant will soon become an essential second appropriate person, and may well be responsible for saving a patient's life. A dental surgery assistant who is unable to carry out the emergency procedures and/or who has not participated in regular practice sessions *cannot* be considered to be a second appropriate person.

Should an emergency occur and the dental surgeon and his assistant are unable to cope, with the result that the patient is injured or even dies, then the dental surgeon will be answerable to his peers for possible professional negligence.

16 COMPLICATIONS WITH INTRAVENOUS SEDATION

Complications with intravenous sedation may be classified as local, systemic or general (including psychological problems).

Local complications

Intravenous injection of any fluid may result in reactions at the site of injection, ranging from transient pain during the actual injection to the delayed response of thrombophlebitis. However, there is no clear distinction between conditions, indeed sometimes they may overlap – which makes their accurate definition vital. Local complications can also include localized accidents, such as the damage that can be caused by the needle itself.

Phlebitis. This underlying inflammatory condition is characterized by reddening, oedema and pain. It is minimal in duration and there is no thrombus formation. When sufficiently marked to warrant reporting, it is often classed as a 'mild thrombophlebitis'.

Haematoma. This complication of intravenous sedation manifests as a swelling containing blood and tissue fluid. In a normal patient it is due to damage to the blood vessel and surrounding tissues resulting from a faulty venepuncture technique. Depending upon the degree of damage and its cause, the blood vessel swells and blood escapes into the surrounding area, producing bruising (**312**).

312
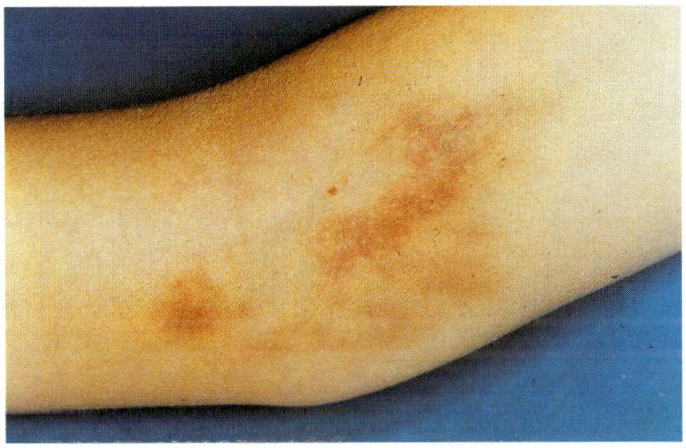

312 Haematoma resulting from a faulty venepuncture technique

313
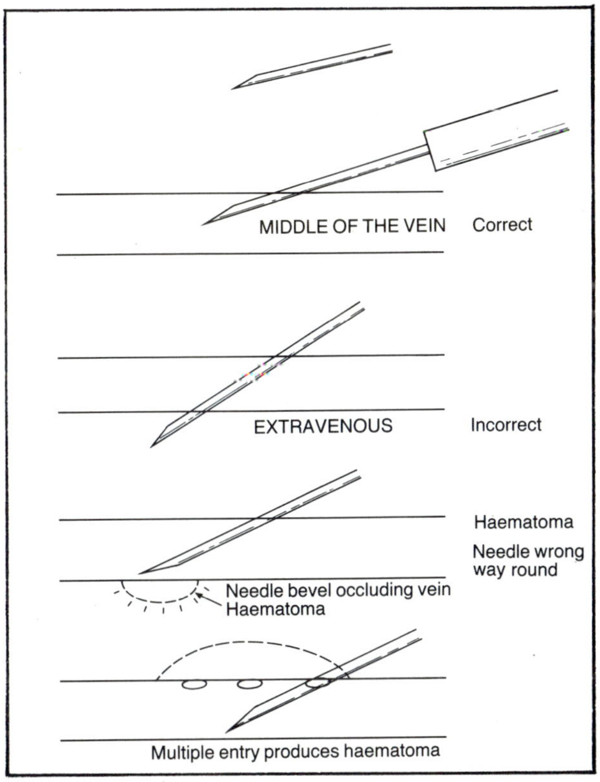

313 Correct positioning of the needle within the lumen of the vein is of prime importance in the administration of drugs in sedation techniques. Note that the needle should never be used upside down

314 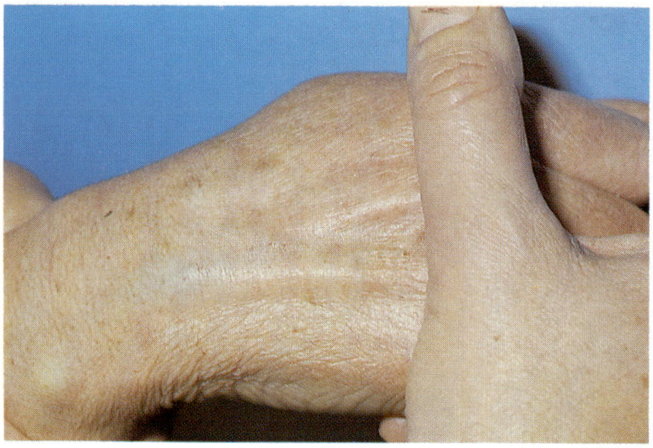 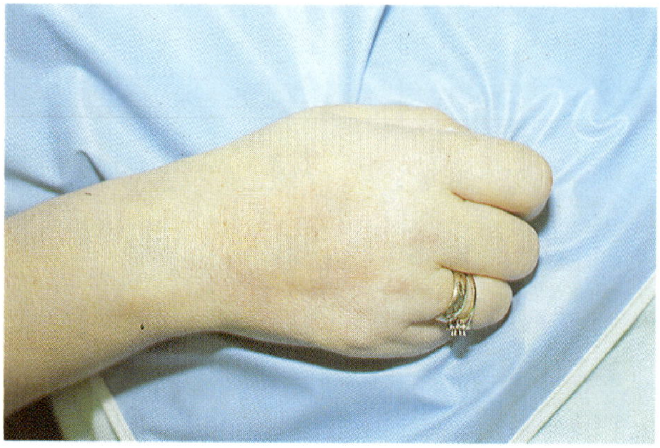 315

314 and **315** Examples of extravenous injection on the dorsum of the hand

To prevent extravenous injection:

1. Make sure the needle is within the vein before injecting the contents of the syringe.
2. If venepuncture fails on two attempts, do not use the same vein for a third attempt.
3. Use as large a vein as possible at the chosen site.
4. Do not persist in venepuncture if you fail a few times. It is better to make another appointment.

Careful observation of the site around the point of venepuncture as the syringe is depressed will usually show whether the needle is intravenous or extravenous, or wrongly positioned against the vein wall.

Treatment of accidental extravenous injection

316 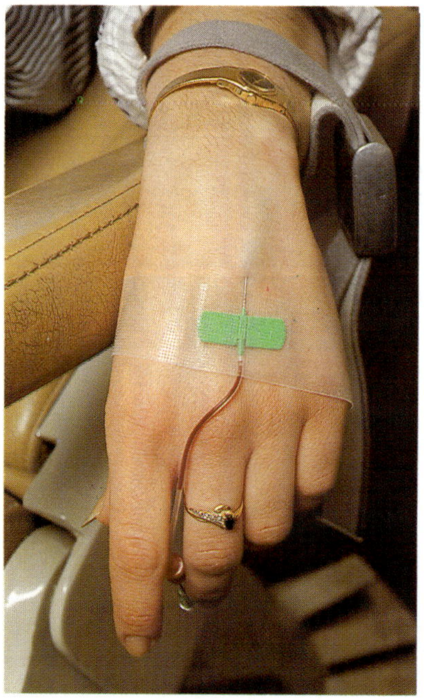 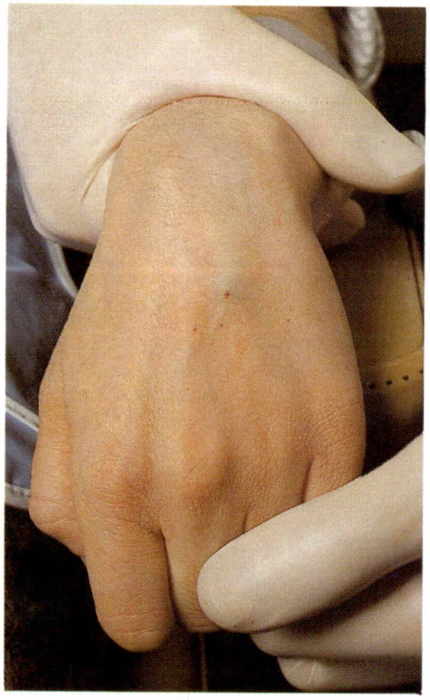 317

316 An extravenous haematoma with the butterfly needle *in situ*

317 The butterfly needle has been withdrawn

1. If the correct intravenous technique is used, an extravenous injection may be detected almost immediately it occurs.
2. The needle should be withdrawn.
3. An isopropyl alcohol swab should be applied to the damaged site. A dressing is then placed over the wound.
4. The patient should be reassured.
5. The damaged limb should be raised straight upwards and held thus for two minutes. This procedure will considerably reduce any swelling or bruising.

Phlebothrombosis. Here there is neither pain nor inflammation, but there is induration, assumed to be caused by an underlying thrombus.

Thrombophlebitis. A combination of the above conditions in which there is oedema, inflammation and tenderness, with a raised, hardened area following the course of the infected vein (**318**). Onset of signs can vary between one or two days and some weeks.

Providing the patient with reassurance – administered in the course of regular visits until the condition improves or disappears – is the best treatment for thrombophlebitis. Some dental surgeons advocate the use of an infra-red lamp to relieve the discomfort.

The incidence of thrombophlebitis with any intravenous drug used for sedation may be lessened by:

318

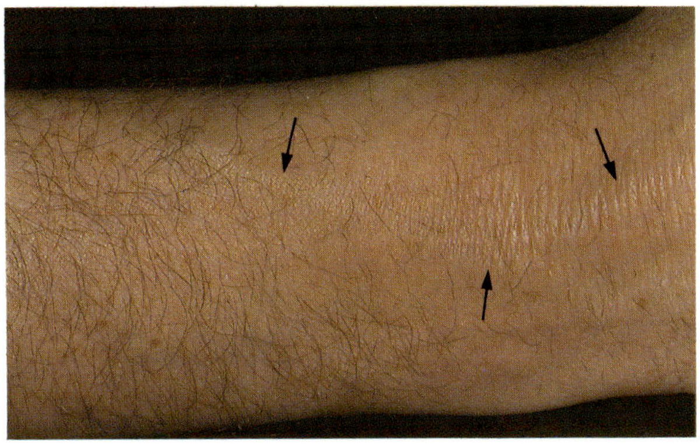

318 Thrombophlebitis – the infected vein is arrowed

1. Selecting a large vein with relatively unrestricted blood flow.
2. Using small-gauge needles to minimize the trauma.
3. Careful venepuncture.
4. Observation of the venepuncture site for swelling suggesting extravascular injection or haematoma on initial intravenous administration of a drug.
5. Slow injection of the intravenous drug.
6. The second appropriate person observing the patient's general condition, i.e. colour, pulse, at all times – especially while the dental surgeon is carrying out the procedures.

There is no record – to the author's knowledge – of a thrombus becoming detached and entering the major venous system; this quite simply does not seem to occur.

Causes of local reactions

It seems that there is no single cause for local reactions but rather a number of contributory factors which predispose towards their occurrence.

For example, the trauma caused by venepuncture may result from:

1. More than one venepuncture in the same vein.
2. A poor intravenous technique.
3. Using a damaged needle.
4. Not holding the overlying skin of the vein taut and so scraping the vein on entry.
5. Too rapid an injection, which can damage the vein's lining.
6. Attempting venepuncture with too large a needle.
7. Attempting venepuncture with too small a needle.
8. Using a drug which contains irritant properties, e.g. propyline glycol in ethanol.

Diazepam itself may also be a causative factor: it is poorly soluble in water and aqueous media, and dilution of the ampoule solution may result in a fine, pale yellow microprecipitate, which increases in turbidity on standing (Rosenbaum, 1982). These properties apply mainly to aqueous diazepam, and can therefore be circumnavigated by using midazolam or diazepam in its emulsified form.

Complications caused by damaged needles

Though rare these have occurred, and it is therefore essential to examine any needle being used for venepuncture before commencing with the procedure.

All butterfly needles should be carefully examined after withdrawal. It is important, where a needle fracture or an accident due to a faulty needle occurs, to retain all the pieces of the damaged needle, together with accurate notes recording what occurred – the latter written at the time of the incident.

319

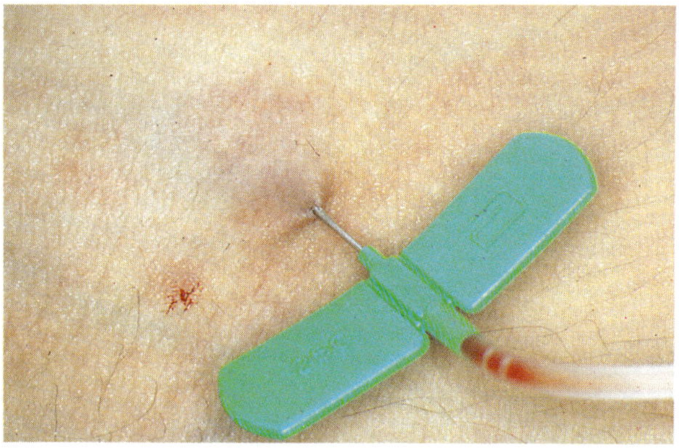

3

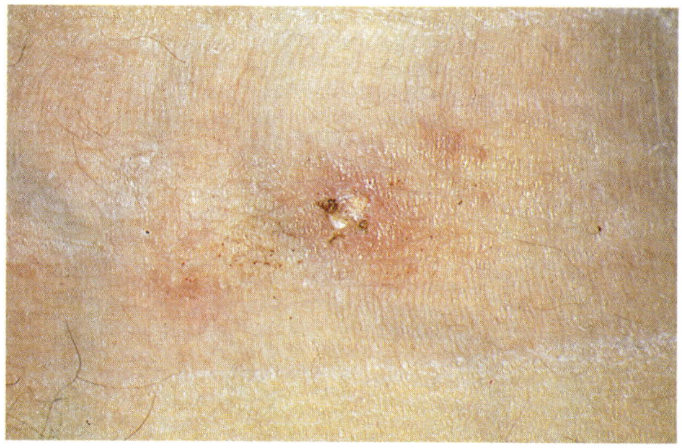

321

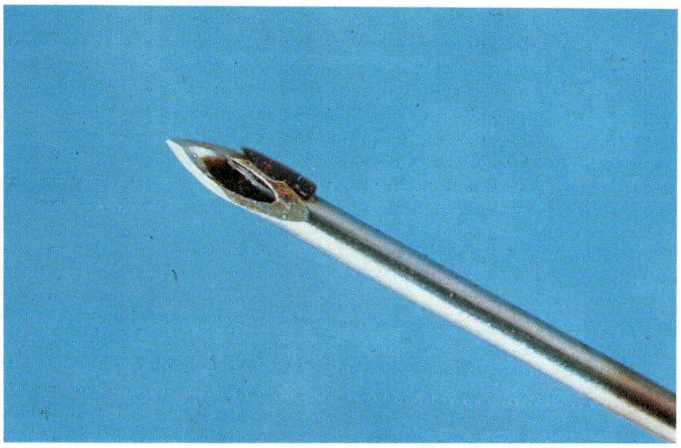

319–321 Difficulty in withdrawing the butterfly needle (**319**) led to its surgical removal by dissection (**320**). The wound was then dressed. Following examination of the butterfly, the needle was found to be faulty (**321**)

322

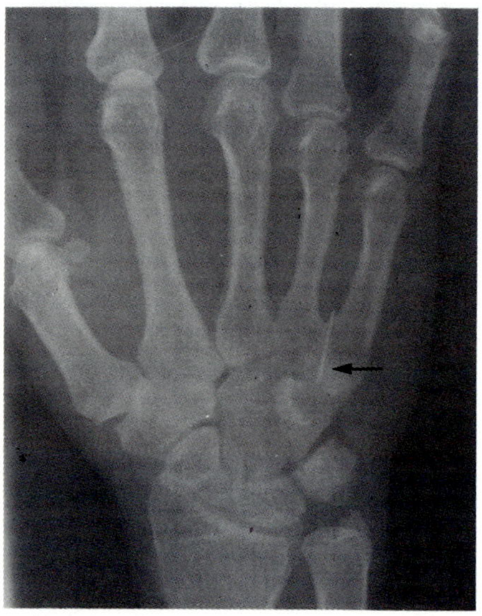

322 A complication affecting a patient undergoing venepuncture on the dorsum of the hand arose with the discovery – some time after the operation – of this metal needle (arrow) embedded in the hand. Although the needle's absence had been noted following removal from the hand of the butterfly, it was only when, a while later, the patient became restless that its location was discovered. It was subsequently removed under a second analgesic without further problems

Local complications following the use of Cryo spray

Some dental surgeons favour spraying the skin area designated for venepuncture, to reduce the discomfort of nervous patients. Ethyl chloride is most commonly employed (**323** and **324**), but care must always be taken not to use too much since, as well as being highly inflammable, its fumes are analgesic. Furthermore, it is unwise to use a Cryo spray for the purpose of painless venepuncture, as it can very easily burn the skin – as can become apparent after the spray has evaporated (**325** and **326**).

323

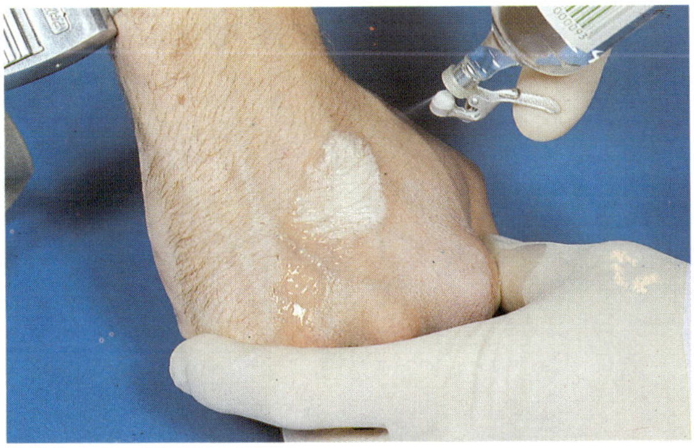

323 The application of ethyl chloride means venepuncture can be carried out painlessly

324

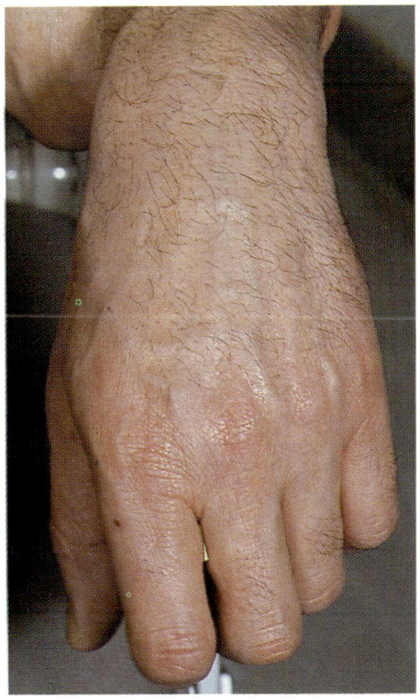

324 After evaporation of ethyl chloride. Note that the hand is undamaged

325

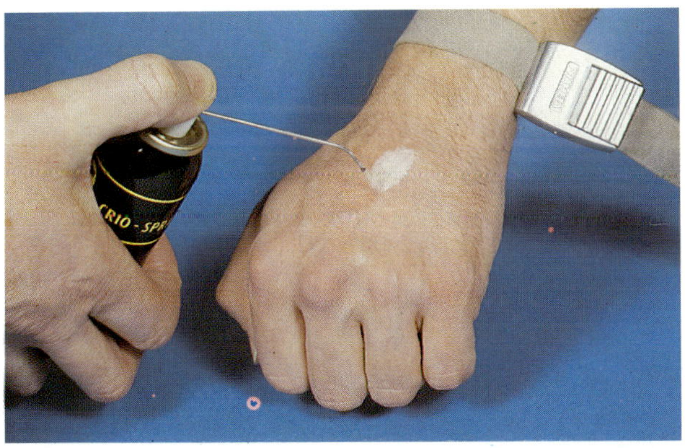

325 Cryo spray is applied

326

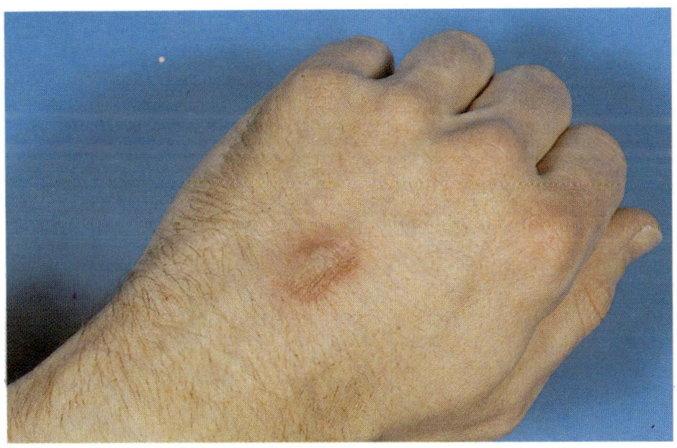

326 Dorsum of the hand following evaporation of Cryo spray. Note burn inflicted

General complications

Respiratory depression – local obstruction

When a patient has any dental or medical condition where the airway is threatened, intravenous sedation is contraindicated. It is important, too, that the basic surgical principle of not injecting into an infected area is strictly observed: not only can an infection be rapidly spread by injection into an infected site, but the resultant swelling can quite easily cause a respiratory obstruction. This type of complication can be avoided by:

1. Correct patient assessment.
2. Controlling an acute infection by drainage and/or antibiotics. Once the infection is controlled and the swelling eliminated, the surgery can be carried out with local analgesia and intravenous sedation if indicated.
3. Urgent surgery carried out under general anaesthesia at an in-patient hospital unit. The anaesthetist is able to establish a safe airway by intubation. Should any problems arise, expert medical staff are at hand.
4. Avoiding injecting into any infected or infected and swollen areas in the mouth. Any swelling on the floor of the mouth, in particular, can lead to respiratory obstruction.

Cases unsuitable for intravenous sedation and local analgesia

The following illustrated conditions (**327–333**) are not suitable for intravenous sedation due to the possibility of obstruction of the patient's airway.

KEY
MH = mylohyoid muscle GG = genioglossus muscle

327

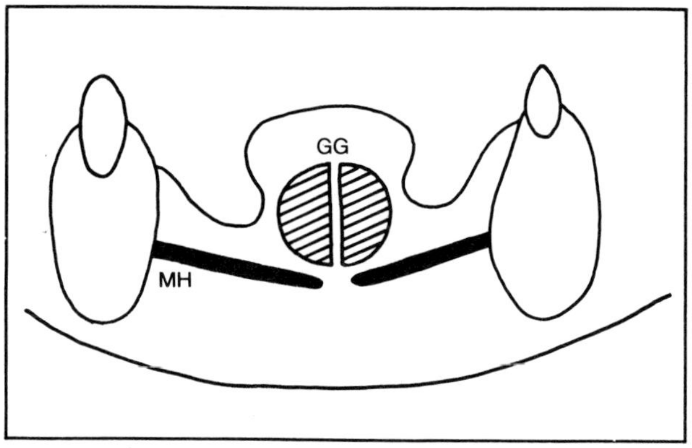

327 An otherwise normal-sized swelling on the floor of the mouth can, as a result of being constricted by the mylohyoid and genioglossus muscles, assume an exaggerated tumescence, such that it can easily cause respiratory obstruction of the oropharynx

328

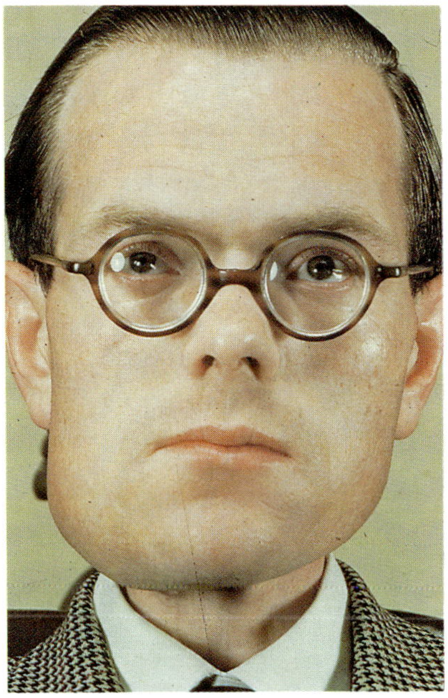

329

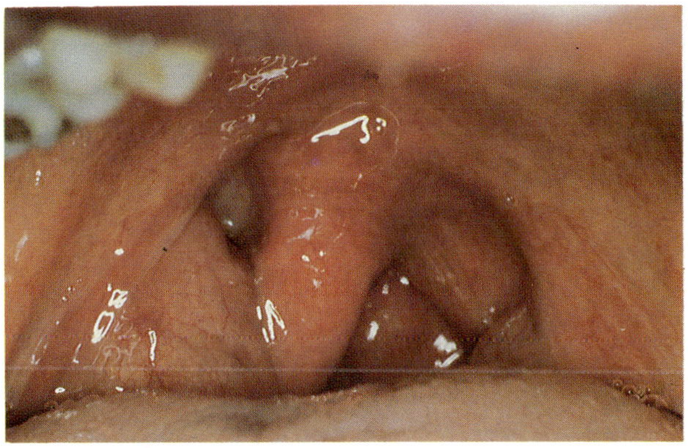

328 The clinical signs of an acutely infected lower right second molar tooth. This patient's condition is a contraindication for using intravenous sedation

329 Unilateral swelling of the pillar of the fauces means respiratory obstruction can easily occur; intravenous sedation is therefore not suitable

330

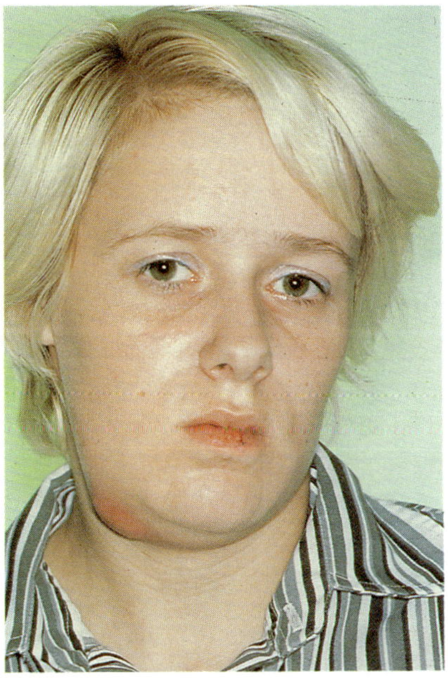

331

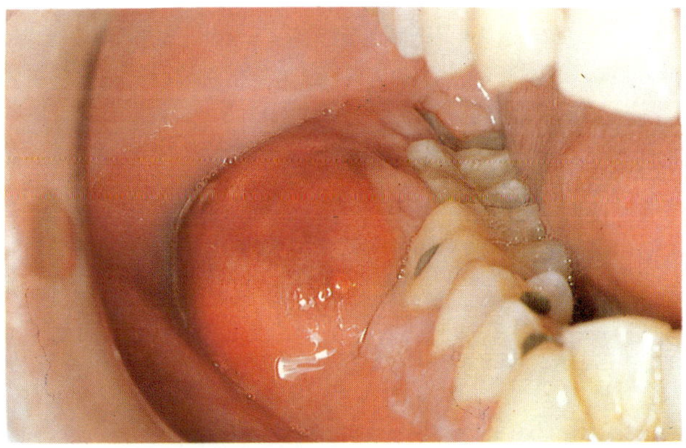

330 Apical abscess. There is extensive swelling, including on the floor of the mouth

331 Paradontal abscess in the $/\overline{78}$ region, with oropharyngeal involvement

332

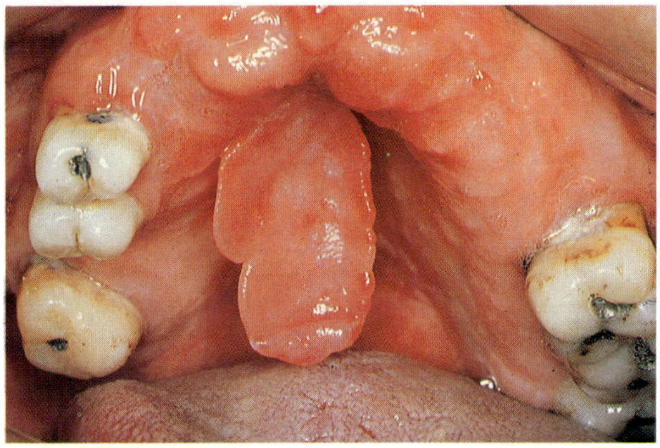

33

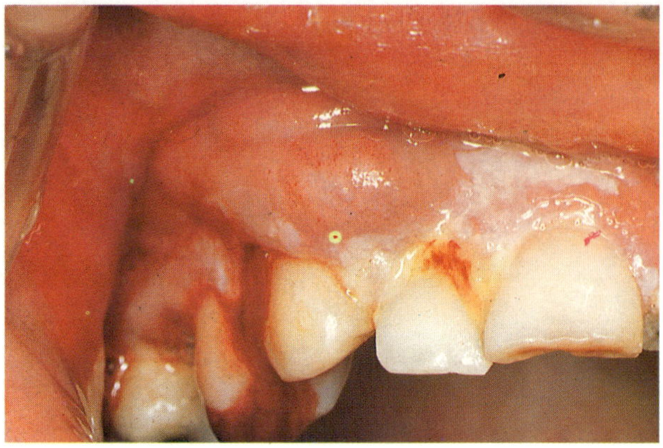

332 Leaf-like granuloma with chronic inflammation from mucofibrous hyperplasia, with swelling of the soft palate

333 Apical infection also involving the palate

Systemic complications

Only minimal cardiovascular effects are produced by the intravenous administration of diazepam in 0.15–0.2mg/kg dosage.

The cardiovascular system changes were demonstrated by Healy *et al* (1970) as a minimal transient tachycardia; Jenkinson *et al* (1974) demonstrated a slight fall in cardiac output due to anxiety; while Allen *et al* (1976) agreed that there were minimal cardiovascular disturbances following intravenous diazepam, but warned of the dangers of combining the drug with known cardiovascular depressants such as methahexitone.

Intra-arterial injections

The injection of a sedation drug into an artery, though uncommon, can have serious consequences when it does occur. The best way to avoid it happening is to perfect a careful venepuncture technique:

1. Use only a well-defined vein. Do *not* use a small vein – especially where older patients are concerned.
2. Avoid the median aspect of the cubital fossa.
3. Always palpate the site of intended venepuncture in case an aberrant artery is related to the vein to be used. Do this even in an anatomical location where an artery is *not* usually present.
4. Following venepuncture – but before depressing the syringe to give an initial dose of the drug being used – always ask the patient if he is comfortable. Ask him again after the initial dose has been administered. (It is not advisable to ask him if he has any pain, as this pre-suggests that problems may arise – and may make an already nervous patient even more anxious.)

Pain or discomfort must be acted upon instantly and no further injection given until the cause of the problem is found. Discomfort may be centrally radiating – indicating a venous problem – while pain may be distally radiating – indicating a possible intra-arterial injection (**334**).

34

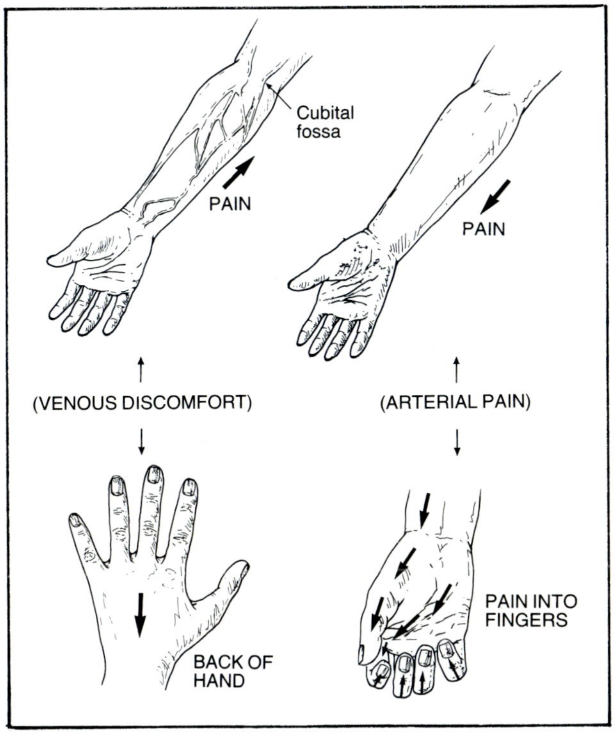

335

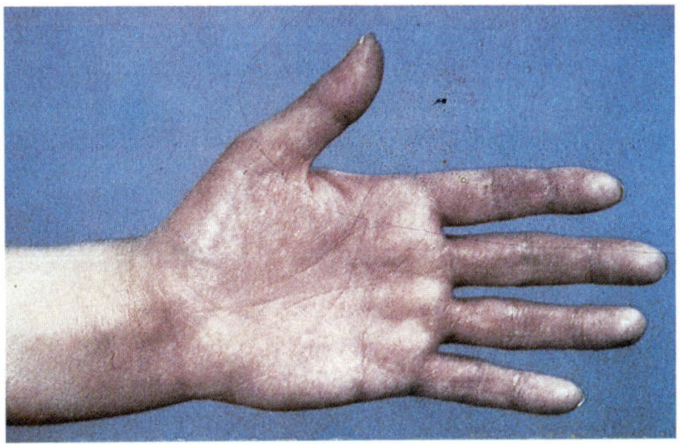

334 The direction of pain and discomfort

335 Acute ischaemia of the hand, caused by the intra-arterial injection of thiopentone. Note the discoloration

36

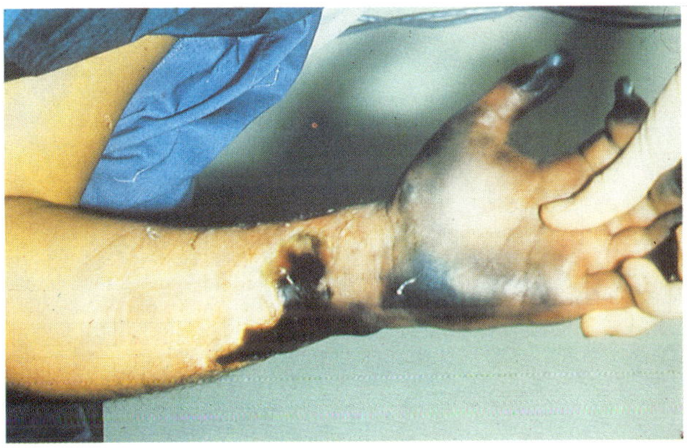

337

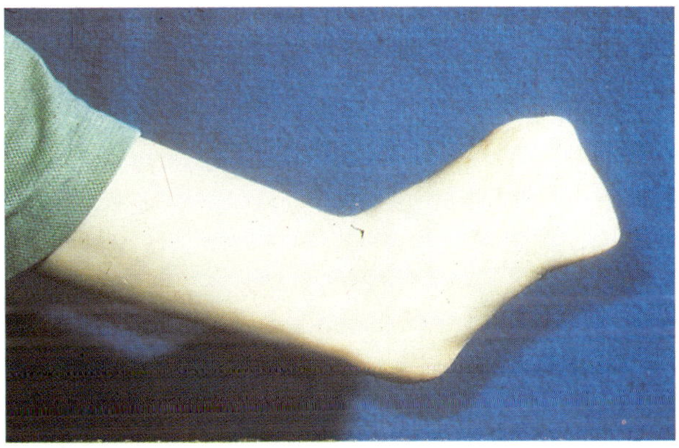

336 and **337** Necrosis of the tissue – gangrene – resulting in distal limb amputation. Although the drug used was not one of sedation, intra-arterial injection could result in severe arterial spasm and have serious effects. Every care must be taken to avoid this situation

Case histories*

1. A 72-year-old man complained of pain in his hand while diazepam was being injected through a cannula on the dorsal and radial aspects of his right wrist, prior to endoscopy. Although the pain soon subsided, by the next day the man had begun to experience intense pain in his thumb and index finger. Initially, there were no abnormal signs, but a day later there was a loss of sensation on the distal aspect of the right thumb and index finger accompanied by discoloration.

Severe ischaemia was confirmed following an operative arteriogram which revealed obstruction of the first and second digital arteries.

2. A 53-year-old woman had 15mg of diazepam injected – prior to general surgery – through a cannula inserted in the middle of the ventral aspect of her left forearm. The following day she complained of pain along the ulnar side of her left hand. No abnormal local signs were present. A diagnosis of cervical spondylosis was made. Two days later the pain was still present; it was accompanied by discoloration of the ulnar side of the middle finger and the radial side of the little finger. Acute ischaemia was diagnosed and it was noted that the venepuncture mark was overlying a superficial pulsating vessel.

The same day, the woman underwent a brachial plexus block with lignocaine and an intra-arterial injection of procaine and heparinized saline via the brachial artery. This produced an improved capillary return. One month later a cervical sympathectomy was performed for persistent pain in the affected digits, and this led to a gradual improvement in power and sensation with no return of pain.

338

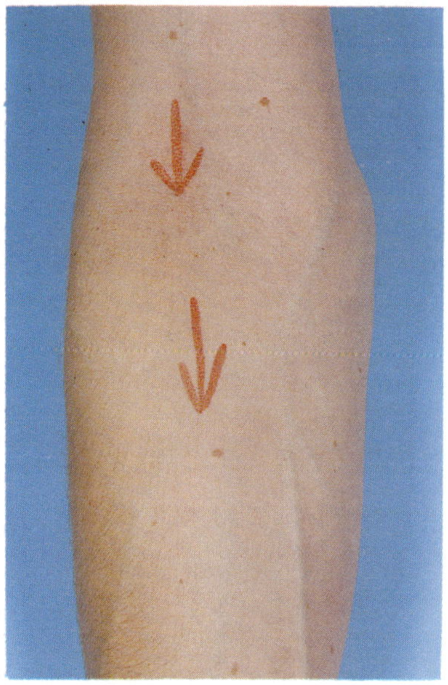

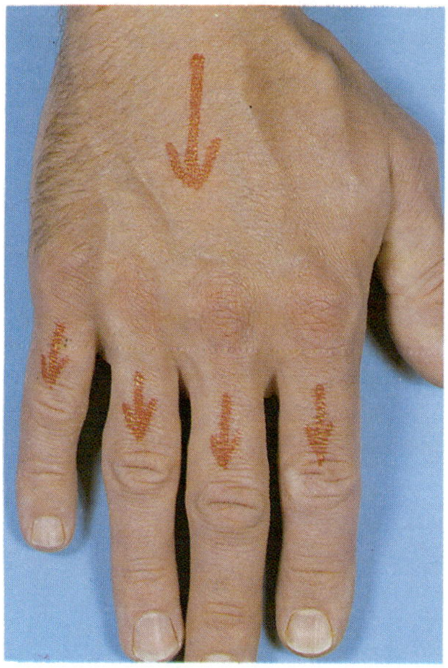

339

338 and 339 Distally radiating pain indicates arterial injection. The accidental intra-arterial injection of a sedation drug (especially diazepam in the formulation of propylene glycol in ethanol) could be the cause – but the clinical signs of ischaemia and gangrene may not be evident for days

Accidental arterial punctures are usually due either to anatomical abnormalities – when the ulnar or radial artery lies superficially – or to technical errors in venepuncture. The intra-arterial injection may also occur as a result of deep vein searching in the cubital fossa.

Do not – in the absence of physical signs of oedema, skin discoloration and sensory loss, which may or may not appear within hours – discount accidental intra-arterial injection, if pain persists.

The procedure, in the light of an accidental

*Both Rees, Dormund, 1980

340 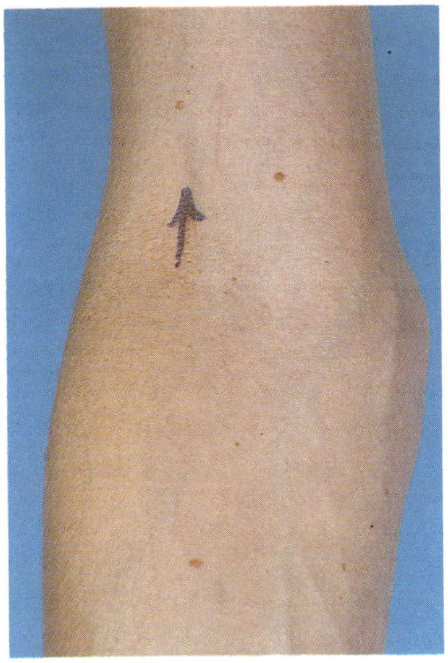 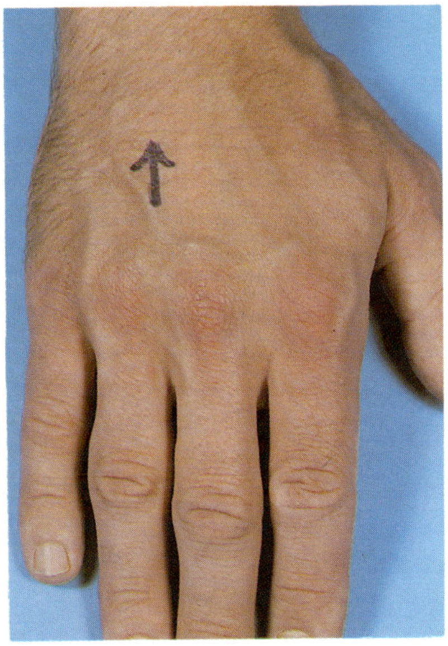 341

340 and 341 Discomfort radiating centrally indicates a venous problem – due, possibly, to:
1. Too fast a rate of injection
2. Too small a vein
3. The employment of an extravenous injection
4. The injection of an irritant or viscous drug
5. The use of a damaged needle

inter-arterial injection occurring in a dental surgery situation, is to discontinue the injection immediately and to accompany the patient to a hospital where specialist treatment will begin straightaway. This might take the form of intravenous heparinization, a surgically administered sympathetic blockade or a local analgesia. Whatever the treatment, it is vital that it is instigated as quickly as possible following the accident – and this is the dental surgeon's responsibility. He should take careful notes of all that occurs and send a report to his Defence Society.

Allergy to diazepam

An apparent allergy to diazepam has occasionally been reported – but whether this was in fact the result of other drugs used in the case, or whether the allergy was actually to the solvent in which the diazepam was dissolved, has not been conclusively proved.

Clarke (1978) states that allergic reactions to diazepam are surprisingly few, the only ones he knows involving Cremophor as a solvent. It is known that Cremophor EL does produce a relatively high incidence of allergic response when used with diazepam. Consequently, diazepam in this formulation should be avoided.

The simple allergic responses reported (Lichfield, 1980) vary in severity. A simple urticarial rash was treated by the oral administration of an antihistamine (pheniramine maleate) postoperatively for a period of three days, after which the rash disappeared. The more extreme allergic reactions produced a typical angioneurotic oedema which had to be treated by 1ml adrenaline (1:1000) i.m., followed by the oral administration of antihistamine (pheniramine maleate) for a few days afterwards.

Treatment of an allergic reaction

Simple allergy. The dental surgeon should immediately stop injecting the drug being used following any sign of an allergic response. If the reaction is mild in nature – as in the case of a mild urticarial rash – a short course of oral antihistamine can be initiated.

Acute allergy. The response here ranges in degree of severity and in rapidity of onset of angioneurotic oedema (Baderman, 1983). In most cases of anaphylaxis, the response is immediate: the patient's face becomes flushed, cyanosed and puffy, and an urticarial rash develops over his – by now, collapsing – body. This condition occurs within minutes of the drug being administered intravenously (and less than one hour following oral or intramuscular administration).

Warning symptoms may present as a tingling, and an itching all over the body – together with a general feeling of tightness in the chest and of suffocation. Coughing and wheezing, and a huskiness of speech, may also occur as the patient becomes anxious and restless. A life-threatening situation may be developing, therefore monitoring of vital signs should be carried out. If the blood pressure begins to fall (due to the escape of fluids within the blood system into the extra-cellular spaces), the patient should be laid flat. Oxygen should be administered through a patent airway and the patient should be reassured. The drug of choice is intramuscular adrenaline, 1ml (1:1000) being gradually injected, followed by an antihistamine injection of 25mg of promethazine hydrochloride. Hydrocortisone 100mg should also be available.

It is advisable to arrange for the patient to see a consultant physician or anaesthetist as soon as possible, depending on the degree of severity of the case.

Drug-induced respiratory depression

This is an uncommon complication of diazepam or midazolam, occurring when either drug is administered in a minimal sedation dosage, alone, to a normal patient. Slow administration of the drug can minimize the depression; patients in high-risk groups can be identified and eliminated beforehand by careful examination of their medical histories. Those particularly susceptible to respiratory depression include:

- Patients suffering from respiratory insufficiency, i.e. emphysema or chronic bronchitis.
- The elderly and the very young.
- Obese, anorexic or debilitated patients.
- Patients on drugs whose mild respiratory depressant effect may be enhanced by the addition of a benzodiazepine. Drugs susceptible in this way include:

  Distalgesic, which is an analgesic consisting of dextropropoxyphene and paracetamol (the former being a narcotic). When high doses of distalgesic are mixed with alcohol, the patient may experience respiratory depression. The same effect may occur with a benzodiazepine and distalgesic combination. Naloxone will reverse the effect of the dextropropoxyphene, but its administration must be accompanied by the maintenance of the airway, breathing and circulation.

  Pentazocine, which is a non-narcotic analgesic and an opiate derivative – being derived from the benzomorphan group (of which the morphine antagonist, nalorphine, is also a member). In common with other narcotics, it can induce respiratory depression, the effects of which – in the event of an overdosage – again, naloxone will reverse.

  Used as an intravenous analgesic, pentazocine is often employed to good effect in a technique designed to lower the dosage of benzodiazepines. However, only dental surgeons with considerable experience of sedation should use this method.

Oversedation or overdosage will also cause respiratory depression (Dixon, 1985), and it is the responsibility of the dental surgeon to administer drugs slowly and in minimal titrated dosages as described in Chapter 9. Until the advent of flumazenil (the antagonist for benzodiazepines), the dental surgeon had to maintain the patient's airway, administer oxygen and keep the patient in a supine position, until the patient recovered.

Forster (1979) stated that the ventilatory and mouth occlusion depression responses to intravenous injection of midazolam or diazepam in equipotent doses are equal, suggesting a direct depression of the central respiratory drive by these drugs. By using minimal sedative doses, McGimpsey *et al* (1983) found that respiratory and cardiovascular effects were minimal. However, the Committee of Safety of Medicines (1985) has warned practitioners of several reported cases of respiratory depression and hypotension following the administration of midazolam.

Although some degree of respiratory depression and hypotension has been demonstrated in certain patients receiving diazepam or midazolam, complications at minimal sedative dosages – though they do occur – are rare. The dental surgeon should nevertheless be aware of this complication.

Case history

A 67-year-old man weighing 85kg received surgical treatment following a road traffic accident. It was decided that intubation was necessary, so the patient was given 2mg of midazolam to facilitate the procedure. He became unconscious in less than two minutes and ventilation ceased. Subsequently the patient made a satisfactory recovery and was weaned from the ventilator on the eighth day.

Vasovagal attack – fainting

The over-anxious patient may undergo a vasovagal attack before or during the administration of intravenous sedation. In such an event, the procedure must be stopped immediately and the patient attended to: lay him out flat on his back with his head below the level of his feet (**342**). Particular attention must be paid to airway, breathing and circulation. Under no circumstances should the sedation procedure continue that day.

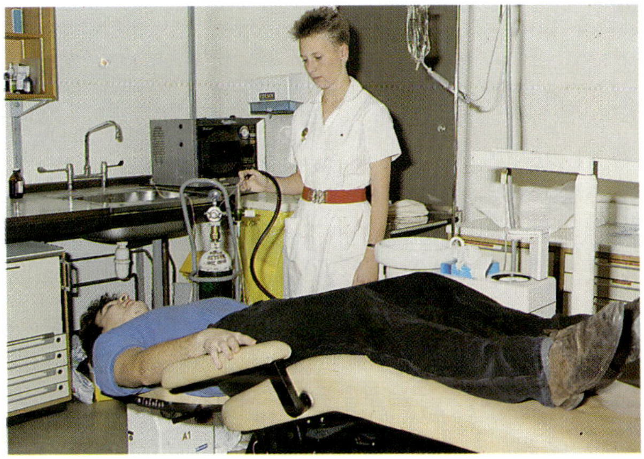

342

342 In the event of a vasovagal attack, the patient is laid out flat on his back, with his head resting below the level of his feet to keep the strain off his heart

Avoiding a faint

The following points should be noted:

1. As a general rule, a healthy patient should be advised not to eat or drink for four hours prior to an intravenous sedation procedure. If the dental surgeon feels there is a danger of hypoglycaemia a small glucose drink may be given to the patient.
2. An effort should be made to see the patient on time, since keeping him waiting may serve to heighten anxiety and stress in what may be an already frightened individual!
3. Possibly the most important factor is the kindness and caring attitude of the dental surgeon and his team.

Overdosage, sensitivity and resistance to diazepam and midazolam

There remains a seemingly indeterminate group of patients for whom it takes only a few milligrams of either midazolam or diazepam for them to become deeply sedated. The dosage administered may bear no apparent relationship to the patient's weight, either – a large patient may sometimes become deeply sedated on just a few milligrams, while a patient small in size and low in body weight may conversely require a higher dosage to become sedated. The intravenous drug must therefore be administered slowly and titrated against the individual patient.

Predictably, there is another group of patients – few in number – who appear not to be affected by benzodiazepines at all. After a 10mg dosage they will look at the dental surgeon and insist they feel normal. Since this response is not unusual in some *sedated* patients too, it is clearly unreliable as a guide to whether or not a patient belongs to the small group of truly resistant cases. However, a patient who performs an EVE Sign Positive and says that he feels normal *is* usually adequately sedated. It should be remembered, too, that the 18–50 age group is less susceptible to the effects of sedation drugs than are older patients (Dundee *et al.*, 1985).

Whatever the facts of the matter, **where an out-patient is concerned the dental surgeon would be unwise to administer more than 10mg of midazolam or 20mg of diazepam intravenously.** In the case of a truly resistant patient, the administration of further large increments of

343

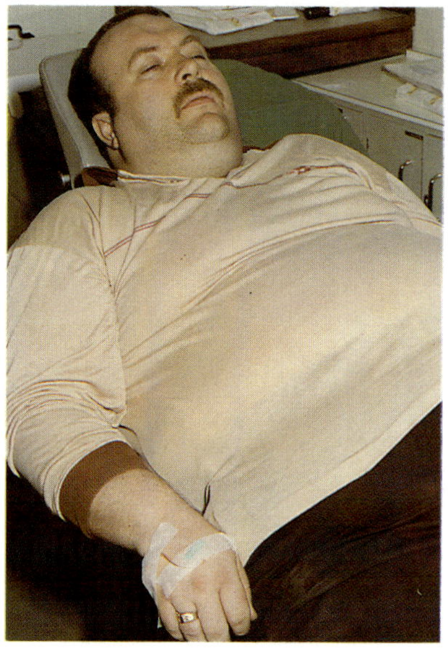

343 This patient, weighing in at nearly 160kg, was adequately sedated via 4mg of midazolam. The dosage necessary is a matter of individual titration and must be determined by the dental surgeon, who is solely responsible for the safety of the patient at all times. Note that it is not advisable to sedate short-necked patients of this size unless the procedure is carried out by a very experienced dental surgeon. Complications involving airway obstruction can occur very rapidly with patients of this build, and may be difficult to deal with

344

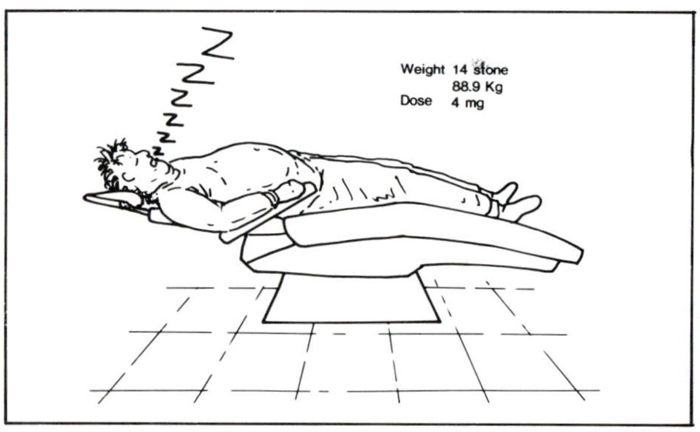

345

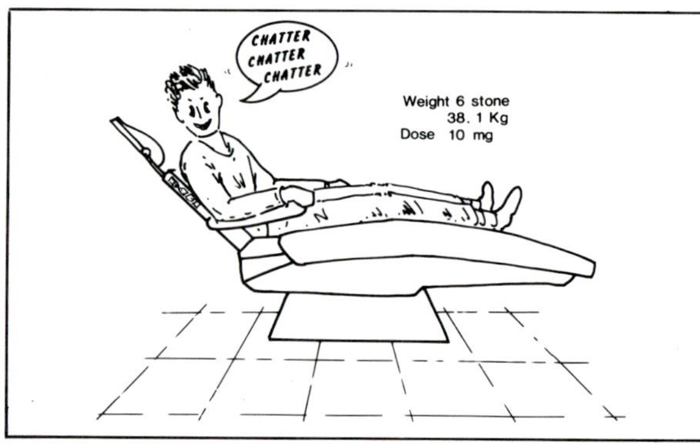

344 and **345** A large patient (**344**) may become deeply sedated on just a few milligrams of midazolam or diazepam . . . while another small in size and low in weight (**345**) may conversely require a higher dosage to become sedated

346
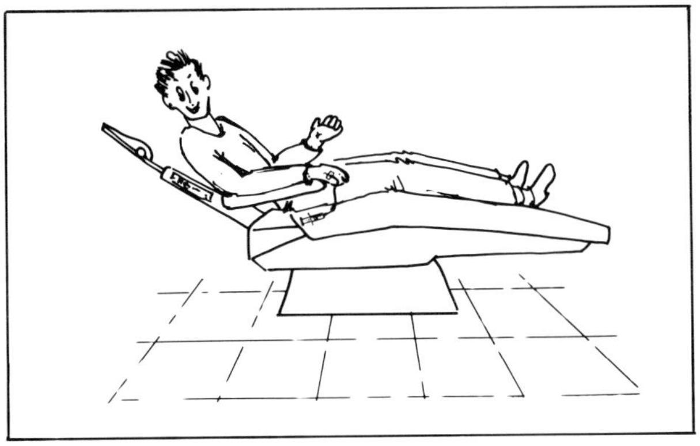

346 After the first incremental dose. Patient: 'Nothing has happened'

347
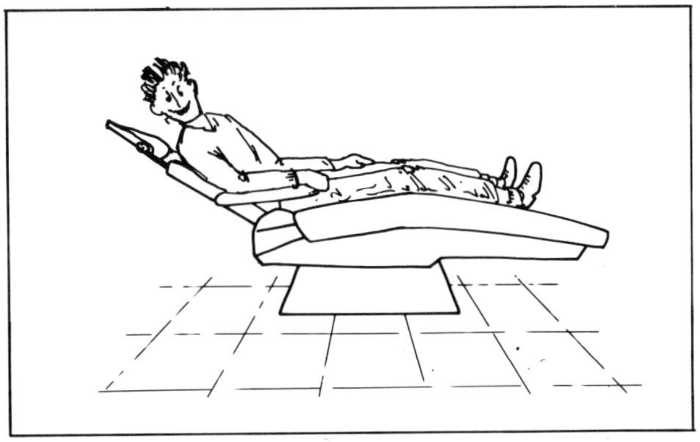

347 After further incremental doses requested by the patient. Patient: 'Nothing has happened'

348
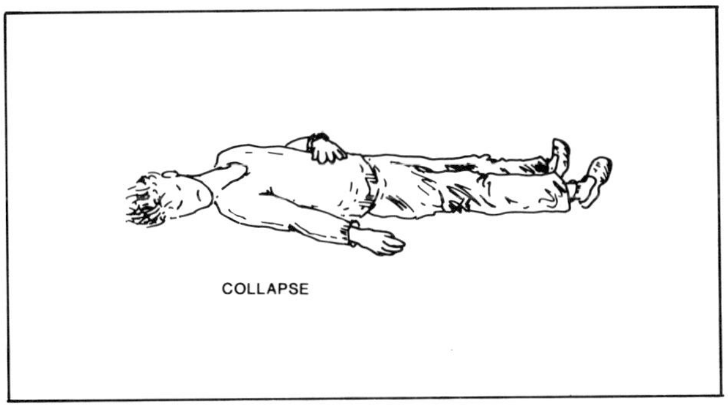

349
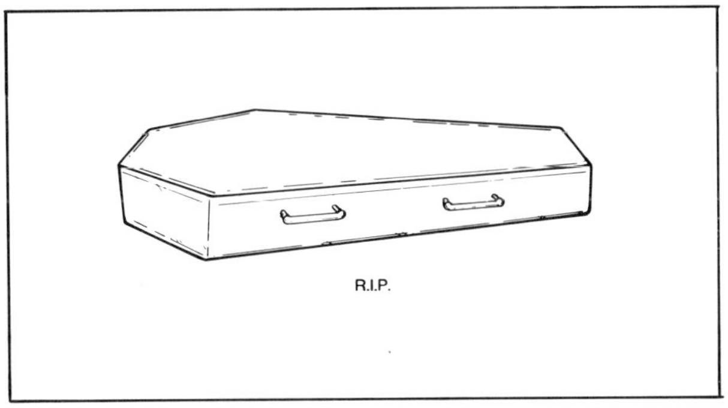

the drug will fail to produce any reaction, other than, ultimately, to induce a state of deep anaesthesia – that is to say, unconsciousness – with potentially fatal consequences. An incautious dental surgeon may yet end up with the dubious distinction of causing death for the first time via a massive overdose of a sedation drug!

It is better for the dental surgeon to discontinue the sedation procedure at a safe dosage level and to treat the patient as a normal post-sedation case; that is to say, the patient should be allowed to rest, before returning home accompanied by his escort. In the case of the drug-resistant patient, alternative arrangements for treatment may be made, i.e. treatment under normal local analgesia or, if necessary, general anaesthesia.

Nausea and vomiting may rarely occur following intravenous sedation, but an attentive dental team can deal with such incidents by the use of aspiration and by turning the patient on his side in the supine position, with the head slightly lower than the body. If necessary, an intramuscular injection of prochlorperazine (Stemetil) 12.5mg or of metoclopramide 10mg may be administered.

General or psychogenic complications of intravenous sedation

It cannot be stressed too strongly that patients who are receiving psychiatric drug therapy and regular medication with benzodiazepines are *not* suitable for intravenous sedation with benzodiazepines.

If the dental surgeon makes it a strict rule to sedate only patients with no questionable medical history and who appear to have a normal psychological profile, he will reduce the risk of psychogenic reaction considerably.

There is a small group of patients who, though otherwise appearing normal in every way, when sedated may exhibit one or other of the following traits (Rood, 1980):

Sobbing. This occurs only rarely during an intravenous procedure, though more often in the course of a recovery. Gentle reassurance by the dental surgery assistant is all that is required in terms of response – although a cup of tea in a pleasant recovery room can also be helpful. The accompanying person should not normally be summoned into the recovery room while the patient is distressed; rather, the patient should be allowed enough time to regain his composure with only the dental surgery assistant present to monitor and reassure him.

Paradoxical rage. Patients may rarely exhibit 'excitation' – and even, possibly, aggression. The dental surgeon should be on guard for this possibility.

Loss of inhibitions. Occasionally, some patients may lose their inhibitions and speak of private matters whilst undergoing sedation. The dental surgeon should do his best to discourage such talk; if this fails, a mouth prop can be placed in the patient's mouth. It would be unprofessional for the dental surgeon to encourage the patient or to speak to him about anything – other than to reassure him with regard to the treatment – apart from trivialities. On recovery some patients will voice their fears of not knowing what they said. They should be immediately reassured and told that speech is impossible whilst under sedation.

Fantasies of indecent assault. Allegations of indecent assault are most commonly made by female patients against male dental surgeons. Occasionally, children are involved – with claims of indecent interference being levelled against dental surgeons of either sex: these can be serious charges indeed.

Patients *can* experience erotic dreams/impressions while undergoing relative analgesia, intravenous sedation or general anaesthesia. If their clothing also becomes disturbed, as a result of the restlessness that often occurs during the sedation procedure, it is not too difficult to see how a susceptible patient might conceive this type of allegation. Misunderstandings can happen.

Innocence alone is not an entirely adequate defence in these matters and **no dental surgeon should do more than make a firm denial of any allegation of indecent assault before seeking advice from his Protection Society.** Neither the Hospital Authority nor the police are entitled to an immediate statement and no person is the best advocate in his own cause. Under no circumstances should the dental surgeon be alone with a sedated patient; the presence of at least one other member of the dental team is essential from the point of view of the safety of the patient, and also serves to safeguard the dental surgeon's reputation (perhaps even his career, too!) in the unlikely event that an accusation of sexual assault arises.

Unless the dental surgeon applies an efficient and ethical approach to the practice of intravenous sedation procedures, he will find that problems of this nature will arise. **He must have a second appropriate person with him at all times during both the sedation and the recovery period of the patient.** It is reasonable for the patient's accompanying person to stay with the patient while he is recovering from a sedation procedure. By his strict observance of the rules, the dental surgeon will protect both himself and the patient.

Case history

A patient for endoscopy was given midazolam for sedation. She had never had the drug before and in the follow-up she stated that she thought she could have been sexually assaulted during the period following administration. She was reassured after it was explained that this was physically impossible, and there were no subsequent problems.

(Dundee, 1986.)

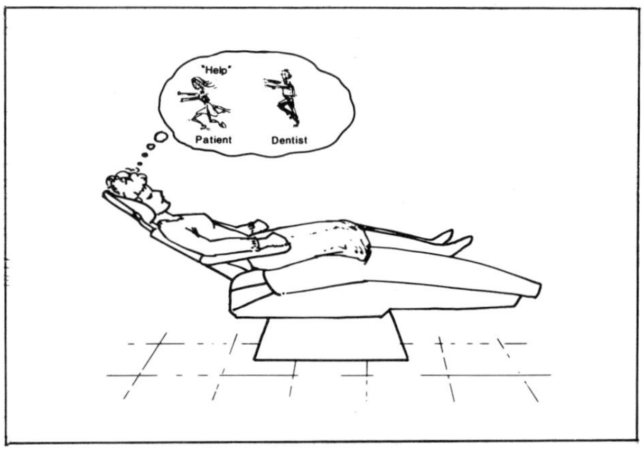

350

During initial studies with midazolam involving medical students and staff, a female volunteer asked to be withdrawn from the study as she was embarrassed by her 'dreams of sexual fantasies'.

Cases have occurred where the dental surgery assistant was asked to leave the surgery during a sedation procedure, to collect an instrument or on some other errand. This is inexcusable if it leaves the dental surgeon alone with the patient, for the outcome can be disastrous for everyone. Under no circumstances should the dental surgeon ever find himself in this situation: there are no apologies for reiterating this point.

Note: If a lightly sedated patient wishes to visit the toilet, the dental surgery assistant should escort the patient there and wait discretely outside the door.

Post-sedation behaviour

In the immediate aftermath of the sedation appointment, the patient will lack his normal mental controls, and will, in effect, be at risk from his own behaviour. It is therefore essential that he is escorted home by a reliable person, and – if possible – he should be kept under observation for the remainder of the day. Under no circumstances should he be given, or be allowed to take, alcohol, drive a vehicle, or act in any way that may involve danger. The last can include preparing a meal on a hot stove or in a hot oven. The accompanying person should be warned that important personal decisions should not be made by the recovering patient.

If the dental surgeon, assisted by an experienced dental surgery assistant, exercises care when taking down the patient's medical history and in the performance of the sedation technique – allowing enough time for the procedure – then the chance of an emergency arising will be reduced, if not eliminated entirely. Regular emergency drills are essential, so that the dental surgeon and his staff will know how to respond in the event of a complication. The actions of a good, experienced dental team may save a life, or at least prevent serious injury befalling a patient. Following a training session in cardiopulmonary resuscitation the staff should sign a training book to show that they have been regularly trained and updated in emergency procedures.

Finally, it is worth noting that accurate details of all cases must be recorded and that, in the event of an incident occurring, the dental surgeon should – as always – inform his Protection Society as soon as possible after the event.

17 CARDIOPULMONARY RESUSCITATION

Introduction

It is reasonable for a patient to be confident that in the event of a life-threatening emergency occurring while he is receiving dental treatment, the dental team will be competent to deal efficiently with it. It is important, therefore, to understand the basic principles of cardiopulmonary resuscitation (CPR) as they may be applied in the dental surgery situation.

It is beyond the scope of this book to cover in detail all the information that a dental team should acquire on the subject before being considered adequately trained. The reading list for Chapter 17 found at the end of the book includes a number of titles on the subject. A wise principal will arrange for all the staff in the practice, from the receptionist to the senior dentist, to receive adequate training in CPR. To this end, also located at the end of the book is a selection of organizations in the UK, the USA, and elsewhere, offering practical courses in the technique of CPR. Following this, a 'hands on' practice should be carried out at regular intervals in the dental surgery.

Many emergencies can be avoided if a careful medical history is taken. Special attention should be given to patients already taking medication, as this fact will give a clue to a possible undisclosed medical history. A patient's attitude and physical appearance can also provide an indication of his state of health.

The possession of adequate equipment in good working order is essential, and a selection of suitable drugs should be readily available. It is of paramount importance that the oxygen-delivery system is tested before the commencement of each intravenous sedation session – and prior to the patient's arrival in the surgery. Drugs for emergencies must also be checked to see that they have not exceeded their expiry date.

All emergency equipment and drugs should be within arm's reach of the dental surgeon and the dental surgery assistant while they are treating the patient in the dental chair. It is ultimately the responsibility of the principal dental surgeon to see that, if an emergency occurs, the dental team is capable of controlling the initial upsetting factor and then is able to carry out a well-rehearsed and efficient CPR procedure which may well save the patient's life.

There are many potential causes of an unexpected collapse in the dental chair, and it is up to the dental surgeon to make a rapid diagnosis to determine which one *is* responsible. The collapse may be due to a simple vasovagal attack; alternatively, it may be the result of a serious myocardiac infarction. The management of the collapse will depend on the dental surgeon: if he is in any doubt at all about the seriousness of the patient's condition, he should put the emergency procedure into operation immediately.

Following a collapse, the dental surgeon should establish the patient's unresponsiveness by gently tapping and shaking him (**352**).

351

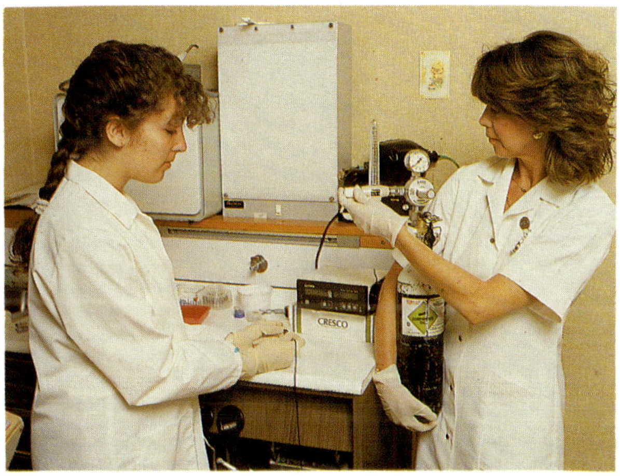

351 Monitoring equipment and oxygen-delivery system must be checked by the dental staff before the sedation session begins. Drugs and drug expiry dates must also be checked regularly

Summoning assistance

If an emergency situation does arise in the dental surgery, either the dental surgeon or the dental surgery assistant should summon help from the receptionist by means of an emergency buzzer or a bell. As already stressed, **the patient must never be left unattended. A minimum of two members of the dental team, one of whom must be the dental surgeon, must be present at all times.**

The receptionist will immediately telephone the emergency ambulance service, and then the local hospital – where a procedure for just such an emergency will already have been arranged. It is also very useful to have a line of direct communication to a consultant anaesthetist or consultant physician. This communication can be effected either by telephone or by a pager system. A list of emergency numbers should be kept within sight of the receptionist.

The ABC of resuscitation

Resuscitation is the saving of life by establishing the three basic requirements for life support, which are: a clear, open airway, breathing, and a heartbeat. This is referred to as the ABC of resuscitation – A being for Airway, B for Breathing, and C for Circulation – and it applies to all unconscious patients, whatever the cause of their condition. (For simplicity, 'the resuscitator' is referred to, here, as 'the dental surgeon' – although, of course, *any* member of the dental team could assume the role, provided she or he has undergone proper training in the essential procedures.

352

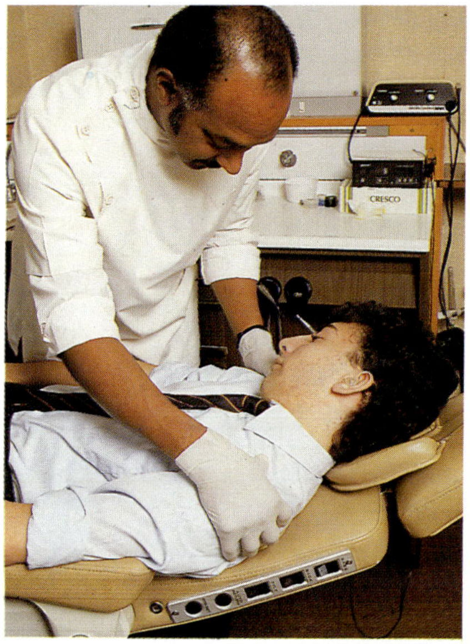

352 Following the patient's collapse, the dental surgeon tries to rouse him by firmly shaking him and shouting at him

AIRWAY For successful resuscitation to take place an immediate opening of the airway is essential.

The commonest cause of obstruction in the unconscious patient is the tongue, which is inclined to fall back (**353** and **354**). To obtain an airway, tilt the head of the patient well back, extending the neck, and hold the chin well forward (**355** and **356**). This simple exercise will move the tongue away from the back of the oropharynx.

353

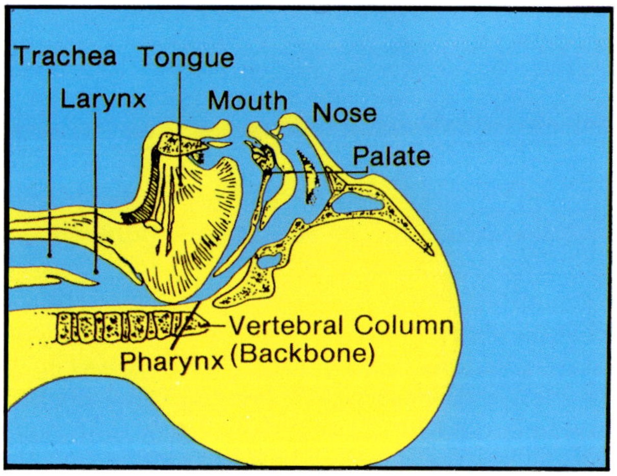

353 In the unconscious patient, the tongue can easily fall back and occlude the airway

354

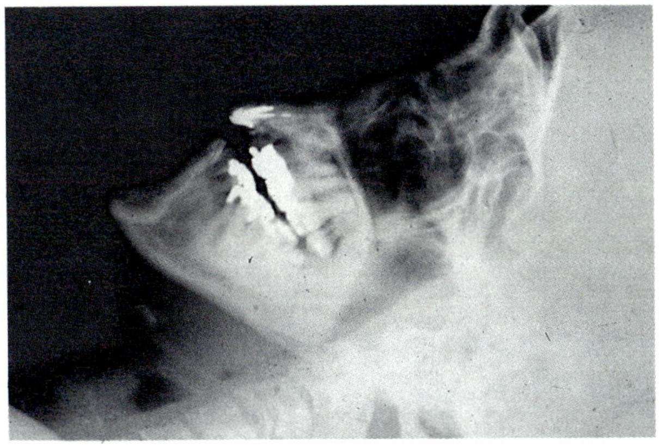

354 Occlusion of the airway. The oropharyngeal space shows as a closed triangle

55

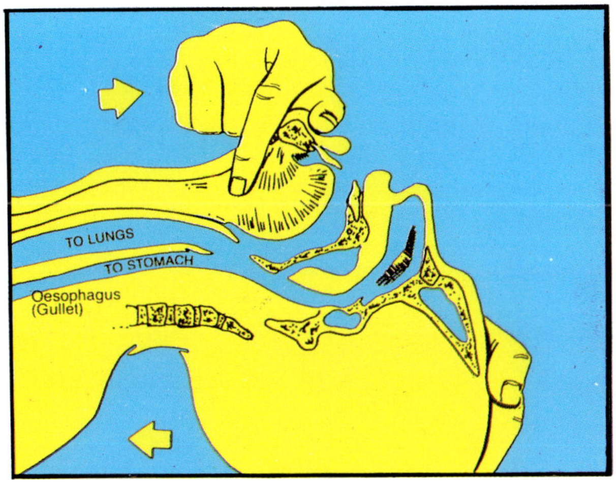

355 The airway is opened by tilting the head backwards and holding the chin forwards

356

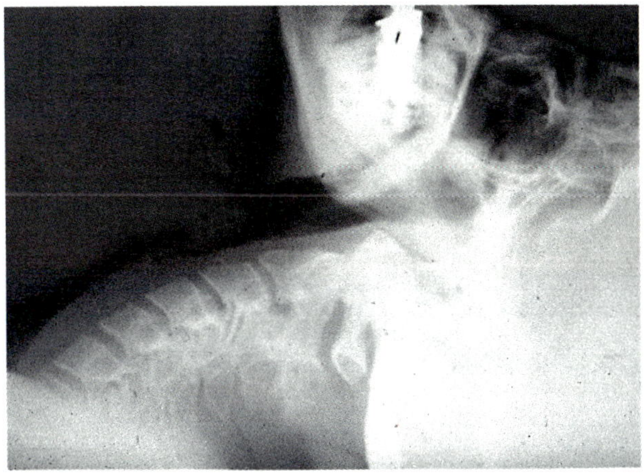

356 Another view of the opening of the airway – compare with **354**

57

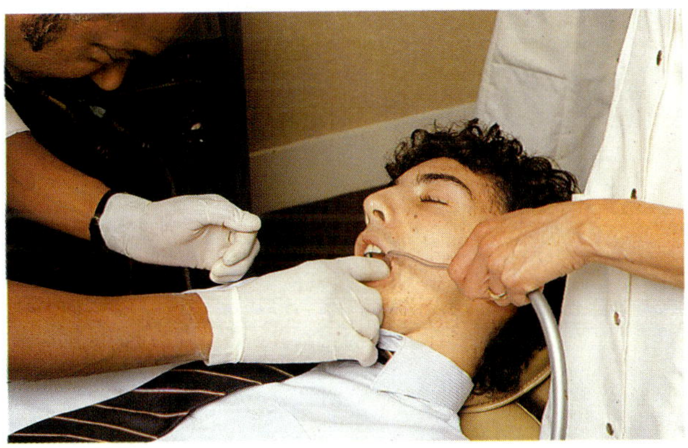

357 The airway cleared, care is taken to see that no foreign body debris is retained in the oropharynx

358

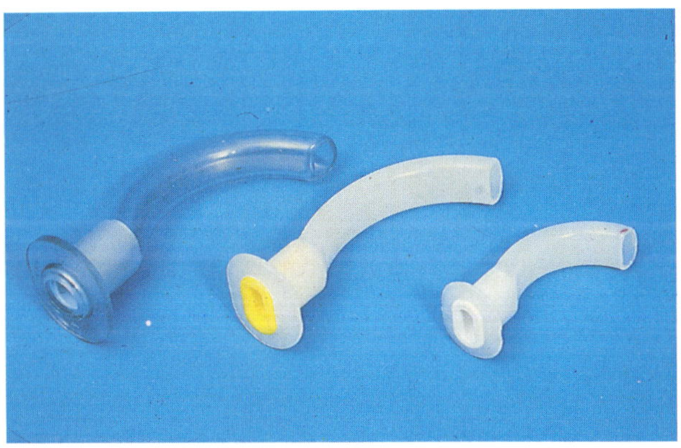

358 The patient's airway may be maintained throughout the resuscitation process by the insertion of a disposable Guedel airway. A selection of correctly sized airways should be kept within arm's reach of the dental surgeon and dental surgery assistant

359

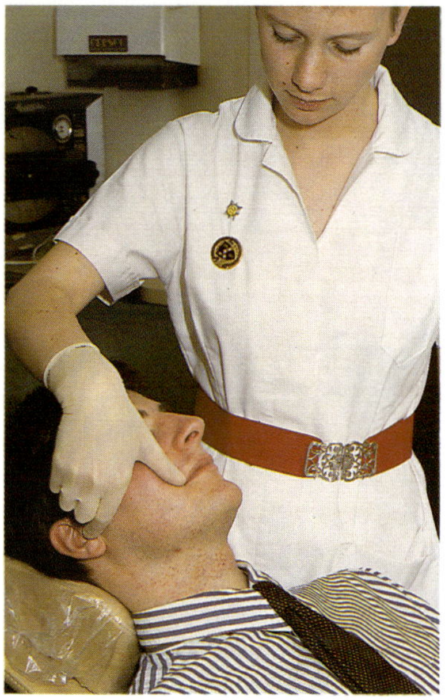

359 A good method of checking the most suitably sized Guedel airway is to measure from the corner of the patient's mouth to the top of his earlobe, and then checking the selected Guedel airway against the side of the patient's cheek

361

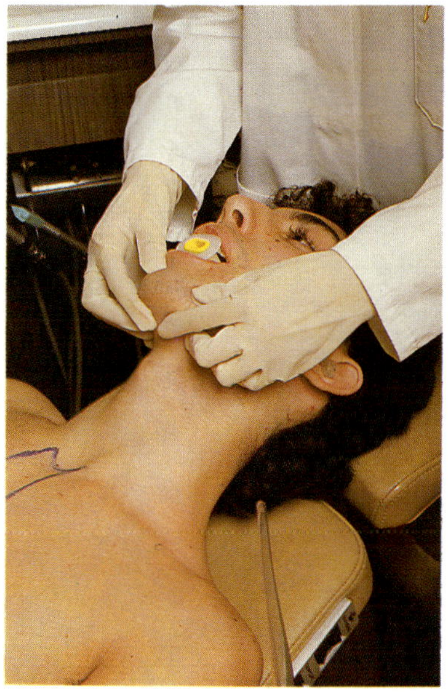

360

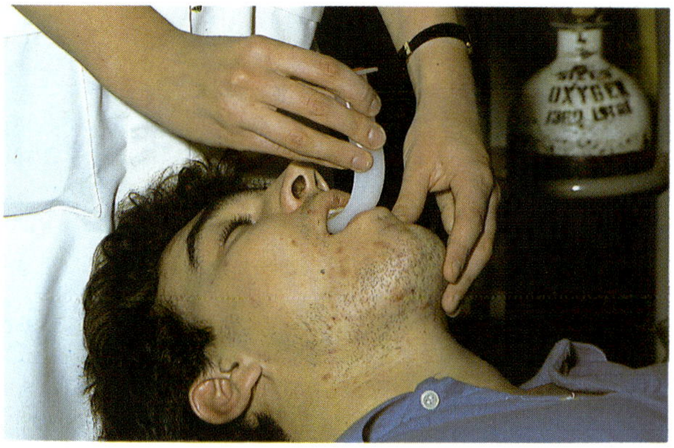

360 and 361 The Guedel airway is inserted into the patient's mouth, so that the flanged end lies inside the lips but outside the teeth. Note that the jaw continues to be supported in a forward position

BREATHING To determine whether or not a patient is breathing, the dental surgeon observes the patient's chest and abdomen, listens for the sound of the patient's breathing, and waits to feel the patient's breath on his cheek (**363**). (LOOK LISTEN FEEL.)

If there is no pulse, the time should be noted: only three minutes remain in which to restore the circulation if irreversible anoxic damage to the brain is to be avoided.

Once it is established that the patient is breathing and that a pulse is present he should be turned on his side to prevent further obstruction (**365**); his vital signs should be monitored continuously thereafter, until he is completely recovered. If the patient is under the influence of intravenous sedation, he will be connected to a monitor already, and it can therefore be instantly established if breathing or circulatory collapse has occurred. Direct physical monitoring by the dental team should augment the electronic form, and should be vigilantly maintained: all electro-

362

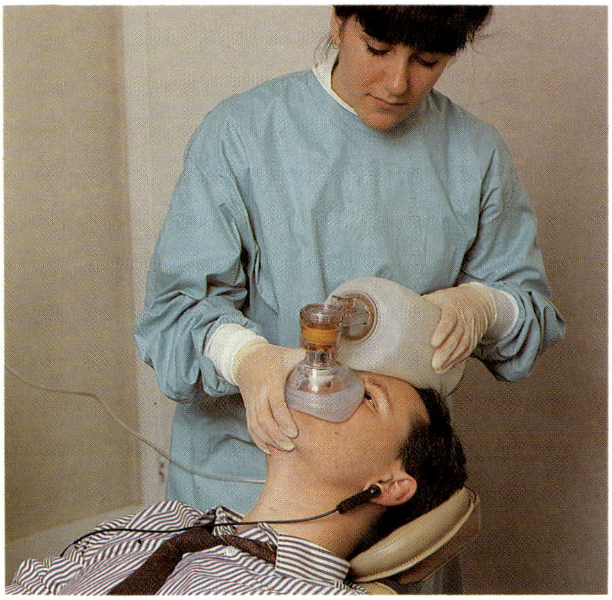

363

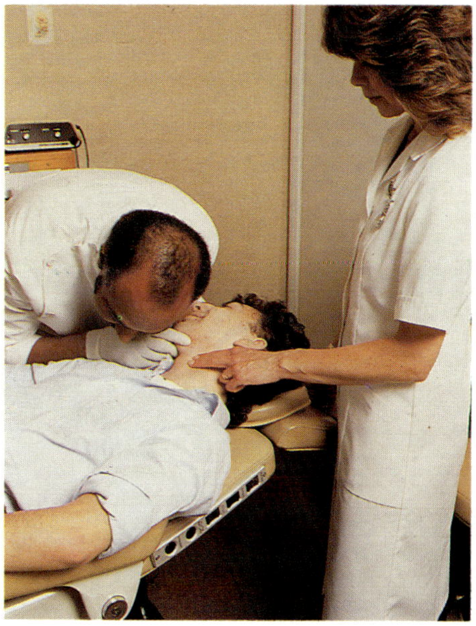

362 The dental surgery assistant uses an oxygen reservoir bag, which is connected to the oxygen supply. The bag is squeezed 12 times a minute for an adult patient – that's one inflation every five seconds. This procedure is continued until the patient starts to breathe on his own

363 Look, listen . . .. The dental surgeon checks for the cause of the emergency, while the dental surgery assistant feels the carotid pulse and calls out the results

364

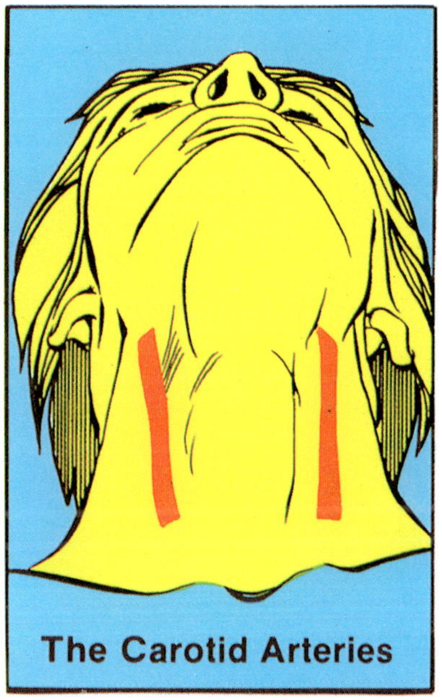

364 The location of the carotid arteries

nic monitoring devices, although desirable, are secondary to that undertaken by the dental surgeon and dental surgery assistant.

The dental surgery assistant should observe the monitoring of the patient and call loud and clear verbal reports to the dental surgeon on the pulse rate, breathing and colour of the patient. While monitoring the patient's vital signs, the dental surgery assistant will also administer oxygen and maintain the airway.

365

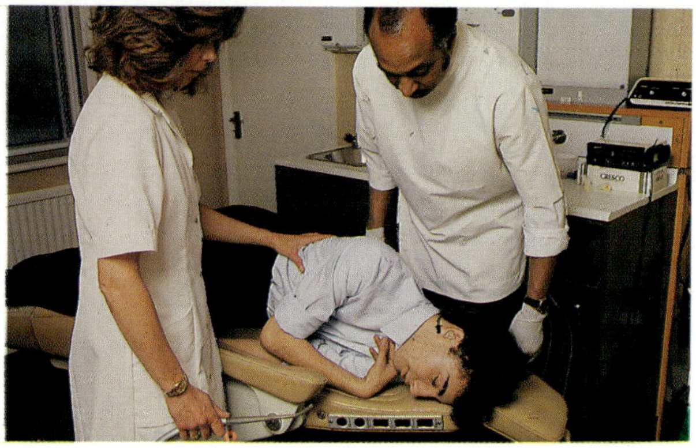

365 The patient's arms are folded and he is then rolled gently onto his side by the dental surgeon and dental surgery assistant

CIRCULATION Adequate oxygenation of the brain by circulating blood is essential to the life of the patient. The dental surgeon will commence External Cardiac Compression when the heart stops and the circulation of blood ceases.

External Cardiac Compression in a dental surgery situation should never be carried out without oxygen resuscitation effected via a reservoir bag connected to an oxygen cylinder.

366

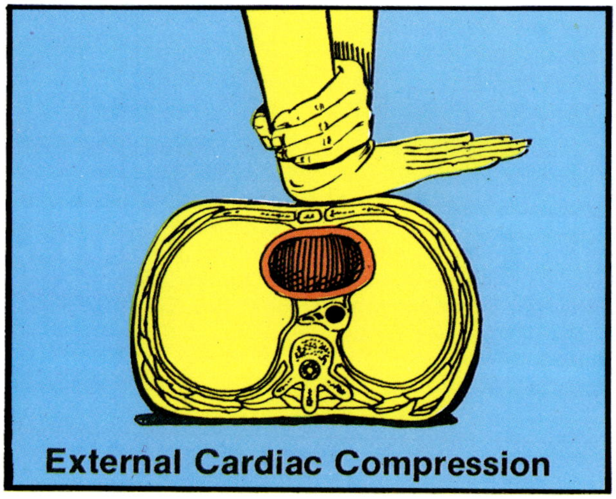

366 By rhythmically compressing the heart between the sternum and the spine, it is possible to provide an artificial circulation. When correctly carried out, External Cardiac Compression will maintain an adequate circulation of blood, thereby sustaining life and preventing brain damage

367

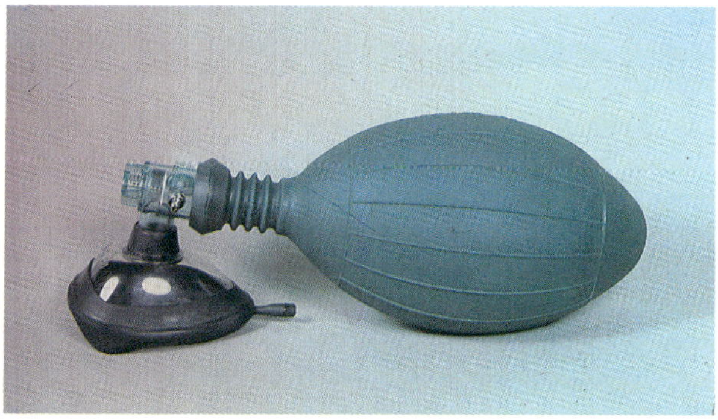

367 Emergency resuscitator – essential in a cardiopulmonary emergency

Identifying the pressure point for the application of External Cardiac Compression

It is essential that dental personnel carrying out External Cardiac Compression know exactly the correct procedure. Pressure incorrectly applied by the resuscitator not only will fail to stimulate the heart, it may also result in a fracture of the xiphoid process. None of the procedures described here can be undertaken with the necessary degree of efficiency unless the would-be resuscitator has participated in regular training sessions held in the dental surgery.

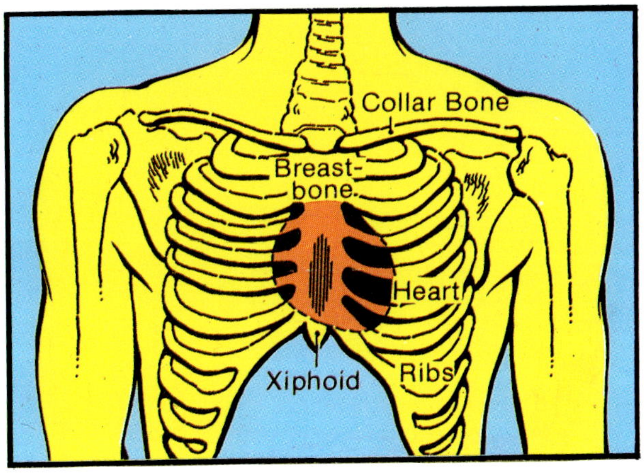

368

368 Anatomy of External Cardiac Compression

369

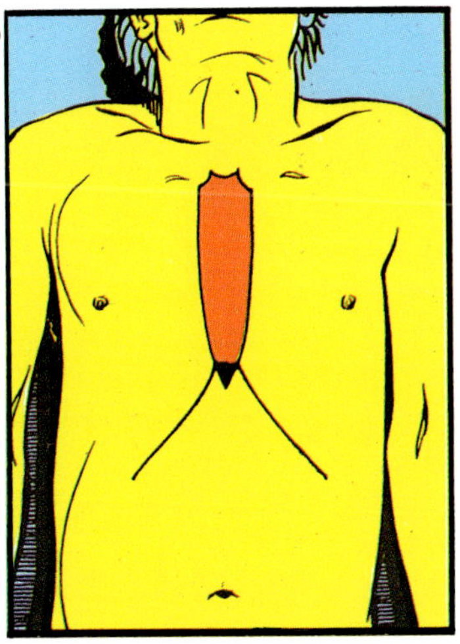

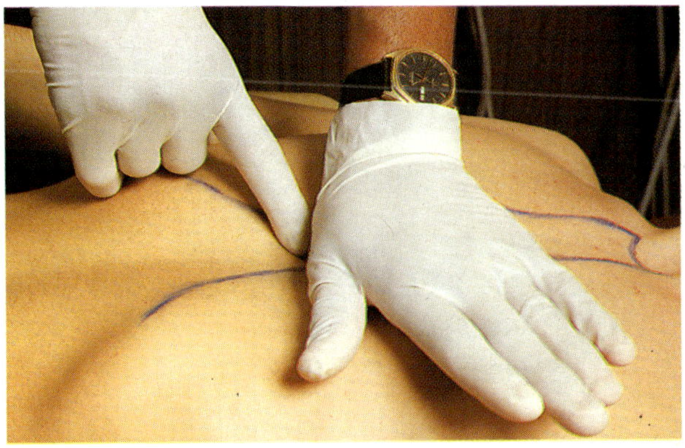
370

369 and **370** The suprasternal notch at the top of the sternum and the xiphoid process at its base are located by touch and identified. Measuring one half of this distance, the lower half of the sternum is the area to which external cardiac massage should be applied

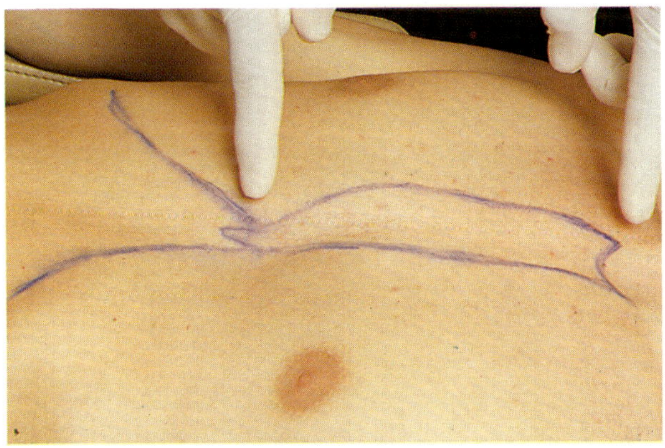
371

371 Another method of identifying the pressure point is by feeling the base of the xiphoid process, measuring two fingers' width above the xiphoid using the pressure point above this point. **Care must be taken not to apply pressure directly over the xiphoid process as this could cause it to fracture. The upper end of the sternum is easy to identify but the lower end requires greater care**

Method of compression

372 The point of pressure for the application of External Cardiac Compression is located – note that the xiphoid process is identified by the dental surgeon/resuscitator. The latter places the heel of one hand onto the compression point, with the fingers straight and slightly raised so no pressure will be applied to the ribs. The other hand is placed firmly and securely on top of it. To prevent slipping, the fingers of the upper hand are hooked around those of the lower one

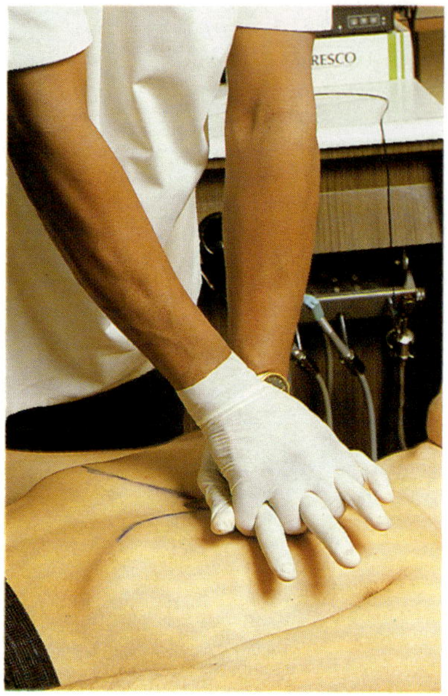

372

Compression is carried out with the dental surgeon's body positioned directly above the patient and with the dental surgeon's arms kept straight – there must be no bending of the elbows (372). In this manner the dental surgeon's body weight assists in the administration of the External Cardiac Compression. Over a long period this correct position is less tiring for the dental surgeon and the External Cardiac Compression is more efficient. Although the dental surgeon should not lift his hands off the patient's chest between compressions, he must release the pressure completely.

Compressions should be rhythmic with equal time for compression and relaxation. The sternum is compressed up to a maximum of 4cm. The ideal rate of compression is 60–80 compressions per minute.

Summary of the technique of artificial circulation

1. Help is summoned.
2. The dental surgeon and dental surgery assistant take up their pre-arranged positions in relation to the collapsed patient.
3. The point of External Cardiac Compression is identified on the lower half of the sternum.
4. The heel of one hand is placed on the pressure point; the other hand is placed on top of the first hand (373).
5. The sternum is compressed towards the spine, about 4cm in adults.
6. The compression should last about one half of a second (half of the rhythmic cycle). Following compression, pressure is released for half a second to allow the blood to flow back into the chest.
7. **Re-apply compression every second; that is: 60 compressions per minute with one ventilation every fifth compression. The pulse must be monitored constantly.** The patient must also be kept in the supine position to allow for venous return.

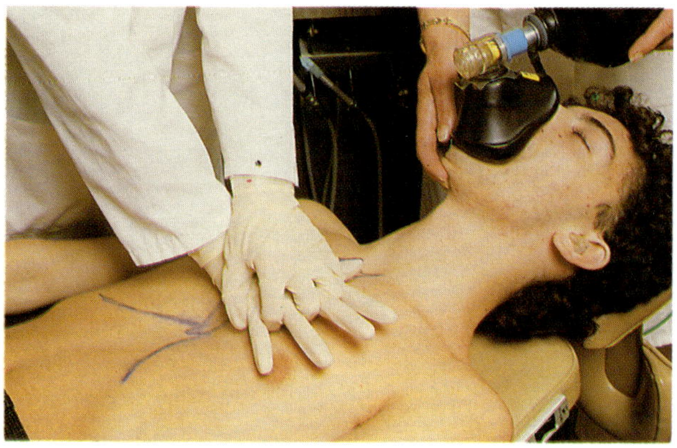

3

373 Artificial circulation: the dental surgeon applies pressure with hands interlocked in the required fashion

Combination of ventilation and sternal compression

Sternal compression carried out on its own will not provide sufficient oxygenation to the lungs; therefore, External Cardiac Compression must be combined with ventilation.

Summary

1. If the patient loses consciousness his head is tilted back and his lower jaw is brought forward to obtain an airway – which must be maintained.
2. If the patient is not breathing, the lungs should be ventilated while the pulse is monitored.
3. If the pulse is present, ventilation should be continued at the rate of 12 per minute (once every five seconds). If the pulse is absent, External Cardiac Compression is started together with oxygen ventilation.
4. The time must be recorded if the pulse stops.
5. The butterfly needle is kept securely attached to the venepuncture site so as to allow easy access in the event of the necessity of drugs being administered (**374**).
6. Procedures are maintained until help arrives or the patient recovers.

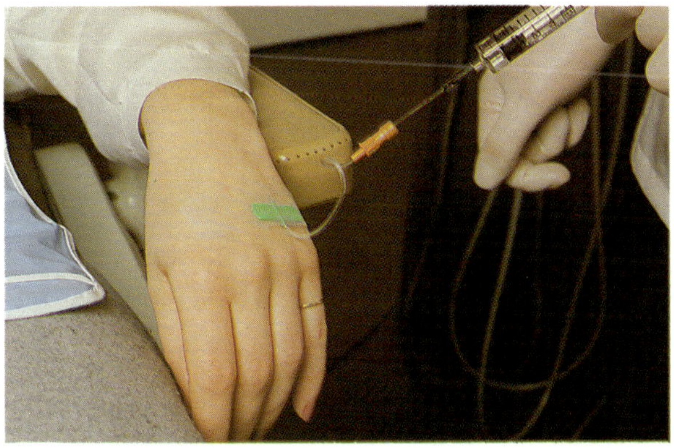

374

374 The butterfly needle attached to the venepuncture site provides for easy access if drug administration becomes necessary

Administration of drugs in an emergency

The administration of drugs in an emergency situation by the dental surgeon is still a subject which is widely debated by senior medical and dental colleagues. It is up to the individual dental surgeon to agree a drug regime with his local consultant colleagues before making up an emergency drug kit. However, it is quite useful for the dental surgeon to stock some emergency drugs which would then be readily available when expert medical help arrives.

18 MEDICO-LEGAL ASPECTS OF INTRAVENOUS SEDATION

Introduction

There has been an increase in the number of cases of litigation brought against dental surgeons in the last few years. At the same time, there has also been a considerable upsurge in the number of patients undergoing intravenous sedation and relative analgesia. In the circumstances, therefore, it would be wise to reflect on certain aspects of these procedures, in an attempt to minimize litigation in a field that can be open to abuse by patient and practitioner alike.

The increase in litigation in the USA has resulted in very high premiums for membership to medical and dental protection societies. This unfortunate trend can happen elsewhere, too, unless dental surgeons take steps to safeguard themselves as well as their patients. It is possible that dental surgeons who practise intravenous sedation will, in the foreseeable future, be asked to provide some evidence of postgraduate training in this speciality. This step, in conjunction with higher premiums, might make some dental surgeons more aware of their responsibilities in a field which is likely to produce problems if procedures are not carried out correctly. Many medico-legal problems that occur are due to lack of knowledge and training on the part of the dental surgeon or dental surgery assistant.

Points to remember

The saying 'Familiarity breeds contempt' is very apt and has led to many a professional man's downfall. No dental surgeon using intravenous sedation techniques should become complacent: sedation procedures and cardiopulmonary resuscitation procedures should be practised and reviewed and, if necessary, updated at regular intervals. Most medico-legal problems arise from lack either of adequate training or of communication between the patient and the dental surgeon. If there is a misunderstanding problems may arise. **All procedures should be carefully explained to the patient in the presence of the dental surgery assistant** (who is also a witness to any written agreement).

It is advisable for the patient to sign a consent form agreeing to the sedation as well as to the dental treatment. First, though, the dental surgeon must decide on the patient's suitability for intravenous sedation, taking the following points into account:

1. There should be no relevant medical history contraindicating intravenous sedation.
2. The patient must be suitably accompanied.
3. Is the dental procedure suitable to be carried out under intravenous sedation?
4. Are the dental surgeon and the second appropriate person suitably trained? Both must be in attendance throughout the procedure.
5. All emergency drugs and oxygen must be within arm's length of the dental surgeon and dental surgery assistant.
6. The availability of all resuscitation equipment and oxygen must be checked prior to an intravenous sedation session.
7. The patient should understand what the intravenous procedure involves and what dental treatment is to be carried out, as well as being briefed as to possible after-effects – for example, pain or bleeding.
8. Where dental treatment will involve the extraction of teeth, the patient should be informed of the fact beforehand, and should also be consulted if it is planned to replace the teeth with a denture.
9. Fees should never be taken from a sedated or recovering patient.
10. The mode of transport home chosen by the patient and his escort should be confirmed to verify its suitability.
11. Avoid polypharmacy if possible, as this increases the possibility of complication.
12. The patient's escort must be given written

and verbal post-operative instructions as to how to look after the patient. The patient should be provided with a night and day telephone number in case of a problem.

13. If all these requirements are observed and the patient signs a consent form, most medico-legal problems can be avoided.

All dental surgeons intending to practise intravenous sedation are advised first to attend a recognized postgraduate course and to obtain some practical guidance. In the event of a problem arising in the surgery relating to intravenous sedation or dental treatment, a written record – in the form of careful and accurate notes – should be produced as soon as is practically possible after the incident. The dental surgeon should then inform his protection society without delay – the incident must not be left unreported. Problems that are left alone tend not to go away; rather, they should be confronted and resolved – preferably with the help and expertise of the protection society.

Despite all reasonable precautions, a dental surgeon may still run into a medico-legal difficulty. Many such problems have nevertheless been settled amicably where the dental surgeon has been able to demonstrate a caring manner and acts correctly. This kind of approach – especially when combined with advice from the dental surgeon's defence society – can often reduce the chances of lengthy and expensive litigation. When intravenous sedation is used and something goes wrong, litigation can always be a possibility. Consider the following examples:

Medico-legal case histories

1. A male dental surgeon was accused of two counts of indecent assault on female patients. The prosecution alleged that the assaults took place while the patients were under sedation to enable conservative dental treatment to be carried out. The first patient received 30mg of diazepam intravenously, a much higher dose than usual, and the second case received 10mg of midazolam intravenously. Despite the dosages, both patients gave a very explicit and detailed description of the alleged assault.

It is unusual for a patient to be able to provide such a detailed statement as was given to the police in this case, after the alleged incident was said to have taken place. Nevertheless, during both sedation procedures, the dental surgery assistant was asked to get an instrument from another part of the dental practice, **leaving the dental surgeon alone with the sedated patient.**

The dental surgeon was duly convicted in a Crown Court on the two counts of indecent assault on female patients. His name was subsequently struck from the dental register.

The points to be learned from this are:

1. Under no circumstances whatsoever should a dental surgeon or a dental surgery assistant be left alone with a sedated patient or, ideally, with *any* patient.
2. If a dental surgery assistant is asked by the dental surgeon to leave the surgery for whatever purpose, the request must be refused unless the dental surgery assistant is replaced by a second appropriate person. **This must be made clear to all dental surgery assistants** who work in practices where intravenous sedation is carried out.

2. A dental surgeon sedated a middle-aged female patient and during the course of the procedure the patient collapsed. The dental surgeon went into a nearby reception area to ask the receptionist to summon help – **leaving the dental surgery assistant alone with a sedated and unconscious patient.** On his return, the dental surgeon attempted cardiopulmonary resuscitation but without success. He then brought in an oxygen cylinder from **outside the surgery** and turned on the oxygen valve. Although the cylinder did contain oxygen, **the oxygen delivery system was faulty and none emerged.**

The dental surgeon next turned to his dental surgery assistant for help in performing cardiopulmonary resuscitation, but the latter had had **no training in the procedure** and was unable to offer any effective assistance.

With the help of another dental surgeon, the dental surgeon then decided to try to **move the unconscious patient** – who had a Guedel airway inserted in her oropharynx – to where there was oxygen available from a delivery pipe. However, the dental surgeon **was unable to avail himself of the oxygen since the pressure was too low.** Cardiopulmonary resuscitation was again attempted; by this time the ambulance had arrived and oxygen was supplied to the patient. The patient was taken to hospital but died shortly after arrival.

The dental surgeon was brought before the General Dental Council and was found guilty of: 1) Failing to obtain enough information relating to the patient's medical condition; 2) Failing to have a second appropriate person present during the administration of intravenous sedation; 3) Failing to take adequate steps to resuscitate the unconscious patient; and 4) Leaving the unconscious patient alone with a dental surgery assistant who did not qualify as a second appropriate person.

The name of the dental surgeon was erased from the dental register.

The key points relating to this case are:

1. The dental surgeon is responsible for eliciting the full medical history of a patient whom he is to sedate. An undeclared medical history does not excuse the dental surgeon from this responsibility, no matter how reticent the patient may be. (In the above case, the patient had a record of thyroid problems and angina of which she did not inform the dental surgeon when he took her medical history.)
2. The dental surgery assistant, being untrained in cardiopulmonary resuscitation, was unfit to act as a second appropriate person.
3. The oxygen and oxygen delivery equipment were not checked before the intravenous sedation session was commenced. The oxygen was not within arm's length of the dental surgeon.
4. Both the dental surgeon and dental surgery assistant were inadequately trained – if trained at all – in the cardiopulmonary resuscitation procedure.

The flagrant disregard of the General Dental Council guidelines by any dental surgeon carrying out intravenous sedation, as well as leading, possibly, to his being found guilty of professional negligence, can also cause the **unnecessary death of a fellow human being.**

Finally, it should be remembered that when a patient seeks dental treatment that requires the administration of intravenous sedation, the dental surgeon bears a special obligation and responsibility to the patient who, while sedated, is unable to care for himself. This responsibility calls for a high degree of professionalism which the dental surgeon should strive to maintain. The dental surgeon and his staff should care for the sedated patient as if it were they themselves who were being treated. Care should be taken to see that the patient does not talk 'privately' to the team while sedated; a mouth prop can sometimes be used to ensure this. Where slightly irrational behaviour results as a side-effect of sedation, this should be dealt with professionally, and care of the patient and confidentiality must be maintained at all times. This high standard of integrity and patient care is especially important in all situations where the patient's normal reactions are temporarily suspended.

The scientific act of administering intravenous sedation should only be undertaken in dental surgeries where trained, experienced and caring staff are present.

GENERAL DENTAL COUNCIL

PROFESSIONAL CONDUCT AND FITNESS TO PRACTISE

NOTICE
FOR THE GUIDANCE OF DENTISTS

NOVEMBER 1989

General Anaesthesia and Sedation

17. Where a general anaesthetic is administered, the Council considers that it should be by a person, other than the dentist treating the patient, who should remain with the patient throughout the anaesthetic procedure and until the patient's protective reflexes have returned.

18. This second person should be a dental or medical practitioner appropriately trained and experienced in the use of anaesthetic drugs for dental purposes. As part of a programme of training in anaesthesia the general anaesthetic may be administered by a dental or medical practitioner under the direct supervision of the said second person.

19. Where intravenous or inhalational sedation techniques are employed a suitable experienced practitioner may assume the responsibility of sedating the patient, as well as operating, provided that as a minimum requirement a second appropriate person is present throughout. Such an appropriate person might be a suitably trained dental surgery assistant or dental auxiliary, whose experience and training enable that person to be an efficient member of the dental team and who is capable of monitoring the clinical condition of the patient. Should the occasion arise, he or she must also be capable of assisting the dentist in case of emergency.

20. For these purposes, the following definition of simple sedation should be understood to apply: 'A technique in which the use of a drug, or drugs, produces a state of depression of the central nervous system enabling treatment to be carried out, but during which communication is maintained such that the patient will respond to command throughout the period of sedation. The drugs and techniques used should carry a margin of safety wide enough to render unintended loss of consciousness unlikely.'

21. Neither general anaesthesia nor sedation should be employed unless proper equipment for their [*sic*] administration is used and adequate facilities for the resuscitation of the patient are readily available with both dentist and staff trained in their use. Resuscitation is very much a matter of skill and timing and dentists must ensure that all those assisting them know precisely what is required of them, should an emergency arise, and that they regularly practise their routine in a simulated emergency against the clock. The Council considers it essential that the equipment necessary for basic life support, including suction apparatus to clear the airway, oral airways to maintain it and positive pressure equipment with appropriate attachments to inflate the lungs with oxygen, must be immediately to hand and ready for use in the operating room.

22. A dentist who carried out treatment under general anaesthesia or sedation without fulfilling these conditions would almost certainly be considered to have acted in a manner which constitutes serious professional misconduct.

19 CONCLUSION

In Part 2 of the book the author has endeavoured to describe and illustrate intravenous sedation techniques that have been safely used over many years in teaching undergraduate and postgraduate courses.

It should be made clear that many techniques exist for the administration of drugs for intravenous sedation. Some may be variations of those described here, others may differ – indeed, opinions may well vary as to some of the techniques included in this book.

Nevertheless, it should be stressed that the intravenous techniques described here are for the basic and fundamental knowledge of undergraduates and postgraduates alike who wish to practise safe intravenous sedation techniques. No graduate should attempt intravenous sedation techniques without first:

1. Reading extensively about the subject.
2. Attending a suitably recognized postgraduate course.
3. Initially practising intravenous sedation only when a more experienced colleague is also present.

The author has been fortunate enough to be involved in the initial clinical trials of diazapam (Diazemuls), midazolam (Hypnovel) and flumazenil (Anexate), and has thus developed his own methods of using these drugs. He has also been involved with cases where problems have arisen as a result of dental surgeons using these drugs incorrectly, or without enough basic knowledge of intravenous sedation techniques. Most problems arise where dental surgeons have not received adequate training – although a basic understanding of relevant techniques is easily acquired via a postgraduate course.

The following extract from the booklet 'Professional Conduct and Fitness to Practise', issued by the General Dental Council in November 1989, should be adhered to by all dental practitioners. It should be remembered that these guidelines are basic levels of acceptable standards of practice. Practitioners should endeavour to reach even higher levels of proficiency and patient care in practice. The extract reads:

7. Every practitioner, in whatever branch of dentistry he or she works, has an ethical obligation to continue professional education for the duration of practice, and failure to do so is tantamount to an abnegation of professional responsibility.

Following qualification every dentist should:

(a) Undergo appropriate vocational training, and thereafter

(b) pursue relevant professional educational activities on a regular and frequent basis.

Dentists who cease to practise (for domestic, health or other reasons) for more than a short period should ensure that they undergo appropriate refresher training before returning to clinical practice.

Drugs for intravenous sedation are not dangerous – people who use them may well be!

Polypharmacy increases the risk of an incident considerably and should be avoided in a general practice situation.

Knowledge of how benzodiazepines work on the body is increasing rapidly, and it is important to keep abreast of the latest developments – for with these will come safer and better advances in the development of drugs for sedation. Doctors and dentists alike owe a great deal to the researchers and to the drug companies who help to make these discoveries possible.

The technique of intravenous sedation offers a great service to those patients who are suitable for its procedures, enabling them to overcome their fears in the knowledge that their pain can be relieved without suffering.

FURTHER READING ETC.*

In a number of cases, either the name of the publisher or the date of publication – or possibly some other detail – was unavailable as we went to press. It is hoped that the list will nevertheless prove useful to all wishing to further their knowledge. *(*Note:* The 'etc.' in the heading above reflects the inclusion, in Chapter 17, of a video.)

Chapter One

Bond, M.R. *Pain: Its nature, analysis and treatment.* London: Churchill Livingstone, 1979.

Melzack, R. and Wall, P. *The Challenge of Pain.* London and New York: Penguin Books, 1982.

Chapter Two

Melzack, R. and Wall, P. *The Challenge of Pain.* London and New York: Penguin Books, 1982.

Wyke, B. The neurology of facial pain. *Br. J. of Hosp. Med.*

Chapter Three

Allen, G.D. *Dental Anaesthesia and Analgesia (Local and General),* 2nd ed. Baltimore and London: Williams and Wilkins, 1979.

Berezowski, B.M., Lownie, J.F. and Cleaton-Jones, P.E. A comparison of two methods of inferior alveolar nerve block. *J. of Dentistry* 1988; **16:** 96–98.

Evers, H. and Haegerstam, G. *Handbook of Dental Local Anaesthesia.* Copenhagen: Schultz, 1981.

Field, E.A., Field, J.K. and Martin, M.V. Time, Steam, Temperature (TST) control indicators to measure essential sterilisation criteria for autoclave in general dental practice and the community dental service, 1988.

Grundy, J.R. Intra Ligamentary Anaesthesia. A survey of use by general practitioners and by staff and students in a dental school. *Conservative Dentistry* 1984; **1:** 36–42.

Howe, G.L. and Whitehead, F.I. *Local Anaesthesia in Dentistry.* Bristol: John Wright and Sons Ltd., 1972.

Khedari, A.J. Alternative to mandibular block injections through intraligamental anaesthesia. *Quintessence International* 2081 1982; **2:** 231–237.

Meecham, J.G. Aspiration during dental local anaesthesia. *Dental Update.* Special Supplement II, 1988, 521–524.

Sowray, J.H. Intraligamentary injections. *Dental Update,* Special Supplement II, 1988; 519–520.

Chapter Five

Allen, G.D. *Dental Anaesthesia and Analgesia (Local and General),* 2nd ed. Baltimore and London: Williams and Wilkins, 1979.

Barber, J., Donaldson, D., Ramras, E. and Allen, G.D. *The relationship between nitrous oxide conscious sedation and the hypnotic state.* 1979.

Guedel, A.E. *Inhalation Anaesthesia.* New York: MacMillan Co., 1953.

Langa, H. *Relative Analgesia in Dental Practice.* Inhalation analgesia with nitrous oxide. London: W.B. Saunders, 1976.

Lindsay, S.J.E. and Roberts, G.J. Methods for behavioural research on dentally anxious children: the example of relative analgesia. *Br. Dent. J.* 1980; **149:** 175–179.

Manford, M.L.M. and Roberts, G.J. Dental treatment in young handicapped patients: an assessment of relative anaesthesia. *Anaesthesia* 1980; **35:** 1157–1168.

Roberts, G.J. Relative analgesia in clinical practice. In Coplans, M.P. and Green, R.A. eds. *Anaesthesia and Sedation in Dental Practice.* Chapter 10. Amsterdam: Elsevier, 1983.

Roberts, G.J. and Wignall, B.K. The laryngeal reflex during oxygen: nitrous oxide sedation. *Br. J. of Anaesth.* 1982; **54:** 1277–1280.

Summers, L. An investigation into the effects of surgical stress on the 'fit' and 'poor risk' patient including the modifying effects of relative analgesia and ß-blockade. *Br. J. of Oral Surg.* 1981; **19:** 3–12.

Chapter Seven

Br. Med. J. 1980; **280:** 910–912.

Committee of Safety of Medicines. Current Problems No. 21.

Chapter Nine

George, K.A. and Dundee, J.W. *Br. J. Clin. Pharmacol.* 1977; **4:** 45.

Greenblatt, D.J. *et al. J. Am. Med. Ass.* 1978; **240:** 1872.

Greenblatt, D.J. and Shader, R.I. *5th Med. J.* (Bgham. Ala.) 1978; **71:** Suppl. 22.

Meffin, P.J. and Wing, L.M.H. *Curr. Ther.* 1980; 21/85.

Chapter Fourteen

Rosenbaum, N.L. and Hooper, P.A. The effects of flumazenil, a new benzodiazepine antagonist, on the reversal of

midazolam sedation and amnesia in dental patients. *Br. Dent. J.* 1988; **165:** 400.
Rosenbaum, N.L. and Hooper, P.A. The use of flumazenil as an antagonist to midazolam in intravenous sedation for dental procedures. *Euro. J. of Anaesthesiology* Suppl. 1988; **2:** 183–190.

Chapter Sixteen

Allen, G.D., Everett, G.B. and Butler, L.A. Human cardiorespiratory and analgesic effects of intravenous diazepam and local anaesthesia. *J. Am. Dent. Assoc.* 1976; **92:** 744.
Baderman, H. Medical or other emergency situations in dentistry. *S.A.A.D. Digest* 1983; **5:** 141–147.
Clarke, R.J.S. Adverse response to intravenous drugs, p. 177. Watkins, J. and Ward, A. Milford. London: Academic Press, 1978.
Committee of Safety of Medicines. Current Problems No. 14, 1985.
Dixon, D. Respiratory depression following midazolam. *Anaesthesia* 1985; Vol. 40, No. 9: 922.
Dundee, J.W. Do fantasies occur with intravenous benzodiazepines? *S.A.A.D. Digest* 1986; **6:** 8.
Dundee, J.W., Halliday, N.J., Loughran, P.G. and Harper, K.W. The influence of age on the onset of anaesthesia with midazolam. *Anaesthesia* 1985; **40:** 441–443.
Forster, A. Respiratory depression by midazolam and diazepam. *Anaesthesiology* 1979; **51:** 383.
Healy, T.E.J., Robinson, J.S. and Vickers, M.D. Physiological responses to intravenous diazepam as a sedative for conservative dentistry. *Br. Med. J.* 1970; **3:** 10.
Jenkinson, J.L., Macrae, W.R., Scott, D.B. and Gould, J.F. Haemodynamic effects of diazepam used as a sedative for oral surgery. *Br. J. Anaesth.* 1974; **46:** 294.
Lichfield, N.B. Complications of intravenous diazepam. *Anes. Prog.* 1980; **6:** 175.
McGimpsey, J.G., Kawar, R., Gamble, J.A.S., Browne, E.S. and Dundee, J.W. Midazolam in dentistry. *Br. Dent. J.* 1983; **155:** 47–50.
Rees, M. and Dormund, J. *Brit. Med. J.* 1980; **281:** 289–290.
Rood, J.P. Anaesthesia in dentistry. *Dental Update* 1980; **7:** 2.
Rosenbaum, N.L. A new formation of diazepam for intravenous sedation in dentistry. *Br. Dent. J.* 1982; **153:** 192–193.
Thurlow, A.C., in Coplans, M.P. and Green, R.A., eds. *Anaesthesia and Sedation in Dental Practice.* Amsterdam: Elsevier, 1983.

Chapter Seventeen

The diagnosis and management of sudden collapse in dental practice. *Br. Dent. J.* 1977; **143:** 196–200.
Emergencies in Dental Practice. DHSS, Alexander Fleming House, Elephant and Castle, London.
First response – newsletter for immediate care. Professional Publ., Vitograph Research Trust, 28a Heytesbury Lane, Dublin 4, Ireland.
JAMA 1980; Vol. 244, No. 5, 453–509.
Page, G., Mills, K. and Morton, R. *A Colour Atlas of Cardio-Pulmonary Resuscitation Techniques.*
Safer, Peter. *Cardio-pulmonary Cerebral Resuscitation.* World Federation of Societies of Anaesthesiologists.
The Surf Life-Saving Training Manual. World Life-Saving Association, British Association, 4 Cathedral Yard, Exeter, Devon EX1 1HJ.
Video of ABC of Resuscitation. CPR Products Div., Vitalograph Ltd., Maids Moreton House, Buckingham MK18 1SW.

Chapter Nineteen

Professional conduct and fitness to practise. General Dental Council 1989; 24, paragraph 7.

USEFUL ADDRESSES

Organizations promoting the study of intravenous sedation and relative analgesia in dentistry

In the U.K.

The Association of Dental Anaesthetists (A.D.A.)
Dr. A. Padfield
Hon. Membership Secretary
351 Fulwood Road
Sheffield S10 3BQ
England.

Society for the Advancement of Anaesthesia in Dentistry (S.A.A.D.)
Hon. Secretary
59 Summerlands Avenue
London W3 6EW
England.

Faculty of Dental Surgery
Course Co-ordinator: Ms. A. O'Mara BA
Royal College of Surgeons of England
35–43 Lincoln's Inn Fields
London WC2A 3PN
England.

College of Anaesthetists
Mr. S.N. Alan Ll.B (Secretary)
35–43 Lincoln's Inn Fields
London WC2A 3PN
England.

Guy's Dental Hospital (U.M.D.S.)
Postgraduate Dental Tutor (Administrator: Miss D. Hogan)
Dr. T.R. Pitt Ford – c/o Conservation Dept.
London Bridge
London SE1 9RT
England.

A comprehensive list of postgraduate dental deans in the U.K. is available on request from:

D.C. Rule FDS, RCS (Eng)
British Postgraduate Medical Federation
33 Millman Street
London WC1N 3EJ
England (tel. 071-831 6222, Ext. 148).

International Federation of Dental Anaesthesiology Societies (I.F.D.A.S.)

President:
Dr. J.K. Grainger MDS, FRACDS (Australia)
President-Elect:
Dr. P.H. Jacobsohn DDS (U.S.A.)

Secretary General:
Mr. P. Sykes LDS, RCS Eng. (U.K.)
Wilmington Lodge
19 Dunstable Street
Ampthill, Bedford MK45 2NJ
England.

Represented in the U.S.A. by:

American Analgesia Society
Dr. A.A. Weiner
1110 North Main Street
Randolph, MA02368.

American Dental Society of Anaesthesiology (A.D.S.A.)
Dr. H.B. Berquist DMD, MSD
1848 Saratoga Avenue (Suite 3)
Saratoga, CA95070.

Dr. N. Trieger
Chief of Dentistry
Montefiore Hospital
111 East 210th Street
New York, NY10467

Dr. H.J. Panuska DDS, MSD
670 Southdale Medical Building
Minneapolis, Minnesota 55435.

American Society for the Advancement of Anaesthesia in Dentistry (A.S.A.A.D.)
Dr. A. Reyes-Guerra
475 White Plains Road
Eastchester
New York, NY10707.

In Australia by:

Australian Society for the Advancement of Anaesthesia in Dentistry (A.S.A.A.D.)
The Secretary – Mr. J. Auld
PO Box 124
Inverell, NSW 2360.

Dr. A.H. Polyblank BDS
Suite One, Bay Lodge Arcade
401 New South Head Road
Double Bay 2028, NSW.

In Germany by:

Dr. W. Jakobs
Bahnhofstrasse 63–65
5522 Speicher.

In Israel by:

Dr. E. Kaufman
Faculty of Dental Medicine
Hadassah Hospital, pob 12000
Ein Karem, Jerusalem.

In Italy by:

Prof. G. Martinelli
1st di Anestesia Rianimazione
Via Massarenti 9
40138 Bologna.

Dr. G. Damia
Via Mascheroni 31
20145 Milano.

In Japan by:

Prof. Hideki Furuya DDS, DMSc, JBDA
Nippon Dental University
1–9–20 Fujumi
Chiyoda-ku, Tokyo 102.

In New Zealand by:

Dr. W.R.E. Laing BDS (Otago)
Flowers Building
Thames Street, Momnsville.

INDEX

Note: page numbers followed by 'f' refer to figure legends, by 't' to tables